HANDBOOK OF GERIATRIC ASSESSMENT

Third Edition

Joseph J. Gallo, MD, MPH
Department of Family Practice and Community Medicine
Department of Psychiatry
University of Pennsylvania School of Medicine
Philadelphia, Pennsylvania

Terry Fulmer, PhD, RN, FAAN
Professor, Director
Center for Nursing Research
Co-Director
John A. Hartford Foundation Institute for Geriatric Nursing
New York University
New York, New York

Gregory J. Paveza, MSW, PhD
Associate Professor
School of Social Work
University of South Florida
Tampa, Florida

William Reichel, MD
Clinical Professor of Family Medicine
Georgetown University School of Medicine
Washington, D.C.
Adjunct Professor of Family Medicine
Brown University School of Medicine
Providence, Rhode Island

AN ASPEN PUBLICATION®
Aspen Publishers, Inc.
Gaithersburg, Maryland
2000

Library of Congress Cataloging-in-Publication Data

Handbook of geriatric assessment / Joseph J. Gallo . . . [et al.]. — 3rd ed.
p. cm.
Includes bibliographical references and index.
ISBN 0-8342-1248-X
1. Aged—Diseasees–Diagnosis Handbooks, manuals, etc.
2. Aged—Psychoogical testing Handbooks, manuals, etc.
3. Aged—Care Handbooks, manuals, etc. I. Gallo, Joseph J.
[DNLM: 1. Geriatric Assessment. WT 30 H2374 1999]
RC953. G34   1999
618.97′075—dc21
DNLM/DLC
for Library of Congress   99-36370
CIP

Orders: (800) 638-8437
Customer Service: (800) 234-1660

About Aspen Publishers • For more than 35 years, Aspen has been a leading professional publisher in a variety of disciplines. Aspen's vast information resources are available in both print and electronic formats. We are committed to providing the highest quality information available in the most appropriate format for our customers. Visit Aspen's Internet site for more information resources, directories, articles, and a searchable version of Aspen's full catalog, including the most recent publications: **http://www.aspenpublishers.com**
Aspen Publishers, Inc. • The hallmark of quality in publishing
Member of the worldwide Wolters Kluwer group.

Editorial Services: Denise Hawkins Coursey
Library of Congress Catalog Card Number: 99-36370
ISBN: 0-8342-1248-X

Printed in the United States of America

1 2 3 4 5

Contents

iii

Contributors

David Carr, MD
Division of Geriatrics and Gerontology
Washington University
St. Louis, Missouri

David J. Doukas, MD
Associate Professor
Department of Family Practice and Community Medicine
Fellow
The Center for Bioethics
University of Pennsylvania School of Medicine
Philadelphia, Pennsylvania

Yolanda B. Esparza, MSW
Social Science Research Associate
Department of Family Practice
University of Texas Health Science Center
San Antonio, Texas

Laurence B. McCullough, PhD
Professor of Medicine and Medical Ethics
Center for Medical Ethics and Health Policy
Baylor College of Medicine
Houston, Texas

Irene Moore, MSW
Director
The University Hospital Geriatric Evaluation Center
Associate Professor
Department of Family Medicine
University of Cincinnati Medical Center
Cincinnati, Ohio

Charles P. Mouton, MD, MS
Assistant Professor
Department of Family Practice
The University of Texas Health Science Center
at San Antonio
San Antonio, Texas

George W. Rebok, PhD
Department of Mental Hygiene
School of Hygiene and Public Health
The Johns Hopkins University
Baltimore, Maryland

James P. Richardson, MD, MPH, AGSF
Chief
Division of Geriatric Medicine
Good Samaritan Hospital
Clinical Associate Professor
Departments of Family Medicine and Epidemiology
and Preventive Medicine
University of Maryland School of Medicine
Baltimore, Maryland

Bruce E. Robinson, MD, MPH
Chief of Geriatrics
Sarasota Memorial Hospital
Internal Medicine, MDC 19
University of South Florida
College of Medicine
Tampa, Florida

Gregg Warshaw, MD
Professor
Department of Family Medicine
University of Cincinnati Medical Center
Cincinnati, Ohio

Preface

The original concept for a book about multidimensional assessment in primary care geriatrics arose from the experience of working with the assessment program of the Baltimore County Department of Health of Baltimore County, Maryland, from 1970 until 1988, and from the experience of establishing a geriatric assessment program at Franklin Square Hospital Center in Baltimore, Maryland, from 1985 to 1986. Since the first edition, geriatric assessment has taken hold as evidenced by a growing literature suggesting that assessing multiple domains is essential in caring for older adults and demonstrating a renewed interest in preventing functional decline.

This third edition of the *Handbook of Geriatric Assessment,* with new and revised chapters, again emphasizes material that has practical application in primary care settings in order to encourage a multidimensional approach in the care of older persons. Chapters on driving evaluation, pain assessment, and considerations in the various settings of care provide expanded treatments of these critical areas. An important chapter on ethnicity and assessment highlights a vital dimension. The social and economic aspects of care are discussed in a new chapter. The chapter on health promotion and disease prevention has been extensively revised to reflect the emphasis on evidence-based recommendations for care. We think all these changes will make the third edition a valuable resource for clinicians.

A major goal of all three editions of the *Handbook of Geriatric Assessment* has been to foster the multidimensional assessment of older adults in all the settings of geriatric care. However, the authors of this book have had to confront the dilemma that there are many words that vary across the professions, including the words used to describe the older people to whom we provide services. Since much of the work of geriatric assessment occurs in medical settings such as hospitals and nursing homes, we generally opted to use the term *patient* in this book. Nevertheless, we recognize that social workers, case managers, home care workers, and other professionals may be more comfortable with the word *client* when referring to older persons receiving services, and we sometimes have used this word. We hope that readers will not be distracted from the central concepts presented that can improve the assessment of older persons by all professionals.

As was the intent of the first edition in 1988 and the second edition in 1995, this third edition fosters a multidimensional approach by discussing the assessment of domains that have a significant bearing on the life of older persons. Although this book was never meant to be a comprehensive guide to all assessment instruments, we wanted to provide readers with instruments, questionnaires, and concepts that can be employed in designing clinical assessment procedures. We have been gratified that many professionals have found previous editions of the *Handbook of Geriatric Assessment* useful in their clinical work. At the same time, the health care system continues to undergo change, driven in part by the pressures of caring for a growing population of older adults. "Guidelines," "evidence-based medicine," "clinical pathways," "managed care," and "disease management" have become commonplace terms. Whether these ideas will have a lasting effect on health care in the future is anybody's guess. The power and promise of the Internet for managing information is likely to play an integral role in how these changes play out. As the roles of nurses and other professional caregivers in the health care system continue to undergo transformation, the notion of multidimensional assessment takes on additional salience. By drawing discussions of the domains of geriatric assessment into one place, we hope that clinicians will continue to find practical and useful ideas to take into their daily work with older people.

1

The Context of Geriatric Care

 t the dawn of the 21st century, the projected growth of the world's aged population is unprecedented. From 1970 to 1997, the proportion of persons aged 65 years and older in the United States has grown from 10% to 13%, and by 2050, 20% of all adults are expected to be 65 years and older.[1] The proportion of persons aged 85 years and older is also growing rapidly.[2] Some estimate that there are more older persons alive on the earth now than have reached old age in all of history.[3] The rate of growth in the proportion of older persons from minority groups is much faster than the rate of growth in the older white population of the United States. This increasing ethnic diversity of the aged will have important implications for how health care is organized and delivered.[4] Aging is a worldwide phenomenon. Each month, of the 1.2 million people around the world who reach later life, 1 million live in developing countries.[5] The age, ethnic, and cultural diversity of the older population suffuses into all the domains of geriatric assessment.

THE CONTEXT OF GERIATRIC CARE

The role of older people in other societies has often been more clearly defined than in modern American culture. In preindustrial society, older persons frequently had considerable wealth and power, which they passed on to the younger members of the group at the appropriate time. Often some special functions were performed by the older members, who knew about family histories and sacred rituals and how to mediate with ancestors. In addition, older persons may have provided some services to the community, such as serving as judges or as experts in child rearing. Even in a technological society, older people are a valuable resource. Contrary to the stereotypes, older people contribute much as informal helpers and unpaid volunteer workers. When all forms of productive activity are combined, the amount of work done by older men and women is substantial.[6,7] Without exposure to productive older people, younger people (including the middle-aged) lose their sense of history. The aging process becomes something to be feared, even a taboo topic, because the values of society place great emphasis on youth. It is tempting to view growing older as something to be ashamed of, as if old age means nothing but static existence or, worse, only decline and deterioration.

On the contrary, older adults have significant developmental work to do. Persons who are successfully aging have made remarkable adaptations and show considerable resiliency. Erikson[8] summarizes this developmental work as the dichotomy of ego integrity versus ego despair: despair, when one looks back on life with regret, not having accomplished what was wanted; and integrity, when one looks back on life and is able to accept it as a unique life in history, one that had to be.

Erikson's first "age of man" relates to the infant's development of "basic trust versus basic mistrust" in the world. The life cycle comes full circle in the relation of ego integrity and basic trust because "healthy children will not fear life if their elders have integrity enough not to fear death."[8] The older person also integrates, in "age-appropriate" ways, the psychosocial themes from previous stages, reflecting back over the entire life cycle. For example, "intimacy and isolation" in young adulthood refers to the development of the ability to be intimate with another versus a failure to develop such relationships. The older adult also faces this issue since the person must deal with the restructuring of relationships.[9]

Growing old marks a time of significant growth for many persons. Among the considerable developmental and adaptive tasks of older adults are dealing with the loss through death or relocation of family and friends, adjusting to changes in living arrangements, retiring, managing with less income, changing social roles, increasing leisure time, and changing sexual and physical functioning; and finally, accepting the inevitability of death. The gracefully aging older person who is able to integrate all these aspects has a great deal to teach younger persons about life.

Successful aging occurs along multiple dimensions, including maintenance of active involvement with life and achieving a sense of psychological well-being.[10] One model of "successful aging" consists of "selective optimization with compensation."[11] *Selection* refers to prioritizing one's activities to the most important or pleasurable and adjusting of expectations; *optimization* refers to maximization of the chosen behaviors through practice and by accommodating conditions to the ability of the older person; *compensation* refers to use of strategies that compensate for aging-related losses. Baltes[11] notes strategies of the pianist Rubenstein as an illustration of selective optimization with compensation. Rubenstein selects a smaller number of pieces to play, rehearses more often, and slows down before allegro movements to give the listener the impression of speed. Perhaps the strategies of successful aging can be taught.[12]

In the future, the role of older adults in society may undergo further development and evolution. Toffler[13] has called the technological revolution that includes the proliferation of computers as the third wave. Contrary to expectations engendered by Orwell's *1984*, this revolution could lead to increased freedom and leisure time. During the first wave (preindustrial society), each household formed an economic unit. The home or the field was the focus of work, and families worked together. Home life and work were intimately related. The second wave was marked by the industrial revolution. Work now took place in the factory. Behavior became dictated by schedules and the division of labor. Consequently, there is less need for older people as repositories of history and culture. The third wave is marked by the advent of the "electronic cottage," with smaller work units and persons working at home. Work again will become less centralized, as it was in the agricultural society of the first wave. Because employees will have the ability to work at home, centralized places of work may become a thing of the past. The implication for the family is that children will once again be near their working parents, a situation that has not been common since the agricultural age. Family roles may then undergo transformation.

Persons may have more than one career over the course of a lifetime. The experience that the elderly have would be invaluable in helping younger workers apply theory to practical problems. Technological change will also demand that education continue throughout life. It may not be unusual for persons to move in and out of formal educational situations at different ages. Older persons may again be seen as "mentors" to the young.[14]

Expectations about medical care will likely be different as well. For example, older adults in the future may have other ideas about the role of the family in caring for the impaired adult. In a mobile society, informal social networks may be strained. Expectations about retirement may be different, so that a lower standard of living or poor health will not be tolerated. Better educated older persons, especially regarding health matters, might question their physicians more than today's older population does and perhaps would want to participate to a greater degree in decisions, seeing themselves as more responsible for the quality of their own health. The World Wide Web has become a source and clearinghouse for health-related information for professionals and patients. In addition, the Internet is providing a forum for discussion and support of caregivers and homebound older adults. At the same time, the health care system is redefining itself. Governments all over the world are grappling with the issue of resource allocation in planning health care services for populations that include greater proportions of older people. It is against this changing backdrop that today's older adults require care.

MULTIDIMENSIONAL ASSESSMENT

Caring for older patients can be a challenging task for clinicians. The clinician is frequently called on to assist older patients and their families in decisions that can have a direct effect on quality of life. Small changes in the ability of an older person to perform daily activities, or in the ability of a caregiver to provide support, can have an impact on major life decisions. Older persons are vulnerable to reversible problems that contribute to disability, but therein lies the clinician's strength since even small improvement in functional status can have significant positive effects. Therefore, caring for the older person requires that the clinician assess functional, social, and other aspects of the patient's condition in addition to the usual focus on medical issues.

The domains of multidimensional assessment, such as mental health, physical health, functioning, and social situation, set the field of geriatrics apart from other fields of medicine. The purpose of this book is to assist health care professionals who work with older patients to include these domains in assessment. The author and contributors are mindful of the primary care practitioner whose time with the patient is limited, and hope that assessment instruments that are useful in everyday practice may become part of routine care, and ultimately save time. Not all older persons who could benefit from multidisciplinary assessment will have access to a team, but practicing physicians and other health care professionals can utilize community expertise and standardized instruments.[15] Instruments found in this book, such as the Folstein Mini-

Mental State Examination[16] and the Instrumental Activities of Daily Living Screen,[17] can be incorporated into the office evaluation of older persons.[18,19] In the concluding chapter, the evidence for a strategy of incorporating geriatric assessment into primary care is reviewed in addition to commenting on a more intensive team evaluation.

A number of strategies can be employed to bring the facets of geriatric assessment into geriatric care despite the time and reimbursement barriers that confront the primary care physician and others who care for older adults.[20] Practitioners should develop relationships with special geriatric assessment teams such as the University of Cincinnati program described in Chapter 12. At the same time, health care professionals working individually can arrive at the same recommendations as a multidisciplinary team, targeting specific problems for intervention.[21,22] Geriatric assessment has reached a stage of development where incorporation into the practices of physicians and other health professionals is practical. The use of computerized assessment capability may facilitate the integration of the components of geriatric assessment into care settings. Approaches described in this book can improve the outpatient recognition and management of functional and medical problems.[19,21–30] The remaining sections of this introductory chapter set the stage for understanding the domains of assessment and the other chapters that follow.

Ethnicity and Assessment

The increasing need to care for older persons from diverse cultures and ethnic groups means that clinicians must consider how assessment and development of a treatment plan are modified to avoid misunderstanding or ineffective care. Users of assessment instruments should be aware of the issues involved when drawing conclusions from test scores for questionnaires derived for persons of a different cultural background from which the instruments were developed and tested. In addition, it is important to try to elicit the beliefs, attitudes, and goals about illness that older adults may have that may differ from what is expected.

Mental Status Assessment

While much can be gleaned from observation of the speech and mannerisms of the patient, formal evaluation with school-like tests of cognitive status can yield valuable information that is accessible to all who use the chart. In the office, use of standardized questions to assess mental function may be particularly important for older patients who are experiencing difficulty in performing certain daily tasks, such as using the telephone or handling money. Mental status testing at the time of admission to the hospital or nursing home serves to establish a baseline and heightens awareness to the onset of delirium. The effect on mental state of depression, substance abuse, adverse effects of prescribed and over-the-counter medications, and other medical conditions should also be considered.

Functional Assessment Including Driving

Functional assessment includes ability of the patient to perform various tasks of daily life, such as dressing and housework, as well as the more cognitively complex and physically demanding tasks such as grocery shopping. Because ability to function is closely tied to quality of life, assessing functioning is a central element of geriatric assessment. Function can be both a signal of illness and a focus for preventive efforts. Aside from specific medical diagnoses, functional status is independently associated with the care the patient needs, the risk for institutionalization, and mortality. The ability to safely drive an automobile is an important but often neglected aspect of functional assessment of older ambulatory patients. The evaluation of the older driver presents one of the most difficult clinical situations faced by the practicing primary care physician for which guidance can be found in Chapter 5, which is devoted to driving assessment.

Social and Economic Status

Older persons often present with problems of daily living and require a comprehensive outlook—one that includes the family of the patient within the physician's purview. In some cases, the health of the caregiver may be of great importance to the patient's well-being. Most long-term care is provided by caregivers who often need physical and emotional support in order to maintain the elder at home. Frequently the caregiver is a woman, especially daughters and daughters-in-law. In contrast to the common myth that families "dump" their older members in institutions, clinical experience shows that families tend to go "above and beyond the call of duty" in providing care for their older relatives. Evaluation of the older person cannot be complete without some assessment of the social support system. Personal finances may have an impact on health, nutrition, and residence. Although clinician inquiry in the area of economic status may not be detailed, the physician should be aware that there are older persons who fail to take prescribed medication or who alter the dosage schedule because of financial considerations. While the economic situation of older Americans has improved considerably in recent decades, medication costs have risen significantly and are often not covered by insurance.

Advance Directives

Older adults are encouraged to plan for uncertainty with regard to their medical care,[31] but few do. Advance directives are legally binding documents that allow individuals to project their wishes about medical treatment into a future period of incapacity. All hospitals, nursing facilities, and home health agencies in the United States must inform patients about their right to make advance directives. Discussion of advance directive options between the well patient and the doctor may someday become an ordinary part of office practice in the care of the elderly, with informed patients having the opportunity to state their wishes, preferences, and values that are relevant to their future medical care. Chapter 7 on eliciting the values of patients discusses a systematic method for addressing issues related to planning for care in the face of incapacity.

Physical Examination

The history and physical examination should be tailored to the older patient with a focus on the discovery of remedial problems. Hearing and vision impairment, restricted mobility, and slowed response time must be considered in the history and physical examination of older persons. The presenting complaint may involve the most vulnerable organ system rather than the organ system expected. For example, congestive heart failure may present as delirium. Consequences of medical diagnoses on each of the domains of multidimensional assessment should be considered in every older patient. How might an additional medication for diabetes affect this patient's mental and functional status? On the other hand, the multidimensional status of the older person should be considered in a larger context when recommending treatment. What value does this patient place on dying at home? Integrating these aspects of assessment and treatment remains a worthwhile goal and a clinical challenge.

Pain Assessment

Knowing how to assess pain in older persons in clinical settings is essential to avoid unnecessary suffering and functional impairment, to monitor the response to therapy, and to achieve freedom from significant pain, which is an important component of quality of life. In Chapter 9, a general approach is recommended that applies when patients with dementia have deteriorated in functioning or appear to be uncomfortable or irritable, but cannot express exactly what is wrong. The adequate assessment of pain is pertinent to the care of ambulatory older persons as well as older adults in specialized settings, such as the nursing home or hospice.

Health Promotion and Disease Prevention

The aspects of mental status, functional status, social situation, values history, and medical considerations act as a *focus* of preventive activities and as a *guide* for highlighting preventive activities that are appropriate for the individual patient. An individualized plan for health promotion and disability prevention grounded in evidence-based guidelines should be based on a multidimensional assessment because older persons vary greatly in their medical and functional status. In Chapter 10, the barriers, ethics, and specific recommendations related to age-appropriate health promotion and disease prevention activities for older persons are discussed. Although age-related changes are frequently associated with physical and physiological decline, health care professionals who treat older adults must avoid the temptation of thinking that older persons are beyond efforts at improving wellness or preventing illness.

The Settings of Care

Because there is considerable functional and ethnic heterogeneity among older persons who are seen in the office, the home, the hospital, the assisted living facility, the hospice, and the nursing home, Chapter 11 provides guidance on issues specifically related to assessment across these settings of care. As a practical matter, geriatric assessment in some settings is mandated in order to improve care planning and to determine the need for additional evaluation.

University of Cincinnati Geriatric Evaluation Center

As in earlier editions of this book, a chapter is included on an exemplary program of geriatric assessment. Describing the activities at Geriatric Evaluation Center of the University of Cincinnati provides the reader with a sense of how a program operates, not only in relation to the process of evaluation, but within the local health care system.

CONCLUSION

Professionals who care for older adults can benefit from reading this book from cover to cover; however, clinicians can also turn to specific chapters to find keys for assessing particular domains. The discussions of the elements of geriatric assessment found here can help in planning the evaluations included in the care of older persons. Technical jargon has been avoided to maximize usefulness for clinicians, but readers with more specialized needs can find additional information on geriatric assessment and instruments in other sources.[32-35]

It should be stated at the outset that assessment findings must be linked to adequate treatment plans. While this requires clinical training and experience, a systematic approach to assessment helps the clinician cover the important issues over time. Since values and circumstances vary from individual to individual and from family to family, specific recommendations based on a given constellation of findings from geriatric assessment cannot be provided. Nevertheless, the domains of assessment must be united in a coordinated whole by the practitioner for the proper assessment of the older patient, whether in the office, the home, the hospital, the assisted-living facility, the hospice, or the nursing home. With a view to the 21st century, the authors and contributors hope that practitioners will glean from this book assessment instruments and ideas useful in the routine assessment of older patients, thereby contributing to their effective and systematic care.

REFERENCES

1. US Bureau of the Census. *Population Projections of the United States by Age, Sex, Race, and Hispanic Origin: 1995 to 2050.* Washington, DC: US Government Printing Office; 1996. Current Population Reports, Series P25–1130.

2. Suzman RM, Willis DP, Manton KG. *The Oldest Old.* New York: Oxford University Press; 1992.

3. Dychtwald K, Flower J. *Age Wave: The Challenges and Opportunities of an Aging America.* Los Angeles: Jeremy P. Tarcher; 1989.

4. Lavizzo-Mourey R, Mackenzie ER. Cultural competence: Essential measurements of quality for managed care organizations. *Ann Intern Med.* 1996;124:919–921.

5. Macfadyen D. International demographic trends. In: Kane RL, Evans JG, Macfadyen D, eds. *Improving the Health of Older People: A World View.* New York: Oxford University Press; 1990:19–29.

6. Herzog AR, Kahn RL, Morgan JN, Jackson JS, Antonucci TC. Age differences in productive activities. *J Gerontol: Soc Sci.* 1989;44:129–138.

7. Herzog AR, Morgan JN. Formal volunteer work among older Americans. In: Bass S, Caro F, Chen YP, eds. *Achieving a Productive Aging Society.* Westport, CT: Greenwood Press; 1993.

8. Erikson EH. *Childhood and Society.* New York: WW Norton and Company; 1963.

9. Erikson EH, Erikson JM, Kivnick HQ. *Vital Involvement in Old Age: The Experience of Old Age in Our Time.* New York: WW Norton and Company; 1986.

10. Rebok GW, Gallo JJ. Successful aging: Optimizing strategies for primary care geriatrics. In: Gallo JJ, Busby-Whitehead J, Rabins PV, Silliman R, Murphy J, eds. *Reichel's Care of the Elderly: Clinical Aspects of Aging.* 5th ed. Baltimore: Lippincott Williams & Wilkins; 1999:622–630.

11. Baltes PB. The many faces of human ageing: Toward a psychological culture of old age. *Psychol Med.* 1991;21:837–854.

12. Baltes PB, Baltes MM. *Successful Aging: Perspectives from the Behavioral Sciences.* New York: Cambridge University Press; 1990.

13. Toffler A. *The Third Wave.* New York: Bantam Books; 1980.

14. Toffler A. *Future Shock.* New York: Bantam Books; 1970.

15. American Geriatrics Society Public Policy Committee. Comprehensive geriatric assessment. *J Am Geriatr Soc.* 1989;37:473–474.

16. Folstein MF, Folstein SE, McHugh PR. Mini-Mental State: A practical method for grading the cognitive state of patients for the clinician. *J Psychiatr Res.* 1975;12:189–198.

17. Fillenbaum G. Screening the elderly: A brief instrumental activities of daily living measure. *J Am Geriatr Soc.* 1985;33:698–706.

18. Applegate WB, Blass JP, Williams TF. Instruments for the functional assessment of older patients. *N Engl J Med.* 1990;322:1207–1214.

19. Lachs MS, Feinstein AR, Cooney LM, et al. A simple procedure for general screening for functional disability in elderly persons. *Ann Intern Med.* 1990;112:699–706.

20. Beck JC, Freedman ML, Warshaw GA. Geriatric assessment: Focus on function. *Primary Care.* 1994;28:10–32.

21. Robinson BE, Lund CA, Keller D, et al. Validation of the Functional Assessment Inventory against a multidisciplinary home care team. *J Am Geriatr Soc.* 1986;34:851–854.

22. Pinholt EM, Kroenke K, Hanley JF, et al. Functional assessment of the elderly: A comparison of standard instruments with clinical judgement. *Arch Intern Med.* 1987;147:484–488.

23. Miller DK, Morley JE, Rubenstein LZ, Pietruszka FM, Strome LS. Formal geriatric assessment instruments and the care of older general medical outpatients. *J Am Geriatr Soc.* 1990;38:645–651.

24. Siu AL, Beers MH, Morgenstern H. The geriatric "medical and public health" imperative revisited. *J Am Geriatr Soc.* 1993;41:78–84.

25. Boult C, Boult L, Murphy C, Ebbitt B, Luptak M, Kane RL. A controlled trial of outpatient geriatric evaluation and management. *J Am Geriatr Soc.* 1994;42:465–470.

26. Boult C, Boult L, Morishita L, Smith SL, Kane RL. Outpatient geriatric evaluation and management. *J Am Geriatr Soc.* 1998;46:296–302.

27. Silverman M, Musa D, Martin DC, Lave JR, Adams J, Ricci EM. Evaluation of outpatient geriatric assessment: A randomized multi-site trial. *J Am Geriatr Soc.* 1995;43:733–740.

28. Reuben DB, Frank JC, Hirsch SH, McGuigan KA, Maly RC. A randomized clinical trial of outpatient comprehensive geriatric assessment coupled with an intervention to increase adherence to recommendations. *J Am Geriatr Soc.* 1999;47:269–276.

29. Valenstein M, Kales H, Mellow A, et al. Psychiatric diagnosis and intervention in older and younger patients in a primary care clinic: Effect of a screening and diagnostic instrument. *J Am Geriatr Soc.* 1998;46:1499–1505.

30. Maly RC, Hirsch SH, Reuben DB. The performance of simple instruments in detecting geriatric conditions and selecting community-dwelling older people for geriatric assessment. *Age Ageing.* 1997;26:223–231.

31. Doukas D, Reichel W. *Planning for Uncertainty: A Guide to Living Wills and Other Advance Directives for Health Care.* Baltimore: Johns Hopkins University Press; 1993.

32. Rubenstein LZ, Wieland D, Bernabei R. *Geriatric Assessment Technology: The State of the Art.* New York: Springer Publishing Co; 1995.

33. McDowell I, Newell C. *Measuring Health: A Guide to Rating Scales and Questionnaires.* 2nd ed. New York: Oxford University Press; 1996.

34. Lezak MD. *Neuropsychological Assessment.* 3rd ed. New York: Oxford University Press; 1995.

35. Bialk BS, Vosburg FL. *Geropsychology Assessment Resource Guide.* Springfield, VA: National Technical Information Service, US Dept of Commerce; 1993. PB 93–213684.

2

Ethnicity and Geriatric Assessment

Charles P. Mouton and Yolanda B. Esparza

INTRODUCTION

The proportion of the US population that is over age 65 years is increasing rapidly. At the same time, the number of older adults from minority groups, such as Hispanics, African Americans, and Asian Americans, continues to rise.[1] For these reasons, it is fitting to begin a book on geriatric assessment by highlighting the need for cultural competence in the assessment of older persons.[2] Cultural competence in health care consists of at least three components: (1) knowing the prevalence, incidence, and risk factors (epidemiology) for diseases in different ethnic groups; (2) understanding how the response to medications and other treatments vary with ethnicity; and (3) eliciting the culturally held beliefs and attitudes toward illness, treatment, and the health care system. Cultural competence in assessment includes sensitivity to changes in meaning and circumstances that were not intended by the developers of a test. All of these areas cannot be covered in this short chapter, but instead some clinical considerations in the assessment of older adults from diverse ethnic groups will be highlighted, setting the stage for the detailed discussions of specific domains that follow in subsequent chapters.

A description of the epidemiology of medical conditions across different ethnic groups would take up a whole chapter[3]; however, in many cases, solid information about the prevalence, incidence, and risk factors even for some common disorders of late life is lacking.[4] For example, there are few credible community-based estimates of the prevalence of Alzheimer's disease in ethnic minorities. Estimates of the prevalence of dementia and Alzheimer's disease in minorities from the few studies that have been done reveal substantial disease burden on the African American and Hispanic communities, with rates of Alzheimer's disease in minorities several times higher than in Whites.[5,6] Although further study is needed on Alzheimer's in ethnic minorities for its own sake, such research also could shed light on why the association of apolipoprotein E with Alzheimer's appears to be attenuated in African Americans.[6,7] Similarly, there is precious little scientific evidence of how medications vary in their effect among ethnic minorities, especially for older adults. Examples of possible differences in response to medications according to ethnicity include the effects of antihypertensives[8] and antidepressants.[9,10]

This chapter focuses on culturally competent assessment in relation to physical function, cognitive impairment, depression, social and economic issues, and ethics in medical decision making. First, some general comments are offered regarding: (1) the heterogeneity of ethnic groups; (2) the reliability, validity, and use of assessment instruments for persons of a different cultural background from which the instruments were developed and tested; (3) enhancing communication between professional caregivers and older adults of diverse ethnic backgrounds; and (4) eliciting beliefs and attitudes about illness.

HETEROGENEITY WITHIN OLDER ETHNIC MINORITIES

Clinicians must confront and question their casual conceptions of race and ethnicity. When socioeconomic factors are considered, apparent differences between older persons from minority groups and other older persons disappear or narrow for many important outcomes. Differences in health and habits ascribed to race often reflect *social* rather than *genetic* differences.[11,12] Older adults are a diverse group, even *within* ethnic categories. It is just as important to understand this heterogeneity *within* ethnic groups as it is to understand the differences *between* ethnic groups.[13] For example, some African Americans were brought to the United States against their will from Africa; others have migrated from the Caribbean.

Hispanic Americans form a heterogeneous group, having cultural origins in Mexico, Puerto Rico, South and Central America, Cuba, and other Spanish-speaking countries. Asian Americans from China, Japan, Korea, and Southeast Asia have differing health practices and beliefs. Native-American older adults derive from over 500 tribes, speaking over 150 languages. Because of this heterogeneity within cultural groups, clinicians should not lose sight of the need to evaluate each older person as an *individual* who has a cultural and personal contextual background that suffuses into every aspect of assessment and care. Clinicians should interpret the information in this chapter as *general guidelines* in assessment of older persons from minority groups, rather than as firm rules to follow when assessing older adults from specific ethnic groups.

RELIABILITY, VALIDITY, AND USE OF INSTRUMENTS FOR ETHNIC MINORITIES

Any assessment procedure is subject to error. Error in measurement can arise because the instrument is inconsistent (poor reliability) or because the instrument does not measure what the clinician thinks it is measuring (poor validity). Neighbors and Lumpkin[14] questioned the assumption that the same construct is measured when instruments developed among Whites are applied to African Americans or other minority ethnic groups. Differing idioms and colloquialisms can cause a translated instrument to have different meanings from those intended by the original developers. Even within ethnic groups, older persons who are recent immigrants may interpret items differently from older persons who have lived in the United States for some time.

At a more subtle level, some constructs may be so different across cultures as to be quite different or even irrelevant. Depressive disorder provides an example of cultural heterogeneity in expression that has drawn attention from anthropologists and medical researchers concerned with its detection and treatment.[15] Some cultures do not have concepts that are equivalent to the Western notion of depression. The Hopi Indians of Arizona, for example, describe an illness similar to major depression but without dysphoria.[16] The Flathead people of Montana express depression as a social phenomenon of loneliness— the feeling that no one cares for you.[17] Neurasthenic patients in China deny dysphoria, but do exhibit the other symptoms of depression, such as psychomotor retardation and somatic complaints.[18] Older African Americans tend to deny sadness, but are more likely to report thoughts of death than older Whites.[19]

In the domain of functional assessment, the willingness of older persons from certain groups to report difficulty taking care of themselves may be powerfully related to fear of admitting their dependence on others. Observed differences in functional status across ethnic groups may represent true differences but could represent measurement error from the instrument used in the assessment of physical function. Physical function assessment generally employs self-reporting instruments that rely on the subjective response of patients. Performance-based measures provide more objective measures of function, but are harder to carry out in the clinical setting and may not always relate directly to performance at home.[20,21] The choice of method generally relates to the clinician's time constraints, training, and need for the most reliable and valid information. A number of instruments are illustrated and discussed in Chapter 4, Functional Assessment, but unfortunately, most of the instruments have not been specifically assessed for their performance in older minorities. An exception is the SF–36 whose reliability or reproducibility has been found to be as high in minority groups as in Whites[22] and which appears to be valid for assessment of functional status in Hispanic Americans.[23]

Finally, literacy and level of educational attainment may be important considerations in assessing older adults, especially ethnic minorities who historically have had less opportunity to advance in school. Older women, in particular, grew up in a period when it was uncommon for girls to finish high school and attend college. The association of ethnic grouping with functional decline and other important health outcomes may have more to do with level of educational attainment than race. At the age of 65 years, persons with 12 or more years of schooling have an active life expectancy (that is, life spent without reported functional disability) that is 2 to 4 years longer than older adults with less education, regardless of ethnicity.[24] Closely tied to educational level attained is literacy, or the ability to understand and use written information. In one study of 144 African Americans over age 65 years living in New York City, half had a reading level below the eighth grade,[25] suggesting that materials designed for older persons must be evaluated for reading level. It remains to be seen whether improved educational opportunities for persons from ethnic minorities will result in older persons with diminished rates of functional impairment when compared to the current cohort of older persons. In clinical work, care should be taken to consider the educational level of clients who may not be accustomed to the type of questions that are asked in many functional and cognitive tests.

Clinicians need not develop their own instruments for assessment of depression, function, or other domains in order to properly assess older adults from different ethnic groups. Instead, in interpreting results from assessment, they should be aware that the reliability and validity of instruments developed, for example, among urban hospitalized patients in the Northeastern United States may not be applicable to a border community in rural South Texas. The selection of instruments and other aspects of assessment should be tailored to the known demographic profile of the practice in which the questionnaires are to be used. As researchers and clinicians become more aware of the cultural context of assessment, it is hoped that there will be more information available to make good decisions about geriatric assessment procedures that are most appropriate to different ethnic groups.

ENHANCING COMMUNICATION WITH ETHNICALLY DIVERSE OLDER ADULTS

The assessment of older adults who do not speak or read English well and who have different world views and goals than those of the health care professional can be a difficult and arduous task. Good communication skills are required for interactions with all older adults. However, social distance, racism, unconscious fears, and similar concerns on the part of patients and professionals may contribute to additional problems in assessment and diagnosis of older adults from varying ethnic groups.[26] Early attention to building rapport will go a long way to facilitating communication. In many cultures, such as among Chinese and Mexican Americans, rapport begins through exchange of pleasantries or chitchat before beginning the business of medical history taking and physical examination.[27,28] Older Hispanic Americans often expect health care personnel to be warm and personal and express a strong need to be treated with dignity.[29] As a sign of respect, older persons should be addressed by their last names. Gesturing should be avoided because seemingly benign body or hand movements may have adverse connotations in other cultures. Clinicians should take care to evaluate whether questions or instructions have been understood, because some persons will nod "yes," while not really comprehending. Since outright questioning of authority is taboo in some cultures, physicians should encourage the patient to ask questions. He or she should tell the patient that even though some things are not normally discussed, it is necessary to do so in order to plan the best care.

ELICITING BELIEFS AND ATTITUDES ABOUT ILLNESS

When caring for older adults, the clinician should make an attempt to elicit beliefs and attitudes about illness. Eliciting beliefs and attitudes about illness that may be rather different from one's own means maintaining an accepting attitude and putting the family and patient at ease that their ideas are valued in developing the care plan. The clinician should ask the patient what he or she thinks is wrong or causing the problem, whether there may be some ways to get better that doctors may not know about, what the patient has done to help the problem, and whether anyone else has been asked to help with the problem. To draw out beliefs about illness, the physician should ask the patient what worries him or her most about the illness, and why the patient thinks he or she is ill now.

Getting into the "assumptive world"[30] of the patient is time well-spent. First, doing so provides useful information about over-the-counter medications or home remedies that might interfere with prescribed medicines. For example, older persons within traveling distance of Mexico obtain pharmacologically active compounds that are not always equivalent to medications bought in the United States.[31] In addition, traditional folk remedies play a central role in health for older Mexican Americans and Asian Americans.[32] In many cases, standard prescriptions may be more acceptable if traditional remedies can continue to be taken. Second, assessing cultural beliefs about illness includes asking about diet. Dietary prescriptions are often a component of traditional healing practices in Native Americans.[33] Third, failure to elicit ideas about illness can result in poor communication, lack of adherence to prescribed therapy, or refusal to undergo tests or therapeutic procedures. For example, the idea that illness is punishment for past deeds may inhibit participation in preventive or therapeutic procedures.[34] Finally, asking and listening about the cultural beliefs of the patient helps establish rapport, shows respect for the older person, and can be one of the most interesting aspects of caring for older adults.

SELECTED DOMAINS OF GERIATRIC ASSESSMENT

Subsequent sections of this chapter will highlight specific considerations in the multidimensional evaluation of older persons from ethnic minority groups. Features of assessment relevant to ethnicity are covered. Readers should refer to other chapters for further information regarding assessments.

Functional Assessment

The functional ability of older African Americans declines more rapidly than other Americans. In the North Carolina Established Populations for Epidemiologic Studies of the Elderly, 9.6% of African Americans older than 65 reported difficulty with two or more activities of daily living (ADL), and 19% reported two or more difficulties on instrumental activities of daily living (IADL).[35,36] Older African Americans were 40% more likely to have trouble getting around and 50% more likely to be confined to their homes than Whites,[37] and the gap between African Americans and Whites appears to be widening.[38] However, in advanced age (the ninth and tenth decades of life), older African Americans appear to function better than Whites probably because only the most hardy individuals survive.[35] Hispanic Americans also have significant burden of functional impairment as assessed by ADL and IADL.[39] Markides and coworkers[40] reported that functional impairment among Hispanics was related to specific medical conditions such as diabetes mellitus, stroke, myocardial infarction, arthritis, and hip fracture. Functional impairment due to these medical conditions was greater in older Hispanic Americans than in Whites.[40-43] Among Asian Americans, comparative data on functional impairment and disability are insufficient to draw firm conclusions. Asian Americans of high socioeconomic status or who came from earlier immigrant groups probably have rates of disability similar to Whites.[44]

Cognitive Assessment

One purpose of evaluating cognitive status in older persons is to detect and manage dementia and delirium. Assessing older adults from ethnic minorities for cognitive impairment, dementia, and delirium presents a number of challenges including finding suitable translators when command of English is poor, understanding the variable beliefs related to cognitive loss with age in different cultures, approaching the decision to institutionalize, and incorporating the ethical issues pertaining to medical decision making.[45] In this section, two commonly used instruments to assess cognitive status with respect to ethnicity are discussed: (1) the Folstein Mini-Mental State Examination (MMSE); and (2) the Short Portable Mental Status Questionnaire (SPMSQ).

African Americans and persons with less than 8 years of formal education tend to be falsely identified as possibly cognitively impaired when using the MMSE.[46-48] Typically, a cutoff score is employed as a way to standardize assessment and determine when cognitive impairment is significant. Among older African Americans, Hispanic Americans, and persons with educational attainment less than high school, a lower threshold score for determination of cognitive impairment has been recommended (less than 18 out of a possible 30 points) to improve sensitivity (82%) and specificity (99%) for the diagnosis of dementia.[49,50] In other words, a standard cutoff of 23 or less to determine cognitive impairment tends to overestimate the number of African American and Hispanics with true impairment of cognitive function. Increasing functional difficulty over time with decreasing MMSE scores was not found among African American women, suggesting that the MMSE may not be a valid predictor of subsequent functional decline; this result is consistent with the idea that the MMSE may misidentify older African Americans as cognitively impaired.[51] The Hispanic Established Populations for Epidemiologic Studies in the Elderly indicated that when the standard MMSE threshold score of 23 was used, 22.3% of Mexican American older adults were classified as cognitively impaired, but this high rate of cognitive impairment may reflect lower educational attainment.[52] In addition to African Americans and Hispanic Americans, Asian American older adults also show decline in MMSE score for lower education and older age.[53] The SPMSQ has been specifically validated in older African American and Hispanic American samples with excellent sensitivity and specificity.[47,54,55]

Depression Assessment

Although the prevalence and incidence rates of depression in African Americans appear to be lower than in Whites,[56] it is not clear the extent to which this relates to a tendency of older African Americans to report somatic symptoms related to depression but not sadness.[19] In clinical samples, as many as 11% to 33% of older African American patients were found to be depressed.[57] Little is known about depression rates in older Hispanic Americans, who also present significant methodological problems when measuring depression.[58] The lifetime prevalence of major depression among Mexican American adults in California was reported to be 7.8%, but this study did not include adults over age 54 years.[59] In other studies using symptom scales, rates of depression in Mexican Americans were reported to be as high as 20% to 30%.[60-62] Suicide rates among older persons tend to be highest in White men and lowest in African American women. Older Chinese women have a suicide rate that is estimated to be up to seven times higher than in White women.[44,63] Japanese women also have higher suicide rates than White women.[44] Rates of suicide among older adults are also very high in Eastern European countries.[64–66]

Because recognition of depression is problematic, standardized assessment instruments have been developed. In most cases, there is little information on how these instruments perform in older ethnic minority groups. Here, two instruments with regard to ethnicity are discussed: (1) the Centers for Epidemiologic Studies Depression Scale (CES-D) and (2) the Geriatric Depression Scale (GDS). The CES-D is a 20-item questionnaire designed to measure depressive symptoms in multiethnic, community-based samples.[67] Reliability estimates for the CES-D are high, ranging from 0.84 to 0.92. Samples of African Americans and other diverse groups have shown that the CES-D can usefully measure depression.[68] The CES-D has a sensitivity of 75% in older African Americans and 94% in older Whites.[47,69,70] The GDS has good sensitivity and specificity in most samples although it appears to have poorer performance among African Americans than among Whites.[68–71] Among Hispanic Americans the GDS was also less sensitive to significant depression.[72,73]

Social and Economic Issues in Assessment

Frequently, it is the family who brings the older patient into the doctor. Therefore, social environment plays an important part in the health of older adults. The quality and density of the social environment are critical factors in maintenance of independent living at home. Adequate social support and interaction are significant predictors of morbidity and mortality in older adults.[74,75] Many cultures have strong traditions of care for older family members. For example, among Hispanic Americans, the concept is called *familismo;* for Japanese families filial piety and family obligation are called *koko.*[29,34] Resistance to accepting help from nonfamily members may reflect an unwillingness to transfer these family obligations to health care professionals. Families of older adults from ethnic minorities may have a great need to participate in the care of their older relatives. African American caregivers report performing more caregiving activities and caring for persons with greater functional and cognitive impairment than did Whites; however, White caregivers reported significantly more burden.[76] In addition to social support from the family, the church is an important source of social and emotional support for older African Americans.[77,78]

At the same time, health care professionals should realize that caring family members may shield their relative from intrusive questions or procedures or may cover up deficiencies in the older patient's performance. Family members must be made aware that adequate assessment of older adults requires that they must act as clear translators of questions and answers, not only of assessment instruments, but also in relation to recommended treatment. Family members may be able to suggest ways that the medical treatment can be integrated with the cultural beliefs and practices of the older person.

Minority older adults tend to show greater levels of financial strain than other Americans.[79,80] Older minorities face "double jeopardy;" that is, the combined effect of age and minority status leads to greater illness burden and greater strain on financial resources.[81-85] Physicians need to consider the financial constraints of older minority patients when developing recommendations for treatment. While direct questioning about finances may be offensive to some older adults, presenting the possibility of a less expensive, but equally effective treatment, shows a depth of understanding that is often appreciated by older persons.

Ethics in Medical Decision Making

Advance care planning and end-of-life discussions are an important component of geriatric assessment. Discussions with older minorities about treatment in the event of serious or terminal illness are often more complex than with middle-class Whites because ethnic, religious, and cultural differences are added to the mix. For example, the core value of personal autonomy may not be as tightly held for some minority groups. Mexican American and Korean older adults rely more heavily on family and physician input for end-of-life decisions than might be typical for Whites. For such persons, physicians will have difficulty if they try to elicit a totally autonomous decision from the patient. In addition, older minorities are more likely than Whites to prefer an aggressive treatment approach, often for fear of abandonment. Even when older persons from minority groups prefer a palliative approach to care, they are less likely to have communicated this to their physicians. Trust and comfort with a personal physician may be two of the most important requirements that will enhance end-of-life discussions.

CONCLUSION

Geriatric assessment is an important component of clinical practice. Assessment can be carried out in a single visit or over a number of visits. Since older ethnic minorities are bound to make up a large proportion of patients in primary care, clinicians should pay special attention to the cultural factors that modify aspects of assessment, including the suitability of specific instruments. Combined with sensitivity to cultural issues and clinical judgment, the health and function of all older adults can be enhanced through careful considerations of the domains of geriatric assessment.

REFERENCES

1. Agree EM, Freedman VA. Implications of population aging for geriatric health. In: Gallo JJ, Busby-Whitehead J, Rabins PV, Silliman R, Murphy J, eds. *Reichel's Care of the Elderly: Clinical Aspects of Aging.* 5th ed. Baltimore: Lippincott Williams & Wilkins; 1999:659–669.

2. Lavizzo-Mourey R, Mackenzie ER. Cultural competence: Essential measurements of quality for managed care organizations. *Ann Intern Med.* 1996;124:919–921.

3. Mouton CP, Espino DV. Ethnic diversity of the aged. In: Gallo JJ, Busby-Whitehead J, Rabins PV, Silliman R, Murphy J, eds. *Reichel's Care of the Elderly: Clinical Aspects of Aging.* 5th ed. Baltimore: Lippincott Williams & Wilkins; 1999:595–608.

4. Gallo JJ, Lebowitz BD. The epidemiology of common mental disorders in late life: Themes for a new century. *Psychiatric Services,* in press.

5. Hendrie HC, Osuntokun BO, Hall KS, et al. Prevalence of Alzheimer's disease and dementia in two communities: Nigerian African and African Americans. *Am J Psychiatry.* 1995;152:1485–1492.

6. Teng MX, Stern Y, Marder K, et al. The APOE-epsilon-4 allele and the risk of Alzheimer's disease among African Americans, Whites, and Hispanics. *JAMA.* 1998;279:751–755.

7. Maestre G, Ottman R, Stern Y, et al. Apolipoprotein E and Alzheimer's disease: Ethnic variation in genotype risks. *Ann Neurol.* 1995;37:254–259.

8. Prisant LM, Mensah GA. Use of beta-adrenergic receptor blockers in blacks. *J Clin Pharmacol.* 1996;36:867–873.

9. Pi EH, Wang AL, Gray GE. Asian/non-Asian transcultural tricyclic antidepressant psychopharmacology: A review. *Prog Neuropsychopharmacol Biol Psychiatry.* 1993;17:691–702.

10. Sramek JJ, Pi EH. Ethnicity and antidepressant response. *Mount Sinai J Med.* 1996;63:320–325.

11. Cooper R, David R. The biological concept of race and its application to public health and epidemiology. *J Health Polit Policy Law.* 1986;11:97–116.

12. Lillie-Blanton M, Anthony JC, Schuster CR. Probing the meaning of racial/ethnic group comparisons in crack cocaine smoking. *JAMA.* 1993;269:993–997.

13. Whitfield KE. Studying cognition in older African-Americans: Some conceptual considerations. *J Aging Ethnicity.* 1996;1:41–52.

14. Neighbors HW, Lumpkin S. The epidemiology of mental disorder in the black population. In: Ruiz DS, ed. *Handbook of Mental Health and Mental Disorder Among Black-Americans.* Westport, CT: Greenwood Press; 1990:55–70.

15. Kleinman A, Good B. *Culture and Depression: Studies in the Anthropology and Cross-Cultural Psychiatry of Affect and Disorder.* Los Angeles: University of California Press; 1985.

16. Manson SM, Shore JH, Bloom JD. The depressive experience in American Indian communities: A challenge for psychiatric theory and diagnosis. In: Kleinman A, Good B, eds. *Culture and Depression: Studies in the Anthropology and Cross-Cultural Psychiatry of Affect and Disorder.* Los Angeles: University of California Press; 1985:331–368.

17. O'Nell TD. *Disciplined Hearts: History, Identity, and Depression in an American Indian Community.* Los Angeles: University of California Press; 1996.

18. Kleinman A. *Patients and Healers in the Context of Culture: An Exploration of the Borderland Between Anthropology, Medicine, and Psychiatry.* Los Angeles: University of California Press; 1980.

19. Gallo JJ, Cooper-Patrick L, Lesikar S. Depressive symptoms of Whites and African Americans aged 60 years and older. *J Gerontol: Psychol Sci.* 1998;53B:277–286.

20. Guralnik JM, Reuben DB, Buchner DM, Ferrucci L. Performance measures of physical function in comprehensive geriatric assessment. In: Rubenstein LZ, Wieland D, Bernabei R, eds. *Geriatric Assessment Technology: The State of the Art.* New York: Springer Publishing Co; 1995:59–74.

21. Guralnik JM, Branch LG, Cummings SR, Curb JD. Physical performance measures in aging research. *J Gerontol.* 1989;44:M141–146.

22. Ware JE, Kosinski M, Keller SD. A 12-item short-form health survey: Construction of scales and preliminary tests of reliability and validity. *Med Care.* 1996;34:220–223.

23. Arocho R, McMillan CA, Sutton-Wallace P. Construct validation of the USA-Spanish version of the SF–36 health survey in a Cuban-American population with benign prostatic hyperplasia. *Quality Life Res.* 1998;7:121–126.

24. Guralnik JM, Land KC, Blazer DG, Fillenbaum GG, Branch LG. Educational status and active life expectancy among older Blacks and Whites. *N Engl J Med.* 1993;329:110–116.

25. Albert SM, Teresi JA. Reading ability, education, and cognitive status assessment among older adults in Harlem, New York City. *Am J Public Health.* 1999;89:95–97.

26. Brangman SA. African-American elders: Implications for health care providers. *Clin Geriatr Med.* 1995;11:15–23.

27. Gallagher-Thompson D, Talamantes M, Ramirez R, Valverde I. Service delivery issues and recommendations for working with Mexican American family caregivers. In: Yeo G, Gallagher-Thompson D, eds. *Ethnicity and the Dementias.* Washington, DC: Taylor & Francis Publishers; 1996:137–152.

28. Elliott KS, Di Minno M, Lam D, Tu AM. Working with Chinese families in the context of dementia. In: Yeo G, Gallagher-Thompson D, eds. *Ethnicity and the Dementias.* Washington, DC: Taylor & Francis Publishers; 1996:89–108.

29. Villa ML, Cuellar J, Gamel N, Yeo G. *Aging and Health: Hispanic-American Elders.* 2nd ed. Palo Alto, CA: Stanford Geriatric Education Center; 1993.

30. Frank JD, Frank JB. *Persuasion and Healing: A Comparative Study of Psychotherapy.* Baltimore: Johns Hopkins University Press; 1991.

31. Greene VL, Monahans DJ. Comparative utilization of community-based long-term care services by Hispanic and Anglo elderly in a case management system. *J Gerontol.* 1984;39:730–735.

32. Espino DV. Medication usage in elderly Hispanics: What we need to know. In: Sotomayor M, Ascencio NR, eds. *Proceedings on Improving Drug Use Among Hispanic Elderly.* Washington, DC: National Hispanic Council on Aging; 1988:7–11.

33. McCabe M, Cuellar J. *Aging and Health: American Indian/Alaska Native Elders.* 2nd ed. Palo Alto, CA: Stanford Geriatric Education Center; 1994.

34. McBride M, Morioka-Douglas N, Yeo G. *Aging and Health: Asian/Pacific Island American Elders.* 2nd ed. Palo Alto: Stanford Geriatric Education Center; 1996.

35. Miles TP, Bernard MA. Morbidity, disability, and the health status of Black American elderly: A new look at the oldest-old. *J Am Geriatr Soc.* 1992;40:1047–1054.

36. Foley DJ, Fillenbaum G, Service C. Physical functioning. In: Cornoni-Huntley JC, Ostfeld AM, Taylor JO, et al, eds. *Established Populations for the Epidemiologic Studies of the Elderly: Resource Data Book.* Washington, DC: National Institute on Aging, National Institute of Health, U.S. Public Health Service; 1990:34–50. Publication no. 90–495.

37. Edmonds MK. Physical health. In: Jackson JS, Chatters LM, Taylor RJ, eds. *Aging in Black America.* Newbury Park, CA: Sage Publications; 1993:151–167.

38. Clark DO. US trends in disability and institutionalization among older Blacks and Whites. *Am J Public Health.* 1997;87:438–440.

39. Andrews J. *Poverty and Poor Health among Elderly Hispanic Americans.* Baltimore: Commonwealth Fund Commission; 1989.

40. Markides KS, Stroup-Benham CA, Goodwin JS, Perkowski LC, Lichtenstein M, Ray LA. The effect of medical conditions on the functional limitations of Mexican-American elderly. *Ann Epidemiol.* 1996;6:386–391.

41. Espino DV, Neufeld RR, Mulvhill MK, Libow LS. Hispanic and non-Hispanic elderly on admission to the nursing home: A pilot study. *Gerontologist.* 1988;28:821–824.

42. Chiodo LK, Karren DW, Gerety MB, Mulrow CD, Cornell JF. Functional status of Mexican-American nursing home residents. *J Am Geriatr Soc.* 1994;42:293–296.

43. Rudkin L, Markides KS, Espino DV. Functional limitations in elderly Mexican-Americans. *Top Geriatr Rehabil.* 1997;12:38–46.

44. Lum OM. Health status of Asians and Pacific Islanders. *Clin Geriatr Med.* 1995;11:53–69.

45. Yeo G, Gallagher-Thompson D. *Ethnicity and the Dementias.* Washington, DC: Taylor & Francis Publishers; 1996.

46. Anthony JC, LeResche L, Niaz U, Von Korff M, Folstein MF. Limits of the 'Mini-Mental State' as a screening test for dementia and delirium among hospital patients. *Psychol Med.* 1982;12:397–408.

47. Baker FM. Issues in assessing dementia in African American elders. In: Yeo G, Gallagher-Thompson D, eds. *Ethnicity and the Dementias.* Washington, DC: Taylor & Francis Publishers; 1996:59–76.

48. Bohrstedt M, Fox PJ, Kohatsu ND. Correlates of Mini-Mental State examination scores among elderly demented patients: The influence of race-ethnicity. *J Clin Epidemiol.* 1994;47:1381–1387.

49. Tangalos EG, Smith GE, Ivnik RJ, et al. The Mini-Mental State examination in general medical practice: Clinical utility and acceptance. *Mayo Clin Proc.* 1996;71:829–837.

50. Crum RM, Anthony JC, Bassett SS, Folstein MF. Population-based norms for the Mini-Mental State examination by age and educational level. *JAMA*. 1993;269: 2386–2391.

51. Leveille SG, Guralnik JM, Ferrucci L, Corti MC, Kasper J, Fried LP. Black/white differences in the relationship between MMSE scores and disability: The Women's Health and Aging Study. *J Gerontol. Series B Psychol Sci Soc Sci*. 1998;53:201–208.

52. Majurin R, Espino DV, Lichtenstein MJ, Hazuda HP, Fabrizio D, Markides KP. Point-prevalence of cognitive impairment in the Southwest US Mexican-American elderly population: A large-scale community survey using the Mini-Mental State examination. *J Gerontol*. Under review.

53. Ishizaki J, Meguro K, Ambo H, et al. A normative, community-based study Mini-Mental State in elderly adults: The effect of age and educational level. *J Gerontol: Soc Sci*. 1998;53:359–363.

54. Pfeiffer E. A short portable mental status questionnaire for the assessment of organic brain deficit in elderly patients. *J Am Geriatr Soc*. 1975;23:433–441.

55. Fillenbaum GG, Heyman A, Williams K, Prosnit B, Burchett B. Sensitivity and specificity of standardized screening tests for cognitive impairment and dementia among elder Black and White community residents. *J Clin Epidemiol*. 1990;43:651–658.

56. Gallo JJ, Royall DR, Anthony JC. Risk factors for the onset of major depression in middle age and late life. *Soc Psychiatry Psychiatr Epidemiol*. 1993;28:101–108.

57. Rosenthal MP, Goldfarb NJ, Carlson BL, et al. Assessment of depression in a family practice. *J Fam Pract*. 1987;25:143–148.

58. Wagner FA, Gallo JJ, Delva J. Depresión en la edad avanzada. ¿Problema oculto de salud pública para México? *Salud Publica Mexico*. 1999;41:189–202.

59. Vega WA, Kolody B, Aguilar-Gaxiola S, Alderete E, Catalano R, Caraveo-Anduaga J. Lifetime prevalence of DSM-III-R psychiatric disorders among urban and rural Mexican Americans in California. *Arch Gen Psychiatry*. 1998;55:771–778.

60. Kemp BS, Staples FR, Lopez-Aqueres W. Epidemiology of depression and dysphoria in the elderly Hispanic population. *J Am Geriatr Soc*. 1987;35:920–926.

61. Munoz E. Care for the Hispanic poor: A growing segment of American society. *JAMA*. 1988;260:2711–2712.

62. Black SA, Markides KS, Miller TQ. Correlates of depressive symptomatology among older community-dwelling Mexican Americans: The Hispanic EPESE. *J Gerontol. Series B, Psychol Sci Soc Sci*. 1998;53:S198–208.

63. Liu WT, Yu E. Asian/Pacific American elderly: Mortality differentials, health status, and the use of health services. *J Appl Gerontol*. 1985;4:35–64.

64. Corin E. From a cultural stance: Suicide and aging in a changing world. *Int Psychogeriatr*. 1995;7:335–355.

65. La Vecchia C, Lucchini F, Levi F. Worldwide trends in suicide mortality, 1955–1989. *Acta Psychiatr Scand*. 1994;90:53–64.

66. Sartorius N. Recent changes in suicide rates in selected Eastern European and other European countries. *Int Psychogeriatr*. 1995;7:301–308.

67. Radloff LS. The CES-D Scale: A self-report depression scale for research in the general population. *Appl Psychol Meas*. 1977;1:385–401.

68. Mouton CP, Johnson MS, Cole DR. Ethical considerations with African American elders. *Clin Geriatr Med*. 1995;11:113–129.

69. Baker FM, Wiley C, Velli SA, Johnson JT. Reliability of the Geriatric Depression Scale and the Center for Epidemiologic Studies of Depression Scale in the elderly [abstract]. Annual Meeting of the American Psychiatric Association, September 24, 1994.

70. Baker FM, Parker DA, Wiley C, Velli SA, Johnson JT. Depressive symptoms in African American medical patients. *Int J Geriatr Psychiatry.* 1995;10:9–14.

71. Baker FM. A contrast: Geriatric depression versus depression in younger age groups. *J Natl Med Assoc.* 1991;83:340–344.

72. Baker FM, Espino DV, Robinson BH, et al. Assessing depressive symptoms in African-American and Mexican-American elders. *Clin Gerontol.* 1993;14:15–21.

73. Baker FM, Espino DV. A Spanish version of the geriatric depression scale in Mexican-American elders. *Int J Geriatr Psychiatry.* 1997;12:21–25.

74. Seeman TE, Kaplan GA, Knudsen L, Cohen R, Guralnik J. Social network ties and mortality among the elderly in the Alameda County study. *Am J Epidemiol.* 1987;126:714–723.

75. Blazer DG. Social support and mortality in an elderly community population. *Am J Epidemiol.* 1982;115:684–694.

76. Fredman L, Daly MP, Lazur AM. Burden among White and Black caregivers to elderly adults. *J Gerontol. Ser B Psychol Sci Soc Sci.* 1995;50:S110–S118.

77. Chadiha L, Morrow-Howell N, Darkwa OK, Berg-Weger M. Support systems of African American family caregivers of elders with dementing illness. *Afr Am Res Perspect.* 1998;4:104–114.

78. Chatters LM, Taylor RJ. Religious involvement among African Americans. *Afr Am Res Perspect.* 1998;4:83–93.

79. Jackson JS, Chatters LM, Taylor RJ. *Aging in African-American America.* Newbury Park, CA: Sage Publications; 1993.

80. The Commonwealth Fund. *National Comparative Survey of Minority Health Care.* New York: The Commonwealth Fund; 1995.

81. Cantor M. The informal support system of New York's inner-city elderly: Is ethnicity a factor? In: Gelfand DE, Kutsik AJ, eds. *Ethnicity and Aging: Theory, Research, and Policy.* New York: Springer Publishing Co; 1979:153–175.

82. Reed W. Health care needs and services. In: Harel Z, McKinney EA, Williams M, eds. *African-American Aged: Understanding Diversity and Service Needs.* Newbury Park, CA: Sage Publications; 1990.

83. Dowd JJ, Bengston VL. Aging in minority populations: An examination of the double jeopardy hypothesis. *J Gerontol.* 1978;33:427–436.

84. Jackson M, Kolody B, Wood JL. To be old and African-American: The case for the double jeopardy on income and health. In: Manuel RC, ed. *Minority Aging: Sociological and Social Psychological Issues.* Westport, CT: Greenwood Press; 1982.

85. Ferraro KF. Double jeopardy to health for African-American older adults? *J Gerontol.* 1987;42:528–533.

3

Mental Status Assessment

any studies since Dr Michael Shepherd and colleagues' seminal work, *Psychiatric Illness in General Practice*, published over 30 years ago,[1] revealed that mental disorders were common in the primary care setting, but that individuals with these disorders frequently went unrecognized, with adverse consequences for them, their family, and the health care system. In the United States, Regier and colleagues have called attention to the de facto mental health services system composed of the general medical services and have highlighted the need for understanding how to integrate general medical care and mental health care.[2] Compared to younger persons, older adults were most likely to receive mental health care from the primary care sector, not from specialists in mental health.[3] The literature dealing with mental health care in primary care settings has been extensively reviewed elsewhere.[4,5]

Mental state assessment is pivotal in evaluating the health of older persons. The accuracy of the medical and social history obtained from an older person will depend on adequate mental and affective functioning. Cognitive impairment predicts poor agreement between self-reported and observer-rated measures of functioning.[6] Assessment of mental status is encouraged in order to detect unsuspected mental impairment and to provide a basis for comparison in future encounters.

29

Most practitioners who deal with older persons have had the experience of treating an elder who is seen by the casual observer to be able to carry on a reasonably coherent conversation, but in whom mental status testing reveals significant difficulties. The person may be able to perform well in a job that has been held for many years as long as the routine is not interrupted. In novel situations, the extent of the deficit may become painfully evident to family or coworkers. The family may not even be aware that behavioral changes are secondary to subtle intellectual deterioration.

Ample evidence reveals that cognitive impairment and psychiatric disorder are often not recognized by health care professionals. Fully one third of older patients admitted to a medical floor in one study of cognitive status in the elderly had significant mental impairment.[7] Other investigators demonstrated that in a 250-bed hospital affiliated with Brown University, only 14 of 65 patients (21%) with cognitive deficits detected on the screening examination had documentation by the patients' physicians that such deficits had been recognized. In only two cases was a mental status examination a part of the patient's record.[8] Other studies have documented the failure of physicians to routinely perform mental status testing on older patients. Significant proportions of demented elders were not diagnosed by their physicians yet were identified by brief mental status screening examination as being impaired.[9,10] Among patients evaluated by a psychiatrist prior to discharge from medical or surgical wards, only 27% of patients with mental impairment were diagnosed prior to discharge; most were believed to have moderate to severe impairment. In outpatient practice, few patients with cognitive impairment are recognized without screening.[11-13] Even among persons with diagnosed dementia whose family members recognized memory problems, only half received a medical evaluation.[14] Physicians may also fail to recognize depression, alcohol abuse, and drug misuse in their patients.[4,15]

The recognition of mental impairment is of more than just academic importance. Patients with abnormal scores on the screening examination had a greater chance of having episodes of confusion during the hospitalization,[8] after discharge,[16] and post-operatively.[17] Cognitively impaired hospitalized patients are less stable with increased morbidity and mortality,[18,19] risk of loss of independence,[16,19-21] post-operative complications,[17] and behavioral difficulties.[22]

The discovery of cognitive impairment should prompt a search for an etiology. The best hope of finding a reversible process may hinge on early recognition by the clinician. Behavioral or personality changes may be placed in context when mental impairment is found to be present. Drugs that impair cognition should be avoided if at all possible. Specific pharmacologic therapy may mandate early detection of dementia.[23] For these reasons, it seems compelling to insist that mental status testing be a part of routine procedure for all older patients, particularly at the time of nursing home or hospital admission.[8,13,24] In other cases, clinical cues or "triggers" should prompt an assessment that may begin with the use of assessment instruments discussed below.

The Agency for Health Care Policy and Research (AHCPR) *Guidelines on Early Identification of Alzheimer's Disease and Related Dementias* presented a number of examples of clinical cues that should prompt an assessment of mental status: namely, difficulty learning and remembering new information, difficulty handling complex tasks, inability to solve problems, trouble with spatial ability and orientation (eg, driving), trouble finding the right words, and behavioral disturbances.[25] The Guideline Panel recommended that mental status testing be interpreted in the context of functional status. Situations in which there is inconsistent information on mental status and functional status (ie, one, but not both, is impaired) call for further neuropsychological assessment and possibly referral for diagnosis and evaluation of dementia. The components of mental status and functional status discussed in this and the next chapter, implemented with the instruments discussed, can assist in evaluation of older adults when the clinical cues for dementia, delirium, depression, or other mental disturbances are present.

The failure of many physicians to perform mental status testing on older individuals is unfortunate. Frequently, it is the person's personal physician who is best able to judge his or her competence, not a consultant who does not have an ongoing relationship with the patient. A periodic assessment of mental status in the chart can be valuable in these circumstances, particularly if legal questions arise.[26] Mental status testing of asymptomatic older adults must be balanced by concerns about falsely labeling the patient as demented. Poor performance on a mental status assessment instrument can arise from many causes. Dementia is a syndrome, a constellation of symptoms and characteristics that require clinical evaluation (discussed in more detail below).

In this chapter, the definition of "mental status testing" includes screening instruments for psychiatric disorder, especially depression. Indeed, cognitive and psychological status are closely related, and it is probably inappropriate to neglect one in discussing the other. Inventories to screen for depression cannot establish a diagnosis, but their use at least keeps the affective disorders in the forefront and imparts to the client a sense that feelings are important to the clinician and appropriate for discussion and consideration. Depression is associated with diminished functional capacity in its own right.[27-31] Since treatment of depression is effective in older persons, a case can be made for careful consideration of the symptoms of depression that underlie somatic complaints or functional decline.[32,33]

THE MENTAL STATUS EXAMINATION

The mental status examination samples behavior and mental capability over a range of intellectual functions (Exhibit 3–1). The shorter standardized examinations to detect cognitive impairment that are discussed later in this chapter attempt to crystallize the examination so that a range of intellectual functions is tested by one or two questions in each area. When the screening instrument detects impairment, further examination is warranted. In clinical settings, this usually means more detailed mental status testing to localize and define the problem. When further characterization of the intellectual functioning is required, neuropsychological testing may be in order. This becomes particularly salient when the individual's cognitive strengths and weaknesses must be delineated to make decisions about supervi-

---

Exhibit 3–1 Components of the Mental Status Examination

Level of consciousness
Attention

Language
  Fluency
  Comprehension
  Repetition

Memory
  Short-term memory
  Remote memory

Proverb interpretation
Similarities
Calculations
Writing
Constructional ability

Source: Adapted with permission from RL Strub and FW Black *The Mental Status Examination in Neurology,* pp 163–172, © 1980 FA Davis Company.

sion and rehabilitative services, in the differential diagnosis of dementia and depression, or after stroke.[34]

Some health care professionals take the mental status examination no further than asking a few questions about orientation, having the person perform calculations, and requiring that he or she remember three items. In some situations, however, a thorough assessment can be crucial in an appropriate diagnosis and hence management. The classic example is an individual with an intracranial hemorrhage who is not making any sense and is mistakenly thought to be psychotic or confused because a specific language disturbance is not recognized. Granted, not every patient needs to be examined in precisely the way described here, but the standard screening mental status instruments discussed later in this chapter are short enough to be used in their entirety to assist in identifying cognitive impairment.

The complete mental status examination encompasses an assessment of the level of consciousness, attention, language, memory, proverb interpretation, similarities (eg, "How are an apple and an orange alike?"), calculations, writing, and constructional ability (eg, copying complex figures). A detailed overview of the mental status examination is provided by Strub and Black in *The Mental Status Examination in Neurology.*[35]

Higher Cognitive Functions

The interview should start with questions of significance to the patient, which also gauge his or her memory and may help allay anxiety. Introductory statements that indicate interest in the older patient as a person (eg, occupation, children, grandchildren, and hobbies) also indicate the patient's current and previous level of mental and social functioning. General appearance and grooming, posture, behavior, speech, and word choice can speak volumes to the careful observer.[36] The examiner should be wary of hearing and visual deficits that may mimic cognitive impairment.

An older patient meeting the physician or nurse for the first time may be anxious about the encounter. He or she may be coming to the interview reluctantly or even coerced by family or neighbors. He or she may worry that the physician or nurse is testing to see if he or she is "crazy." Even in a nonthreatening environment, the interview can cause anxiety, thereby resulting in apparent confusion, inaccurate or incomplete reporting of information, and poor performance on testing. There is fear of error, and the patient may become hesitant to perform requested tasks. Disturbances of memory and intelligence exhibited during the examination may be a reflection of psychic stress and depression rather than dementia. It is wise to intersperse questions that are stressful or that focus on disability with others that are not and to end the interview on a positive note.[37]

The higher cognitive functions that may be specifically tested include the patient's fund of information and ability to reason abstractly and perform calculations (Table 3–1). Once some preliminary questions about personal history are discussed, the patient may be asked questions regarding current events in the news (eg, "Who is the president now?") or commonly known historical information (eg, "When did World War II end?") to assess the fund of information. In evaluating responses, it is critical to know the level of educational attainment and whether English is the patient's first language.

Assessment of insight and judgment has important implications for considering driving skills and independence. Accidents and burns may be more common among cognitively impaired persons with poor insight and judgment.[38] Observe the patient's responses to mental status testing and conversation to note whether statements belie lack of insight into deficits.[38]

Proverb testing and similarities shed light on the patient's reasoning ability, intelligence, and judgment. The examiner needs to be careful

Table 3–1 Higher Integrative Functions

Location	Assessment
Frontal lobes	Points finger each time the examiner makes a fist and makes a fist when the examiner points
Temporal lobes	*Dominant:* standard aphasia testing (spontaneous speech, repetition, comprehension, writing, and naming) *Nondominant:* interprets affect (names affects shown in photos of faces or conveyed in examiner's voice)
Parietal lobes	*Dominant:* names fingers, knows left and right, performs calculations on paper, reading *Nondominant:* constructs copy of matchstick figure made by the examiner
Occipital lobes	Matches colors and objects if unable to name them

Source: Adapted with permission from EC Shuttleworth, Memory Function and the Clinical Differentiation of Dementing Disorders, *Journal of the American Geriatric Society*, Vol. 30, pp. 365–366, © Lippincott Williams & Wilkins.

that the patient is not repeating the meaning of a proverb from memory rather than reasoning what an abstract interpretation might be. The Cognitive Capacity Screen[7] and the Kokmen Short Test of Mental Status,[39] discussed below, are examples of screening instruments that include a test of reasoning with similarities, a task requiring the subject to think in abstract categories to discover how two concepts are alike. An example of a similarity is: "How are a poem and a novel alike?" It has been suggested that the use of similarities is better than the use of proverb testing for the assessment of abstraction ability.[40]

The ability to perform calculations may be tested with serial 7s (ie, "Take 7 away from 100 and keep subtracting 7 from the answer all the way down"), serial 3s (ie, "Take 3 away from 20 and keep subtracting 3 from the answer all the way down"), or with simple math problems. Corrected mistakes should not be counted as errors. Calculation ability also requires substantial memory and concentration ability. Occasionally, patients who have difficulty with serial 7s will handle the subtractions flawlessly if the problem is expressed in dollar terms (ie, "If you had $100 and took away $7, how much would you have left?").

Memory

Of all the components of the mental status examination, memory assessment most commonly engenders anxiety, and understandably so. It sometimes puts the patient at ease when the examiner prefaces the evaluation, particularly when using a standard questionnaire, with an explanation such as the following: "I'm going to ask you some questions. Some are easy. Some may be hard. Please don't be offended, because it's the same routine I use for everyone." The examiner should give positive reinforcement during the examination with expressions such as "that's OK" or "that's fine."

Memory can be thought of as comprising three components. First and most fleeting is immediate recall. This can be assessed with digit repetition. Normal older persons can correctly recall five to seven digits.[41,42] The second component of memory is short-term memory, ranging over a period of minutes to days. This is usually tested by asking the person to remember 3 to 4 objects or abstract terms and then requesting him or her to recall them 5 or 10 minutes later after an intervening conversation or other testing. Examples of words used are "apple, table, penny"[43] and "brown, honesty, tulip, eyedropper."[35] The memory of aphasic persons may be tested by asking them to recall where items have been hidden in the room. It has been suggested that older persons do not use mnemonics when given a memory task and that this in part accounts for their failure to recall items.[42] Also, there is some evidence for increased processing time in older persons, and this may interfere with learning.[44] A third component of memory is remote or long-term memory. In one study, older adults were able to recall 80% of a catechism that had been learned some 36 years before.[45]

In general, older persons' self-reports of memory difficulty correlate poorly with objective measures of memory function. Not uncommonly, persons who complain fervently of memory loss are depressed, whereas someone with Alzheimer's disease may be oblivious to profound memory deficit. Early in the course of the disease, however, Alzheimer's patients may complain of memory loss.[46] Normal middle-aged or older persons may complain of memory difficulties, but their memory symptoms fit what has been called benign senescent forgetfulness or more recently, age-associated memory impairment[47,48] or aging-associated cognitive decline.[49,50] These patients may be aware of a problem and apologize. They may not recall details of an experience, but certainly remember the experience itself. The forgetfulness fluctuates so that details not recalled at one time may be remembered at another.

Patients with more significant memory loss often have accompanying intellectual deficits. Kral referred to this as malignant memory loss because the patients in his original series with this type of memory decline had greater mortality than a group who did not.[48] Patients with malignant memory loss not only forget details of an event but may not recall the experience itself, or may confabulate about forgotten details.[41,48]

New nomenclature is emerging to describe the memory decline that is associated with normal aging, to replace the term "benign senescent forgetfulness." Some middle-aged and older persons exhibit memory dysfunction due to age in the routine tasks of daily life, such as trouble remembering items on a shopping list or forgetting telephone numbers. To fulfill the criteria for age-associated memory impairment, the person must have objective evidence of impairment on a memory function test, such as the Wechsler Associate Learning Subtest, but also must have absence of dementia (the diagnosis of which would imply a more global intellectual impairment), as evidenced by the Folstein Mini-Mental State Examination (MMSE).[47,51] Subjects with a family history of Alzheimer's dementia who met criteria for age-associated memory impairment did not have evidence of altered glucose metabolism.[52] Criteria for aging-associated cognitive decline will stimulate further developments on subthreshold dementia.[52,53] The fourth edition of the *Diagnostic and Statistical Manual (DSM-IV)* includes research criteria for mild neurocognitive disorder characterized by memory and other cognitive impairment that is due to a general medical condition but does not meet full criteria for dementia.[54]

Attention and Level of Consciousness

Before an examiner can test and comment on the higher intellectual functions of the brain, including memory, some assessment (even if informal) must be made of the patient's level of consciousness. Obviously, functions such as orientation and memory cannot be tested in a comatose patient.

Orientation to surroundings is a fundamental beginning to mental status testing, but unfortunately, in routine clinical situations, the mental status evaluation often ends there. Questions regarding orientation to time, place, person, and situation are basic. Most people continually orient themselves by means of daily routines, clocks and watches, calendars, news media, and social activities. Older persons, on the other hand, particularly those living alone or in nursing homes, may not experience these activities and as a result may have poor orientation to time and events.[37,55]

Once it is determined by observation that the person is alert enough for mental status testing to proceed, his or her attentiveness is assessed. Assessing attentiveness is important because a person who is easily distracted and unable to attend to the examiner will have poor performance on mental status testing solely because of inattention. Special note must be taken of the person who is inappropriately distracted by environmental noise or talking in the hallway. In such a case, specific examination for attention deficit indicative of delirium may be warranted. Tests of attention sometimes used include digit repetition and the "A" test of vigilance. The length of a string of digits able to be repeated immediately after presentation tends to remain stable with age. A normal 90-year-old should be able to repeat four digits, perhaps even seven or eight, after the examiner.[41] In the "A" test, the patient is asked to tap the table when the letter "A" is heard while the examiner presents random letters at a rate of one letter per second. The examiner observes for errors of commission and omission.

Neglect is a form of inattention in which the individual does not attend stimuli presented from a particular side, and it occurs most commonly with nondominant hemisphere lesions (usually the right). The examiner needs to avoid interviewing such a person from the neglected side if communication is to be effective.

Language

Language should be observed and tested in a comprehensive mental status examination.[56] Spontaneous speech is observed during the initial interview. Does the patient make errors in words or grammatical construction? Persons with dysarthria, who have difficulty in the mechanical production of language, use normal grammar. Do spoken words flow smoothly? Fluency is one of the features that is used to differentiate the aphasias.

A simplified approach to aphasia divides the spoken language functions to be tested into three areas: comprehension, fluency, and repetition. Comprehension can be tested by asking the patient yes-or-no questions. If there is doubt about the responses, the patient may be asked to point to objects in the room. The task may be made more difficult by having him or her try to point to objects in a particular sequence or after the examiner has provided a description of the item rather than the item's name.

Fluency is a characteristic of speech that describes the rate and rhythm of speech production and the ease in initiating speech. Patients may be asked to name objects and their parts such as a wristwatch and its band, buckle, and face. Repetition is tested with easy expressions (eg, "ball" or "airplane") progressing to more difficult ones (eg, "Methodist Episcopal" or "Around the rock the rugged rascal ran").

The aphasias can be organized around the three characteristics of comprehension, fluency, and repetition (Figure 3–1). The person in whom the entire language neural substrate is destroyed, for example, due to infarction and edema after a stroke, has a global aphasia, and, indeed, may be mute. All three language parameters are impaired in such a case. After a period of recovery, some language function may return.

Wernicke's aphasia is characterized by impaired comprehension and repetition. Speech is fluent but marked by paraphasia (ie, words or sounds that are replaced by other sounds, such as "wife" or "car" for "knife") and neologisms (ie, nonsense words). Persons with this type of aphasia have severe difficulty with comprehension and may not even be aware that their own speech output is incoherent, which can be a considerable obstacle in rehabilitation. The person with Wernicke's aphasia may describe a picture of a boy reaching into a cookie jar this way: "It's a barl, a boil, oh, you know, getting the thing, the thing, it's just the top, boy, you know."

Persons with Wernicke's aphasia may improve significantly in their comprehension but continue to exhibit fluent speech with paraphasia. This condition is called conduction aphasia. The neurologic lesion in

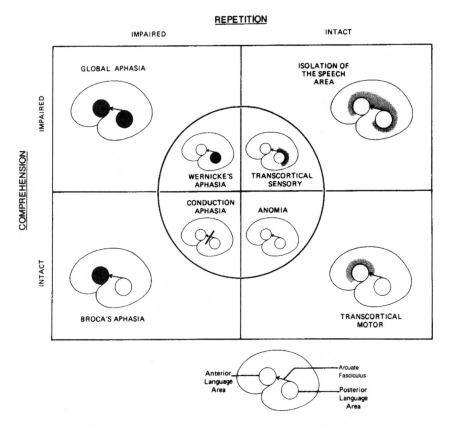

Figure 3–1 Aphasia diagram: The three components of language function to be tested are comprehension, fluency, and repetition. Aphasias depicted within the central circle are the fluent aphasias. *Source:* Reprinted from J Gallo et al., Mental Status Assessment, Handbook of Geriatric Assessment, 2nd ed., p. 19, © 1994 Aspen Publishers, Inc.

conduction aphasia may involve the arcuate fasciculus, the connection between the anterior (motor) and posterior (sensory) language areas. Persons with conduction aphasia usually do not demonstrate the amount of verbal output noted in those with Wernicke's aphasia. They may be able to read well for comprehension but cannot read aloud.

Persons with an initial Wernicke's aphasia may continue to improve beyond a conduction type of aphasia (ie, they will have better comprehension) and ultimately be left with an anomic aphasia. With anomic aphasia, persons have difficulty finding words but show fluent speech, good repetition, and good comprehension.

Patients with relatively preserved comprehension, impaired repetition, and severely limited verbal output consisting of mostly nouns and verbs (ie, telegraphic speech) have Broca's aphasia. Although repetition is impaired, it may be clearer than the person's spontaneous speech. Since his or her speech contains mostly nouns and verbs, he or she may have difficulty with the expression, "No ifs, ands, or buts." Broca's aphasia involves an anterior brain lesion, and if the nearby motor strip is affected, a concomitant hemiplegia occurs. The person with Broca's aphasia may describe a picture of a boy reaching into a cookie jar this way: "Boy . . . yes, ah . . . jar, cookie."

Patients with global aphasia, Wernicke's aphasia, conduction aphasia, and Broca's aphasia have in common impaired repetition ability. There are rarer syndromes of aphasias, called transcortical aphasias, in which repetition function is remarkably preserved out of proportion to the disability in comprehension and fluency.

Isolation of the speech area is a transcortical aphasia that occurs when a zone of infarction extends around the boundaries of the speech areas so that they are isolated from the associative regions of the brain. This may occur in so-called watershed infarcts because of hypotension and resultant ischemia in the "watershed" zone between the areas of distribution of the anterior and middle cerebral arteries. Such a lesion can also be found after carbon monoxide poisoning or following prolonged hypoxia. Persons with isolation of the speech area can repeat words and phrases perfectly, even words from foreign languages they have never heard. Their spontaneous speech is sparse and nonfluent, and comprehension is impaired (see Figure 3–1).

Partial transcortical syndromes, isolating only part of the speech apparatus, are probably more common than complete isolation of the speech area. The anterior (ie, transcortical motor) or posterior (ie, transcortical sensory) language areas may be isolated from the associative cortices of the rest of the brain.

Comprehension is relatively preserved in persons with transcortical motor aphasia. Their speech is similar to that of someone with Broca's aphasia, which is an aphasia that also involves anterior portions of the cortex. Persons with transcortical sensory aphasia have fluent speech and impaired comprehension, similar to those with Wernicke's aphasia. Both transcortical sensory aphasia and Wernicke's aphasia involve posterior portions of the cortex. The spontaneous speech of the individual with transcortical sensory aphasia is filled with paraphasic errors (ie, word substitutions), but repetition is preserved. Sorting out aphasia is easier when the three domains of fluency, comprehension, and repetition are kept in mind. Other language syndromes include reading difficulty only (ie, alexia), alexia with writing difficulty (ie, agraphia), and Gerstmann's syndrome (ie, acalculia, agraphia, right/left disorientation, and finger agnosia or inability to name the fingers).

Writing and Construction Ability

The components of the mental status examination discussed to this point can smoothly follow the history interview since it is primarily a verbal examination. At this point in the examination, the patient may be presented with a blank sheet of paper for subsequent tests.

The patient is asked to write his or her name at the top of the page. Although the signature is usually overlearned and can be intact even with writing difficulty for more complex tasks, this action acclimates the patient to the idea that he or she is going to be asked to do some writing, and the signature is a nonthreatening way to begin. Below the signature the patient is asked to write a complete sentence, perhaps about the weather. While the person has the blank sheet of paper and pen in hand, construction ability may be tested. The ability to reproduce the line drawings of the examiner represents construction ability. This can be a very sensitive test of parietal lobe damage and is an early abnormality in dementia. Trouble with construction ability is not something most persons will complain of specifically, but testing constructional ability can be revealing. The testing begins with simple figures such as a triangle or square and progresses to more complex drawings such as a cube, house, or flowerpot. Mattis reminds that testing the ability to copy figures is not specific to dementia because trouble with this test may reflect motor incoordination or apraxia.[40]

Asking the patient to draw a clock showing the numerals and time (eg, "10 minutes past eleven o'clock") can act as a single item screen for cognitive impairment. The examiner draws a large circle on a blank sheet of paper and asks the patient to fill in the numbers as on a clock. This task is thought to be a sensitive test of parietal lobe dysfunction. Persons with primarily right or nondominant hemisphere dysfunction write the numbers correctly but plan poorly. Those with primarily left or dominant hemisphere dysfunction have trouble writing the numbers but execute the general plan of the clock correctly, perhaps placing lines where the numbers should be. Clock drawing has been used to screen for cognitive impairment[57] as well as to follow progression of diagnosed Alzheimer's disease.[58] Several scoring methods for the clock drawing task are available.[57-61] The examination of higher integrative functions is summarized in Table 3–1.[62]

DIFFERENTIAL DIAGNOSIS OF DEMENTIA

In considering the differential diagnosis of cognitive impairment, the primary distinction that must be made by the clinician is among dementia, delirium, or a specific neurologic deficit, such as aphasia or amnesia. At the outset, it must be emphasized that older adults may exhibit delirium superimposed on dementia. The aged central nervous system may be especially vulnerable to dysfunction brought about by metabolic disturbances. Decline in function of persons with dementia should prompt a search for potentially reversible conditions.

Dementia is a syndrome characterized by loss of intellectual capacity involving not only memory but also cognition, language, visuospatial skills, and personality. All five components need not be impaired, but they frequently are to varying degrees. Dementia implies intellectual impairment in clear consciousness, and may be progressive, stable, or remitting. The term "organic mental disorder" has been dropped in the *DSM-IV.*[54] Criteria for several subtypes of dementia are delineated in *DSM-IV:* dementia of the Alzheimer type, vascular dementia, dementia due to human immunodeficiency virus, dementia due to head trauma, dementia due to Pick's disease, dementia due to Creutzfeldt-Jakob disease, dementia due to other medical general conditions, substance-induced persisting dementia, and dementia due to multiple etiologies.

Delirium is marked by clouding of consciousness, usually of acute onset (ie, in hours or days). Persons who are delirious may be agitated or lethargic, and levels of activity may vary throughout the day. Agitated delirium calls attention to the person, while that of those persons who are quietly delirious may go unrecognized and unattended. It cannot be overemphasized, however, that delirium is a syndrome, not a diagnosis. The recognition of delirium, like fever, requires further explanation.[63] A standardized schedule to detect delirium has been published,[64] but short instruments that assess cognitive function may serve this purpose as discussed later in this chapter.

Once the clinician determines that global intellectual impairment is present and consistent with dementia, a consideration of the specific etiology is in order. Although the chance of finding a remedial condition seems remote, the list of diagnostic possibilities is so large, and the scope of the problem in an aging society is so great, that dementia and any concurrent conditions need to be assessed thoroughly.

The notion of searching for a "reversible" dementia (implying that nothing can be done to help the person with an "irreversible" dementia) is only helpful in so far as it prompts a consideration of the myriad causes of intellectual decline. In a study of 107 demented older persons, 16 improved 6 months after their initial assessment.[65] Eleven were patients with "reversible" dementia, but they showed a deteriorating course typical of Alzheimer's disease on further follow-up. The five remaining patients with "irreversible" dementia who improved did so after concurrent conditions, such as congestive heart failure, depression, and anemia, were addressed. Classifying dementia as reversible (treatable) or irreversible (not treatable) may unnecessarily compromise patient management. Instead, all demented persons must be considered to be at increased risk for secondary treatable conditions,[65,66] not to mention that caregivers require attention in the care of dementia patients.

One helpful scheme (Exhibit 3–2) that organizes the differential diagnosis of dementia and aids the clinician's memory was suggested by Cummings and Benson.[67] By considering a hierarchy of clinical features, the dementias can be systematically reviewed in the clinician's mind.

Exhibit 3–2 Classification of the Major Causes of Dementia Based on the Occurrence of Features of Cortical and Subcortical Dysfunction

Cortical dementias
- Alzheimer's disease
- Frontal lobe degeneration

Subcortical dementias
- Extrapyramidal syndromes
  - Parkinson's disease
  - Huntington's disease
  - Progressive supranuclear palsy
  - Wilson's disease
  - Spinocerebellar degeneration
  - Idiopathic basal ganglia calcification
- Hydrocephalus
- Dementia syndrome of depression
- White matter diseases
  - Multiple sclerosis
  - Human immunodeficiency virus encephalopathy
- Vascular dementias
  - Lacunar state
  - Binswanger's disease

Combined cortical and subcortical features
- Multi-infarct dementias
- Infectious dementias
  - Slow-virus dementias
  - General paresis
- Toxic and metabolic encephalopathies
  - Systemic illnesses
  - Endocrinopathies
  - Deficiency states
  - Drug intoxications
  - Heavy metal exposure
- Miscellaneous dementia syndromes
  - Post-traumatic
  - Post-anoxic
  - Neoplastic

Source: Adaped with permission from JL Cummings and DF Benson, *Dementia: A Clinical Approach,* Woburn, MA, Butterworth-Heinemann, © 1983.

First, are the features consistent with a cortical dementia such as Alzheimer's or Pick's disease? Alzheimer's disease is characterized by an insidious onset with a progressive deteriorating course. Typically, memory is affected early on. Clinical criteria for the clinical diagnosis of Alzheimer's disease reported by McKhann and associates aid in the evaluation of patients with dementia.[68] Of course, definite diagnosis of Alzheimer's disease requires histopathologic evidence obtained at autopsy, but a diagnosis of probable and possible Alzheimer's disease can be made clinically using the criteria set forth by the National Institute of Neurological and Communicative Disorders and Stroke-Alzheimer's Disease and Associated Disorders Association Task Force on Alzheimer's Disease. Probable Alzheimer's disease may be diagnosed with the following criteria[68]:

1. dementia established by clinical examination and by the MMSE or similar examination
2. deficits in two or more areas of cognition
3. progressive worsening of memory and other cognitive functions
4. no disturbance of consciousness (to distinguish from delirium)
5. onset most often after age 65
6. no systemic disorder or other brain disease that could account for the findings

The diagnosis of Alzheimer's disease is supported by progressive deterioration in specific functions such as language, impaired activities of daily living, and evidence of cerebral atrophy on computed tomography (CT) scan. DSM-IV criteria for dementia of the Alzheimer type include multiple cognitive deficits (eg, memory impairment, aphasia, apraxia, agnosia, and disturbance of executive function) and interference with social and occupational roles (Exhibit 3–3).[54]

A scale developed as a tool to assist in the differential diagnosis of dementia, specifically for the diagnosis of Alzheimer's disease, is the Inventory of Diagnostic Clinical Features of Dementia of the Alzheimer Type.[69] A maximum score of 20 is possible, attained by persons with uncomplicated dementia of the Alzheimer type. The higher scores (14 or greater) reflect greater consistency with the diagnosis of Alzheimer's disease and lower scores with other diagnoses.

In retrospective and prospective studies, the inventory was highly accurate in differentiating persons with Alzheimer's disease from those who have dementia from another etiology. This inventory (Exhibit 3–4) gives greater weight to loss of intellectual functions than to motor abnormalities. Atypical presentations of dementia of the Alzheimer type

Exhibit 3–3 Diagnostic Criteria for Dementia of the Alzheimer Type

---

A. The development of multiple cognitive deficits manifested by both:
   (1) memory impairment (impaired ability to learn new information or to recall previously learned information)
   (2) one (or more) of the following cognitive disturbances:
       (a) aphasia (language disturbance)
       (b) apraxia (impaired ability to carry out motor activities despite intact motor function)
       (c) agnosia (failure to recognize or identify objects despite intact sensory function)
       (d) disturbance in executive functioning (ie, planning, organizing, sequencing, and abstracting)
B. The cognitive deficits in criteria A1 and A2 each cause significant impairment in social or occupational functioning and represent a significant decline from a previous level of functioning.
C. The course is characterized by gradual onset and continuing cognitive decline.
D. The cognitive deficits in criteria A1 and A2 are not due to any of the following:
   (1) other central nervous system conditions that cause progressive deficits in memory and cognition (eg, cerebrovascular disease, Parkinson's disease, Huntington's chorea, subdural hematoma, normal-pressure hydrocephalus, or brain tumor)
   (2) systemic conditions that are known to cause dementia (eg, hypothyroidism, vitamin B_{12} or folic acid deficiency, niacin deficiency, hypercalcemia, neurosyphilis, or HIV infection)
   (3) substance-induced conditions
E. The deficits do not occur exclusively during the course of a delirium.
F. The disturbance is not better accounted for by another Axis I disorder (eg, major depressive disorder or schizophrenia).

Source: Reprinted with permission from the *Diagnostic and Statistical Manual of Mental Disorders*, Fourth Edition. Copyright 1994 American Psychiatric Association.

---

or mixed diagnoses may fail to be identified because of the absence of multiple areas of intellectual impairment assessed by the inventory.[69,70] The scoring scheme of the inventory reflects the generally normal results of motor examination of persons with Alzheimer's disease and the early impairment of language and memory. Demented persons who present with signs or symptoms of a movement disorder should suggest to the practitioner a diagnosis other than primary degenerative (cortical) dementia.

Patients with Pick's disease, the other primary cortical dementia, have personality changes with poor judgment and social graces, but with strikingly preserved memory, language, and visuospatial skills early in the course of the dementia. Pathologic changes in Pick's disease occur primarily in the temporal and frontal lobes of the brain.

Exhibit 3–4 Inventory of Diagnostic Clinical Features of Senile Dementia of the Alzheimer Type

Mental Functions	0	1	2
Memory	Normal or forgetfulness that improves with cues	Recalls one or two of three words, spontaneous, incompletely aided by prompting	Disoriented, unable to learn three words in 3 min, recall not aided by prompting
Visuospatial	Normal or clumsy drawings, minimal distortions	Flattening, omissions, distortions	Disorganized, unrecognizable copies of models
Cognition	Normal or impairment of complex abstractions and calculations	Fails to abstract simple proverbs and has difficulty with mathematical problems	Fails to interpret even simple proverbs or idioms, acalculia
Personality	Disinhibition or depression	Appropriately concerned	Unaware or indifferent, irritability not uncommon
Language	Normal	Anomia, mild comprehension deficits	Fluent aphasia with anomia, decreased comprehension paraphasia

Motor Functions	0	1	2
Speech	Mute, severely	Slurred, amelodic, dysarthric	Normal hypophonic
Psychomotor speed	Slow, long latency to response	Hesitant responses	Normal, prompt responses
Posture	Abnormal, flexed, extended, or distorted	Stooped or mildly distorted	Normal, erect
Gait	Hemiparetic, ataxic, apractic, or hyperkinetic	Shuffling, dyskinetic	Normal
Movements	Tremor, akinesia, rigidity, or chorea	Imprecise, poorly coordinated	Normal

Source: Adapted with permission from J Cummings and D Benson, Dementia of the Alzheimer Type: An Inventory of Diagnostic Clinical Features, *Journal of American Geriatric Society,* Vol. 34, pp. 12–19, © 1986, Lippincott Williams & Wilkins.

Is there evidence of a halting progression to the disorder with spotty mental status deficits, associated with a history of hypertension or strokes? Vascular dementia, which is thought to be the result of strokes or cerebrovascular disease,[71] may be more common than previously appreciated.[72,73] Several lines of evidence now suggest that cognitive impairment in older adults is associated with vascular lesions in the central nervous system, even without dementia.[73-82] Some individuals exhibit changes of Alzheimer's disease occurring in the context of multiple infarcts (mixed dementia). Small infarcts, strategically located, may be associated with increased vulnerability to Alzheimer's disease.[83] Thus, the relationship between cardiovascular disease risk factors, such as lipid and apolipoprotein profiles, dementia, and stroke, is complex indeed.

Vascular factors have long been thought to influence mental health in late life. For example, describing changes in the brains of patients with dementing illness, one influential writer, Dr Benjamin Ball, wrote in 1881, "localised softening caused the more severe states of cognitive impairment."[84] Even as late as the 1960s, many of the mental disturbances of late life were ascribed to atherosclerosis.[84,85] The realization that most dementia appeared to be related to neuropathologic changes described by Alzheimer in 1906 largely discredited the notion of atherosclerotic dementia. Now recent evidence has rekindled interest in the role of vascular factors in dementia,[86] including Alzheimer's disease,[87-89] and even in depression arising in late life.[90] Medicine is in the early stages in the investigation of how cardiovascular disease risk factors, such as hypertension, diabetes, high cholesterol, smoking, and atrial fibrillation, contribute to cognitive impairment in late life.

In the clinical examination of the person with vascular dementia, the practitioner should look for spasticity in the limbs, hyperreflexia, plantar extensor reflexes, and an abnormal gait. The personality is relatively preserved. The CT scan reveals evidence of infarcts in only half of patients suspected of having vascular dementia.[91] Criteria of *DSM-IV* for vascular dementia are similar to the criteria for dementia of the Alzheimer type except that focal neurologic signs and symptoms are present or imaging studies reveal cerebrovascular disease.[54]

Senile dementia of the Binswanger type, described over 100 years ago, is a type of vascular dementia more commonly recognized because of new imaging techniques, particularly magnetic resonance imaging.[92] Patients with this type of dementia have an insidious onset of dementia with gait disturbance, urinary incontinence, and neurologic signs early in the course of the illness. Diagnostic criteria include at least two of the following: hypertension or other known cardiovascular risk factors; evidence of cerebrovascular disease; evidence of subcortical features, such as abnormal gait or muscular rigidity; and subcortical attenuation of white matter on brain scan.[93] The pathologic condition relates to infarctions in the white matter just below the cortex, resulting in isolation of cortex from deeper structures. Risk factors (eg, diabetes and hypertension) for small artery disease may predispose persons to senile dementia of the Binswanger type.[94,95]

Recognition of vascular dementia assumes particular importance when considered with hypertension treatment or modification of other cardiovascular risk factors. Some investigators believe there is a "therapeutic window" within which blood pressure should be controlled. When blood pressure was lowered below this optimal range, the persons with vascular dementia exhibited further cognitive decline.[96] In contrast, persons who stop smoking benefit by showing less cognitive decline.[96] The Hachinski Ischemic Score (Exhibit 3–5) has been devised to help distinguish vascular dementia from other types of dementia. Persons with a score of 7 or more are said to be more likely to have vascular dementia or at least a vascular component to their dementia.[97] An extensive review of the literature by Liston and associates led the authors to conclude that a low Hachinski Ischemic Score could help rule out vascular dementia because ischemic lesions severe enough to produce a dementia would be expected to be severe enough to cause the associated neurologic changes and elevate the score.[98]

Is there evidence of a movement disorder? Parkinson's disease is a subcortical process associated with a dementia. The person's intellectual processes seem to be "slowed" along with his or her movements.

Exhibit 3–5 Hachinski Ischemic Score

1. Abrupt onset (2)
2. Stepwise deterioration (1)
3. Fluctuating course (2)
4. Nocturnal confusion (1)
5. Relative preservation of personality (1)
6. Depression (1)
7. Somatic complaints (1)
8. Emotional incontinence (1)
9. History of hypertension (1)
10. History of strokes (2)
11. Evidence of associated atherosclerosis (1)
12. Focal neurologic symptoms (2)
13. Focal neurologic signs (2)

The score for each feature is noted in parentheses. A score of greater than 7 suggests a vascular component to the dementia.

Source: Adapted with permission from VC Hachinski et al., Cerebral Blood Flow in Dementia, *Archives of Neurology* Vol. 32, p. 634. Copyright © 1975, American Medical Association.

Frequently there is a superimposed depression. Subcortical dementias classically are associated with abnormalities of the motor system, such as stooped posture, increased muscle tone, and abnormal movements and gait.[67] Other subcortical dementias are associated with Huntington's chorea, progressive supranuclear palsy, and Wilson's disease. The concept of cortical and subcortical types of dementia is not as clear-cut as it would seem. Some of the features generally reported to be characteristic of one type may be found in the other, such as aphasia being present in persons with subcortical dementia.[99] Dementia with Lewy bodies is characterized by pathology in the cortical region,[100] but results in features that include movement disorder. In peoples with Lewy body dementia, deficits in memory and visuospatial ability occur as in Alzheimer's disease, but so do fluctuating cognition, recurrent visual hallucinations, and motor features resembling Parkinson's disease.[101]

Is there an affective component to the dementia? Persons who vigorously complain of memory impairment often are depressed (or have early Alzheimer's disease, or both). Those suffering from dementia syndrome of depression, on close continued observation, may be able to learn new facts and might give a detailed account of their memory loss. Depression as a precursor of intellectual impairment is discussed more fully later in this chapter.

Is the classic triad of normal pressure hydrocephalus present? Normal pressure hydrocephalus is characterized by the triad of gait disturbance, urinary incontinence, and dementia. Physical examination reveals spasticity in the legs with hyperreflexia and plantar extension reflexes. Of course, the classic triad need not be present. The CT examination shows dilated ventricles, but there may be considerable overlap with other dementias.[102]

Is there evidence of a toxic process? Prescription medications are among the greatest offenders, but hidden alcohol abuse must be considered as well.[103–108] Commonly used medicines (eg, propranolol or digoxin) may cause an altered mental state as the only side effect. Some medicines (eg, the benzodiazepines) can precipitate a delirium or seizures when discontinued.

Is there evidence of a metabolic abnormality? Electrolyte imbalance, such as hyponatremia, can result in a confused mental state. Calcium abnormalities can cause lethargy. Hypoxia or hypercarbia, as could result from pulmonary or cardiac disease, may also cause confusion.

Is there evidence of an endocrine abnormality? Testing for apathetic hyperthyroidism or for occult hypothyroidism should be part of the complete workup for dementia. Are the electrolytes suggestive of an adrenal problem? Is there evidence of a nutritional deficiency, such as deficiency of thiamine, niacin, or vitamin B-12? Thiamine deficiency, which is associated with alcohol abuse, may result in Wernicke's encephalopathy or organic amnestic syndrome. Niacin deficiency is associated with dementia. Vitamin B-12 deficiency may result in psychological changes without concomitant macrocytosis.

Is there evidence of an infection such as meningitis? Of course, reliable diagnosis would require lumbar puncture. Lumbar puncture probably is not very helpful applied indiscriminately to the diagnosis of dementia; it should be reserved for specific circumstances, such as acute deterioration with fever. Neurosyphilis is an unusual cause of dementia today but can be present even with a negative rapid plasma reagin test. Creutzfeldt-Jakob disease is a rapidly progressing dementia caused by a slow virus and characterized by myoclonus in its late stages and a burst-silence pattern on electroencephalography. Dementia secondary to human immunodeficiency virus is perhaps the newest addition to the list. The acquired immune deficiency syndrome could be important to keep in mind, particularly when risk factors, such as sexual exposure to high-risk persons or the use of blood products, are present.[109,110]

Are there focal neurologic signs suggestive of an intracranial process such as a neoplasm or a chronic subdural hematoma? Is there a history of trauma followed by changes in mental state? A complete mental status examination may reveal deficits that point to involvement of an otherwise "silent" area of the brain. Cranial CT rarely may find a mass lesion presenting as dementia when focal signs are absent.

Finally, is there more than one process occurring simultaneously? Are there concurrent medical illnesses that could be more optimally treated? In other words, is an overlying delirium resulting in deterioration of the mental status with preexisting dementia? Over 30% of persons with dementia have more than one disorder contributing to the persistence of the dementia.[111] The need to consider alternative conditions rather than ascribing the changes to a deterioration of dementia cannot be overemphasized when persons who carry a diagnosis of dementia have acute changes in their ability to function.

MENTAL STATUS ASSESSMENT INSTRUMENTS

Many short mental-status screening instruments have been devised to assist clinicians. Some screening instruments for intellectual functioning were devised for the sole purpose of assessing mental status, and others form part of a total instrument that includes measures of functional status and/or psychiatric illness. Further information on instruments to assess mental state may be found in the *Geropsychology Assessment Resource Guide*[112] and in *Measuring Health: A Guide to Rating Scales and Questionnaires.*[113] Instruments that are commonly endorsed for clinical practice will be reviewed, bearing in mind that other strategies are being developed to achieve the goals of a brief and accurate scale to assess mental status (see Froehlich et al[114] and Solomon and Pendlebury[115]).

The sensitivity and specificity of a test are used to assess performance of the test at specific cut points. Sensitivity and specificity are characteristics of tests that do not change with the prevalence of the disease in a population. Simply stated, the sensitivity of a test is the proportion of those persons with a disease who are detected by the test. Specificity is the proportion of those who are free of disease who are identified as such by the test. A related concept is the predictive value of a test result. The predictive value of a positive test is the proportion of persons who have a positive test and truly have the disease. The rest of the group, those with a positive result but without disease, are considered to have false-positive results. The predictive value of a negative test is the proportion of persons who have a negative test and truly do not have the disease. The rest of the group, those with a negative result but with the disease, have false-negative results.

The predictive value of a test varies as the prevalence of the disease in the population varies. The more common the disease is in the population to be tested, the greater is the predictive value of a positive test; but as the predictive value of a negative test goes down, the number of false-negative results increases. This makes intuitive sense because it would seem that the more common the disease, the more likely it is that a positive test result is true. Conversely, it will be less likely that a negative test represents a "true" negative. In a nursing home, for example, where the prevalence of dementia is presumably higher than in the general population, the predictive value of a negative screening test is diminished compared with the value of a negative test in community-dwelling older adults.

In contrast is the case of a less common disease. The lower the prevalence of the disease in the population to be tested, the greater is the predictive value of a negative test, but the predictive value of a positive test goes down; the number of false-positive results increases. Again, it would seem intuitive that the rarer a disease is, a positive test is more likely to be wrong rather than truly indicating someone with the rare illness.

In addition to simple detection of the demented state, the mental status assessment instruments can stratify persons with regard to the severity of dementia. Many of the instruments designed specifically for this purpose also include some assessment of functional ability, the dementia rating scales, to be discussed in Chapter 4. Because a score is generated by some of the mental status assessment instruments discussed in this section, stratification is possible merely on that basis. Mental status assessment instruments may exhibit threshold or ceiling effects. In other words, persons beyond a certain level of severity of dementia score the same despite some differences in degree. In a population with a predominance of severely demented persons, for example, an instrument would not be useful for following change if all severely affected individuals performed equally poorly. By the same token, in a population of relatively well elders, an easy test will be insensitive to mildly demented persons, who may be able to perform well on it, whereas on a more discriminating test they would have difficulties. This is vividly illustrated by the case of a patient who studied for the MMSE. She was being admitted to a retirement home and was disappointed when the physician did not ask her "those questions" her friend had told her about. She had studied the "answers" to the examination based on information from her friend, who was a resident in the home.[116]

Folstein Mini-Mental State Examination

The MMSE[117] is one of the most widely employed tests of cognitive function, and is one of the best studied.[118,119] Population-based norms are readily available according to age and educational level.[25,119] The MMSE consists of two parts (Exhibit 3–6). The first part requires verbal responses only and assesses orientation, memory, and attention. The three words used to test memory are left up to the examiner, leaving the possibility that this question could vary in difficulty. The items "apple, table, penny" were used in the Epidemiologic Catchment Area Program.[119] In addition to serial 7s, the individual is asked to spell "world" backwards, and the best score may be taken for calculating the total score. A "chess-move" strategy is used to score the "world" item (ie, the number of transpositions required to spell "DLROW" yields the number of errors).[120] The second part evaluates the ability to write a sentence, name objects, follow verbal and written commands, and copy a complex polygon. The maximum score is 30. The test is not timed. A telephone version of the MMSE is available for special purposes.[121]

In the original work with the MMSE, normal older persons scored a mean of 27.6. Patients with dementia, depression with cognitive im-

Exhibit 3–6 The Folstein Mini-Mental State Examination (MMSE)

Maximum Score	
	Orientation
5	What is the (year) (season) (date) (day) (month)?
5	Where are we (state) (county) (town) (hospital) (floor)?
	Registration
3	Name three objects: one second to say each. Then ask the patient all three after you have said them. Give one point for each correct answer. Repeat them until he or she learns all three. Count trials and record number.
	Attention and calculation
5	Begin with 100 and count backward by 7 (stop after five answers). Alternatively, spell "world" backward.
	Recall
3	Ask for the three objects repeated above.
	Language
2	Show a pencil and a watch and ask the patient to name them.
1	Repeat the following: "No ifs, ands, or buts."
3	A three-stage command: "Take a paper in your right hand, fold it in half, and put it on the floor."
1	Read and obey the following: (show written item) CLOSE YOUR EYES
1	Write a sentence.
1	Copy a design (complex polygon).
30	Total score possible

Source: "MINI-MENTAL STATE." A PRACTICAL METHOD FOR GRADING THE COGNITIVE STATE OF PATIENTS FOR THE CLINICIAN. *Journal of Psychiatric Research,* 12(3):189–198, © 1975, 1998 Mini Mental LLC. The copyright in the Mini Mental State Examination is wholly owned by the Mini Mental LLC, a Massachusetts limited liability company. For information about how to obtain permission to use or reproduce the Mini Mental State Examination, please contact John Gonsalves, Jr., Administrator of the Mini Mental LLC, at 31 St. James Avenue, Suite I, Boston, Massachusetts 02116—(617)587-4215.

pairment, and affective disorders formed a continuum with the mean scores for these groups of 9.7, 19, and 25, respectively. Not only did the demented persons score the lowest and the depressed ones the highest, but after treatment for depression the depressed persons with cognitive impairment showed improvement in their scores. The demented individuals had no change, as would be expected.[117]

The MMSE was administered to patients undergoing cranial CT scanning referred from neurologic and psychiatric services at the University of Iowa. Patients whose CT scan showed no cerebral atrophy had a mean score of 26.4. Those with focal brain lesions scored 25.3, which was not significantly different from the group without atrophy.

Patients with atrophy alone had a mean score of 18.0. Thus, the MMSE correlates to some degree with structural changes in the brain.[122] Although one report failed to show a difference in sensitivity between the MMSE and the Short Portable Mental Status Questionnaire (SPMSQ),[123] others have suggested that the sensitivity of the MMSE is better than that of the SPMSQ,[124,125] with an ability to pick up cognitive impairment closer to 90% rather than 50% (Table 3–2). The sensitivity of an instrument such as the MMSE, which, unlike the SPMSQ, tests recent memory, written and spoken language, and construction ability (drawing), in addition to orientation, would be expected to be better because a broader range of intellectual functions is sampled.

In any case, when the MMSE reveals the individual is impaired, additional diagnostic testing and mental status examination are indicated to further define the disorder, as would be true for any brief screening instrument. This is acceptable practice in general medical settings using the MMSE as part of a routine screen of older persons.[11]

The sensitivity of the MMSE was 76% when 126 patients on neurosurgical and neurologic wards were tested, and a cutoff score of 23 was used to differentiate impaired from normal patients.[126] The mean age of these patients was 49.9. Patients with bilateral hemispheric damage or with left

Table 3–2 Sensitivity, Specificity, and Predictive Value of the Folstein Mini-Mental State Examination (MMSE)

	Clinical Examination Consistent with Dementia	Clinical Examination Not Consistent with Dementia	
Score indicates impairment	Agrees	False positive	Predictive value of a positive test is 60%–93%
Score indicates no impairment	False negative	Agrees	Predictive value of a negative test is 77%–95%
	Sensitivity is 50%–87%	Specificity is approximately 90%	

A cutoff score of 24 is used to indicate dementia.

Sources: Adapted from *Journal of Neurology, Neurosurgery, and Psychiatry,* © 1984, Vol. 47, pp. 496–499, with permission from the BMJ Publishing Group; *Psychological Medicine,* Vol. 12, No. 2, pp. 397–408, © 1982; *Journal of the American Geriatric Society,* Vol. 28, No. 38, pp. 381–384, © 1980, Lippincott Williams & Wilkins.

hemispheric damage scored around 23, whereas control subjects and patients with right hemispheric damage scored around 28. Thus, the instrument detects left hemispheric dysfunction better than it does right hemispheric dysfunction. This asymmetrical detection of dysfunction was also shown to be true for the Cognitive Capacity Screen, to be discussed later in this chapter.[127] In the study of Dick and associates, there was excellent agreement between the results of the MMSE and those of the Wechsler Adult Intelligence Scale.[126] Dropping the cutoff score to 20 or 21 decreased the sensitivity of the instrument but allowed a greater number of normal persons to be classified correctly.

There is some question as to the adjustment of scores on mental status screening instruments based on the educational level of the subject. A low score may imply more severe intellectual impairment among persons with high educational attainment. As the education level increases, one expects the specificity of an instrument to rise; an abnormal test result probably really is abnormal because one would expect better performance from an educated person. Conversely, sensitivity goes down as educational level increases; a "normal" or "negative" test result occurs in an impaired person. For example, the sensitivity of the MMSE was 93% in a population with less than an eighth-grade education but fell to 71% for the individual with more than eight grades of schooling.[125,128]

Lower scores may occur among patients with less education who are not demented.[119,129] Normative data on the MMSE based on age and educational attainment were provided by Crum and her colleagues[119] and in the report from AHCPR.[25] Among persons with 0 to 4 years of education, a cutoff point of 19 represents the 75th percentile (in other words, 75% of community-dwelling adults with 0 to 4 years of education would score below 19 on the MMSE). Corresponding cutoff points are: for persons with 5 to 8 years of schooling, 23 and below; for 9 to 12 years of schooling, 27 and below; for schooling at the college level and beyond, 29 and below.[119] The person should be asked how much schooling he or she has had to assist in interpreting scores. It should be remembered that the MMSE and other mental status instruments serve as only one component in assessment of dementia, along with criteria in Exhibit 3–3.

Short Portable Mental Status Questionnaire

One of the simpler tests widely used to assess mental status is the SPMSQ developed by Pfeiffer.[130] This test comprises 10 questions dealing with orientation, personal history, remote memory, and calculations (Exhibit 3–7). The Kahn-Goldfarb Mental Status Questionnaire[131] is also a 10-item instrument; it is the prototype of short mental state examinations and is similar to the SPMSQ.

The final error score of the SPMSQ is modified by various factors. The number 1 is subtracted from the error score if the person has less than a high school education. More than three errors would identify the person as impaired. In the administration of this test, the examiner must keep in mind that the date must be exact, the birth date must be exact, the mother's maiden name does not require verification, and calculations must be done in their entirety and correctly.

A questionnaire such as this is compact, is easy to use, and requires no special materials. It would appear to meet the minimal criteria for face validity, being a mental status examination covering orientation, remote memory, and calculation. There is no task to assess short-term memory. How well the instrument performs for the assessment of cognitive functioning in clinical situations needs to be determined. Compared with a neuropsychiatric examination, how does the SPMSQ fare?

To evaluate the SPMSQ, it is necessary to return to the statistical concepts of sensitivity, specificity, and the predictive value of a positive or negative test discussed previously. When administered to community-dwelling older adults, the specificity is found to be better than 90%.[123,132] The sensitivity, the ability of the test to detect impairment, is not as great and may be as low as 50%.[123] This means that although

---

Exhibit 3–7 Short Portable Mental Status Questionnaire (SPMSQ)

1. What is the date today?
2. What day of the week is it?
3. What is the name of this place?
4. What is your telephone number? (If the patient does not have a phone: What is your street address?)
5. How old are you?
6. When were you born?
7. Who is the president of the United States now?
8. Who was the president just before that?
9. What was your mother's maiden name?
10. Subtract 3 from 20 and keep subtracting 3 from each new number you get, all the way down.

Source: Adapted with permission from E. Pfeiffer, A Short Portable Mental Status Questionnaire for the Assessment of Organic Brain Deficit in Elderly Patients, *Journal of the American Geriatric Society*, Vol. 23, pp. 433–441, © 1975, Lippincott Williams & Wilkins.

90% of normal elders are identified correctly as not impaired, as few as half of the demented persons are detected. Thus, there are few false-positive results, but many false-negative results. In another study, the sensitivity was found to be 82%, but the SPMSQ could not clearly differentiate mildly impaired from normal elders.[133] Other studies have found good performance of the SPMSQ in clinical settings.[134,135] Fillenbaum and colleagues examined the performance of the SPMSQ in a large community sample of the elderly, finding that SPMSQ scores were less affected by ethnicity and educational level when scoring adjusted for these factors.[136]

If one wished to be sure to detect as many cases of dementia as possible for further assessment, more stringent test requirements might be used. Fewer errors than the recommended four would then be acceptable as indicating a positive test. This was suggested in a Finnish study, which demonstrated that by using three errors as indicative of a positive test, sensitivity increased from 76% to 86%.[132]

Unlike the sensitivity and specificity, the predictive value of a positive and of a negative test result will vary depending on the prevalence of cognitive impairment in the study or practice population. In published data,[123,130] the predictive value of a positive test is around 90%; that of a negative test is 70% to 80%. Thus in older populations, a positive test, indicating impairment, has a 90% probability of being correct, whereas a negative test has about an 80% chance of being correct (Table 3–3).

Put another way, of those who are determined to be impaired by their score on the SPMSQ, 90% are indeed found to be impaired by a "gold standard," namely, a complete mental status examination and psychiatric evaluation. The predictive value of a normal (ie, negative) SPMSQ is about 80% in a community-dwelling population of elderly; 20% will have detectable cognitive impairment on more thorough testing. In a nursing home setting, where the prevalence of dementia is presumably higher, the predictive value of a negative test falls to around 70%; thus, 30% with a satisfactory score do not have normal cognitive functioning.

The SPMSQ is entirely verbal and easy to memorize. The clinician may consider supplementing the SPMSQ with the written parts of the mental status examination (eg, signing name, writing a sentence, and drawing) discussed earlier in this chapter, particularly if the instrument is used as a periodic screening assessment of mental status. A more complete examination would be done if the SPMSQ detects intellectual impairment or if the presenting complaint is related to confusion or personality change. In either case, knowledge of the prior performance of the individual is clearly of value.

Table 3–3 Sensitivity, Specificity, and Predictive Value of the Short Portable Mental Status Questionnaire (SPMSQ)

	Clinical Examination Consistent with Dementia	Clinical Examination Not Consistent with Dementia	
Score indicates impairment	Agrees	False positive	Predictive value of a positive test is up to 90%
Score indicates no impairment	False negative	Agrees	Predictive value of a negative test is 70%–80%
	Sensitivity is 50%–82%	Specificity is approximately 90%	

Four errors are used as a cutoff score to indicate dementia.

Sources: Data from the *Journal of the American Geriatric Society,* Vol. 23, pp. 433–441, © 1979; Vol. 27, pp. 263–269, © 1979; Vol, 28, pp. 381–384, © 1980, Lippincott Williams & Wilkins.

Orientation and Nonorientation Items

The SPMSQ and the MMSE rely heavily on questions of orientation. As indicated by the low sensitivity of both tests, the common practice of using orientation-type questions to screen for dementia may miss as many as half of such persons. A brief example illustrates this pitfall of using an interview heavily weighted toward orientation-type questions: A 66-year-old woman presented at the request of her family because of difficulty with memory. The patient's daughter stated that on several occasions the patient had forgotten the names of some family members and friends. The patient was still driving, keeping her checkbook, cooking, and performing the usual activities of daily living. Her SPMSQ score was 10 (no errors). Further mental status testing revealed she could not recall three items, copy a simple diagram, or write an organized sentence. Thus orientation-type questions alone failed to identify a problem. Had just the SPMSQ been given, the intellectual deficits would have remained undetected.

Klein and associates reported on the sensitivity and specificity of various components of the MMSE.[137] The components of the examination were divided into two broad categories: orientation items (ie, Does the person know the day, month, year, city, and hospital?) and nonorientation items (ie, Can the person subtract 7 serially from 100, spell the word "world" backward, and recall 3 items after 5 minutes?).

Items of orientation had uniformly low sensitivity. Demented persons not uncommonly were oriented and therefore would have been missed by the unwary examiner using this type of question exclusively. Examiners need to recall that low sensitivity means a low proportion of those with dementia is actually detected by the test. On the other hand, nonorientation items were highly sensitive in detecting dementia, but since many normal elders also encountered difficulty with these items, the specificity was low. Recall that low specificity means a low proportion of normal persons is identified as "normal" by the test. The clinical importance of this distinction between orientation and nonorientation items lies in interpreting the answers to the items (Table 3–4). The individual who knows where he or she is and the date may still be intellectually impaired.

Cognitive Capacity Screen

A 30-question Cognitive Capacity Screen[138] was used in the detection of "organic brain syndromes" in patients with medical illness (Exhibit 3–8). Those patients with scores less than 20 (maximum score of 30) were more likely to meet clinical criteria for dementia. A low test score could reflect a condition other than dementia, of course, such as a low educational level. Conversely, a high test score would not rule out the possibility of a focal abnormality. Most psychiatric patients tested scored greater than 20 on the test. The scale is a bit more cumbersome than the SPMSQ or the MMSE but includes some areas not tested by others, such as abstraction ability. (Questions 18 and 19 deal with similarities.)

A high proportion of hospitalized patients given the Cognitive Capacity Screen were found to be impaired, as indicated by a score of less than 20. The same study found that 11 patients in the control group (18%) also scored less than 20; however, when these patients were examined carefully, only one met the criteria for dementia.[139] The investigators did not examine the patients with a normal score to see if any demented patients were missed.

On a neuropsychological service, the Cognitive Capacity Screen had a sensitivity of 49% and a specificity of 90%.[127] The sensitivity was increased when the examination was combined with a Memory for Designs test, which identified the patients with right hemispheric lesions missed by the Cognitive Capacity Screen. It was suggested that the Cognitive Capacity Screen misses right hemispheric lesions (only

Table 3–4 Sensitivity and Specificity of Orientation and Nonorientation Items of the Mental Status Examination

Item	Sensitivity (%)	Specificity (%)
Orientation items		
Day	52.8	91.7
Month	56.9	96.5
Year	51.4	98.6
City	15.3	100.0
Hospital	20.8	100.0
Nonorientation items		
Serial 7s (to 79)	97.2	50.0
"World" spelled backward	94.4	61.8
Recall of all three items	97.2	43.1
Recall of at least two items	80.6	74.3
Serial 7s (to 79) or "world" backward and recall of at least two items	100.0	49.3

Source: Reprinted with permission from LE Klein et al., Univariate and Multivariate Analyses of the Mental State Examination, *Journal of the American Geriatric Society*, Vol. 33, pp. 483–488, © 1985, Lippincott Williams & Wilkins.

two of the seven patients with such lesions were detected by the test). Patients with diffuse brain injury may be easier to detect with screening instruments since patients with focal lesions may have deficits that the test does not elicit.[127]

The propensity to miss structural lesions was emphasized in a study comparing results on the Cognitive Capacity Screen with those found on neurologic examination. The sensitivity in consecutive admissions to a neurologic service was 73%; the specificity was 90%.[138] The predictive value of a positive test was 93%; that of a negative test was 67%. Of nine patients with a false-negative test, five were found to have a moderate degree of dementia, and all nine had focal (or multifocal) cerebral disease such as brain tumor or abscess. Seven of these patients had obvious neurologic deficits, such as hemiparesis.

Kokmen Short Test of Mental Status

The Kokmen Short Test of Mental Status attempts to sample a wide range of intellectual tasks, including some not tested by the SPMSQ and the MMSE, such as abstraction.[39] This assessment instrument

Exhibit 3–8 Cognitive Capacity Screen

---

1. What day of the week is this?
2. What month?
3. What day of the month?
4. What year?
5. What place is this?
6. Repeat these numbers: 8 7 2.
7. Say them backward.
8. Repeat these numbers: 6 3 7 1.
9. Listen to these numbers: 6 9 4. Count 1 through 10 out loud, then repeat 6 9 4. (Help if needed. Then use numbers 5 7 3.)
10. Listen to these numbers: 8 1 4 3. Count 1 through 10 out loud, then repeat 8 1 4 3.
11. Beginning with Sunday, say the days of the week backward.
12. 9 plus 3 is?
13. Add 6 (to the previous answer or "to 12").
14. Take away 5 ("from 18").

    Repeat these words after me and remember them; I will ask for them later: HAT, CAR, TREE, TWENTY-SIX.

15. The opposite of fast is slow. The opposite of up is _____ .
16. The opposite of large is _____ .
17. The opposite of hard is _____ .
18. An orange and a banana are both fruits. Red and blue are both _____ .
19. A penny and a dime are both _____ .
20. What were those words I asked you to remember? (HAT)
21. (CAR)
22. (TREE)
23. (TWENTY-SIX)
24. Take away 7 from 100, then take away 7 from what is left and keep going: 100 minus 7 is ____ .
25. Minus 7 ____ .
26. Minus 7 ____ . (Write down answers; check correct subtraction of 7)
27. Minus 7 ____ .
28. Minus 7 ____ .
29. Minus 7 ____ .
30. Minus 7 ____ .

    Total correct (maximum score: 30) ____ .

Source: Reproduced, with permission from: J Jacobs et al., Screening for Organic Mental Syndromes in the Medically Ill, *Annals of Internal Medicine,* © 1977; 86: pp. 40–46, American College of Physicians.

(Exhibit 3–9) was given to 93 "nondemented" patients on a general neurologic consult service and to 87 demented persons living at home. The latter group included 67 individuals with Alzheimer's disease. When a score of 29 points or less was used to classify a patient as de-

mented (total maximum score is 38), the sensitivity to detect dementia was 95.5% and specificity was 91.4%. The Kokmen Short Test of
Mental Status as well as the next instrument to be discussed were included with others as recommended tools in the AHCPR guidelines on
Alzheimer's disease.[25]

Orientation-Memory-Concentration Test

A 6-item Orientation-Memory-Concentration (OMC) Test (Exhibit
3–10) with weighted items has shown that 90% of older persons without mental impairment have a weighted error score of 6 or less.[140]
Weighted error scores of ten or more were consistent with the presence
of dementia in most patients. The memory phrase and the months
backward questions are among the first items to be answered wrong as
dementia develops. The OMC Test certainly is an example of a test that
is short and convenient for use by the primary care practitioner. In a
comparison with the SPMSQ, the OMC Test performed favorably but
identified more older persons as cognitively impaired.[136]

Category Fluency

The test of category fluency, or the set test, is a simple test in which
one asks the person to name as many items as he or she can in each of
four sets or categories.[141] The four sets are fruits, animals, colors, and
towns. A maximum of 10 is allowed in each set for a maximum score
of 40. The test is not timed. A score of less than 15 is abnormal, and
80% of demented older persons scored in this range. Conversely, no
one with an affective disorder scored less than 15 and only 2 of 146 os-
tensibly normal elders did so (1%). This certainly compares favorably
with the tests outlined earlier.

The value of the set test was demonstrated in a University of Iowa
study.[142] Simply stated, eight psychological tests were given to a group
of normal elders and to a group with the diagnosis of dementia. The
investigators then proceeded to determine which tests best differenti-
ated the two groups. Two items stood out in discrimination ability.
One was the ability to remember designs, and the other task was a variation of the set test (ie, the production of a list of words beginning
with a given target letter). Presented as a "school-type" test in the examination of the nervous system, the set test would seem to be less

Exhibit 3-9 The Kokmen Short Test of Mental Status

Orientation
Full name, address, building, city, state, day of the week or month, month, year.
Score one point for each correct response.
Maximum: 8

Attention
Digit repetition (start with five, go to six and then seven if correct). Record the
best performance and score the number of digits repeated forward correctly.
Maximum: 7

Learning
Remember the following: apple, Mr. Johnson, charity, tunnel. Give a maximum
of four trials to learn all words and record the number of words learned and the
number of trials to learn them. Score one point per word learned but subtract one
less than the number of trials to do so from the number of words learned.
Maximum: 4

Arithmetic calculation
Do the following: 5 times 13, 65 minus 7, 58 divided by 2, and 11 plus 29. Score
one point for each correct answer.
Maximum: 4

Abstraction
How are the following alike? An orange and a banana, a horse and a dog, a table
and a bookcase. Score one point for each definitely abstract answer.
Maximum: 3

Information
Who is the President now?
Who was the first President?
How many weeks are there in a year?
Define "island."
Score one point for each correct answer.
Maximum: 4

Construction
Draw the face of a clock showing 11:15 and copy a picture of a three-dimen-
sional cube (which the patient may view while copying). Score, for each drawing,
two points for an adequate conceptual drawing, one for a less than complete
drawing, and zero if the patient is unable to perform the task.
Maximum: 4

Recall
Recall the four items from the learning task. Score one point for each word recalled.
Maximum: 4

Source: Adapted with permission from E Kokmen et al, *Mayo Clinics Proceedings*, Vol. 62, pp.
282–283, © 1987, Mayo Foundation.

Exhibit 3–10 Orientation-Memory-Concentration Test

Items	Maximum Error	Score	Weight	Total
1. What year is it now?	1	_____	× 4	_____
2. What month is it now?	1	_____	× 3	_____
Memory phrase. Repeat this phrase after me: John Brown, 42 Market Street, Chicago				
3. About what time is it? (within one hour)	1	_____	× 3	_____
4. Count backward from 20 to 1.	2	_____	× 2	_____
5. Say the months in reverse order.	2	_____	× 2	_____
6. Repeat the memory phrase.	5	_____	× 2	_____
			Total score:	_____

Score one point for each incorrect response; maximum weighted error score equals 28. Over 90% of normal elders have a weighted score of 6 or less. Scores greater than 10 are suggestive of mental impairment.

Source: American Journal of Psychiatry, Vol. 140, p. 739, 1983. Copyright © 1983, the American Psychiatric Association. Reprinted by permission.

likely to offend most elderly patients. Category fluency is sometimes considered a measure of executive functioning; that is, indicative of frontal lobe functioning.

Clock-Drawing Task

In the clock-drawing task, the individual is presented with a pen and a piece of paper on which a 4- to 6-inch circle is drawn and asked to write the numbers and draw the hands of the clock to show "10 past 11." While there are several versions of the clock-drawing task (for example, differing in whether the circle outline is provided or must be drawn by the person and the time to be represented), the clock-drawing task may be useful in eliciting some signs of cognitive impairment and assessing persons with dementia.[57–61,143–145] The clock-drawing task no doubt taps into multiple cognitive and motor functions rather than attempting to assess specific domains, such as memory, and serves as a practical method of screening and assessment that is acceptable to most people. Patients with left-sided hemispheric damage may tend to get the "gestalt" of the clock correct (eg, there are lines at the 12, 3, 6, and 9 o'clock positions, but no numbers) because of language deficits. Right-sided lesions may result in clocks with readable numbers that are grouped all to one side. Clocks drawn by persons with Alzheimer's disease may exhibit all of these and other features, such as perseveration (repetition of the same number all around the clock).

A qualitative evaluation of changes noted by reviewing the dated drawings in the medical record will be sufficient in most clinical applications. However, investigators have provided scales to rank the drawing for completeness and correctness[58] or to rate specific components of the clock drawn and combine the ratings into a score. The clock-drawing interpretation scale recommended by Mendez and colleagues[59] falls into this latter category (Exhibit 3–11). Other scoring methods are found in other sources.[60,61,145] Simplified and more objective methods than the Mendez scoring criteria have been suggested,[61,145] but none is standard.

Persons with Alzheimer's disease and other dementias score significantly worse than older adults without dementia,[57-59] and when a scoring threshold is used, the clock-drawing task shows good sensitivity and specificity in comparison with a diagnosis of dementia.[61] Unfortunately, the clock drawing task may not be immune to an effect of the level of educational attainment of the patient. Mean scores of patients with more education were higher than scores of persons with less than 9 years of schooling.[143] There is a need for more standardization of the administration and scoring of the clock-drawing task. This task may be thought of as a supplement to other mental status assessment instruments such as the MMSE.[145]

Summary of Mental Status Assessment

Assessing mental status of patients is important, especially on initial work-up for an older adult admitted to a hospital or nursing home, and whenever behavior, mental status, or level of functioning is a cause for concern. Changes in mental state can be more confidently assessed when a baseline has been established. Assessment of mental status must be considered within the context of the individual's functional status, the physical examination (especially vision and hearing), the history from an informant, and the total clinical picture. Mental status questionnaires can be used in combination with the written parts of the mental status examination to provide a record of performance for the medical chart; the record can then be used for following the progression of cognitive impairment or as a baseline assessment.

Exhibit 3–11 Clock-Drawing Interpretation Scale

Ask the patient to draw a clock and indicate the time as "ten after eleven." Score
one point for each item.

1. There is an attempt to indicate a time in some way.
2. All marks or items can be classified as part of a closure figure, a hand, or a symbol for clock numbers.
3. There is a totally closed figure without gaps (closure figure).

Score only if symbols for clock numbers are present.

4. A "2" is present and is pointed out in some way for the time.
5. Most symbols are distributed as a circle without major gaps.
6. Three or more clock quadrants have one or more appropriate numbers: 12–3, 3–6, 6–9, and 9–12 per respective clockwise quadrant.
7. Most symbols are ordered in a clockwise or rightward direction.
8. All symbols are totally within a closure figure.
9. An "11" is present and is pointed out in some way for the time.
10. All numbers 1–12 are indicated.
11. There are no repeated or duplicated number symbols.
12. There are no substitutions for Arabic or Roman numerals.
13. The numbers do not go beyond the number 12.
14. All symbols lie about equally adjacent to a closure figure edge.
15. Seven or more of the same symbol type are ordered sequentially.

Score only if one or more hands are present.

16. All hands radiate from the direction of a closure figure center.
17. One hand is visibly longer than another hand.
18. There are exactly two distinct and separable hands.
19. All hands are totally within a closure figure.
20. There is an attempt to indicate a time with one or more hands.

Source: Adapted with permission from MF Mendez et al., Development of Scoring Criteria for the Clock Drawing Task in Alzheimer's Disease, *Journal of the American Geriatric Society,* Vol. 40, pp. 1095–1099, © 1992, Lippincott Williams & Wilkins.

Some persons will need more careful delineation of mental status and would benefit from formal neuropsychological testing, particularly when presentation or course does not follow expected patterns.

ASSESSMENT OF MOOD

Mood is to affect as climate is to weather.[54] The mood disorders include major depression, dysthymia, and bipolar (manic-depressive) disorder. Publication of *Diagnosis and Treatment of Depression in Late Life: Results of the NIH Consensus Development Conference* called attention to depression in late life in primary care by including a chapter highlighting the primary care setting.[33] The Consensus Panel update on depression in late life continued to emphasize the importance of the primary care sector for older adults who are depressed.[146] *Clinical Practice Guideline for the Detection, Diagnosis, and Treatment of Depression in Primary Care*, published by AHCPR, points out that the course of major depression among the elderly, as well as other poorly characterized mood disturbances, is not well understood.[147] The Institute of Medicine's report, *The Second Fifty Years: Promoting Health and Preventing Disability*, observed that a better definition of depression in older adults would facilitate effective studies of depression in late life in the community.[148] Finally, *Healthy People 2000*, a report from the Department of Health and Human Services, acknowledged the role that the primary care sector plays in maintaining good health of older persons.[149] Clearly, if intervening in depression and suicide in late life is possible, primary care physicians, and other health professionals in primary care, are in a position to do so.[150–152]

Clinical studies and epidemiologic studies using symptoms scales, like the ones discussed in the following sections, show that the prevalence of depression *increases* with age, while epidemiologic studies using the standard criteria show a decrease in prevalence of depression with age.[153] At the same time, suicide rates *increase* with age.[154] Thus depression in older persons presents a paradox; depression prevalence in epidemiologic studies decreases with age, while suicides increase with age. While many factors contribute to suicide in the aged, it seems that: (1) the criteria for major depression are not age-specific, (2) medical problems and functional impairment contribute to preoccupation with death and suicide, and (3) hopelessness, not sadness, may be more pertinent in predicting suicide risk.

Older persons may not feel comfortable raising concerns of a psychological nature to their physicians. An older person may believe it is an imposition on the physician's time that should be occupied with "real" problems. The primary care provider, who has an intimate knowledge of the older person and family, should assess the person for the possibility of depression. Asking about feelings indicates that feelings are appropriate subjects for discussion and are not a waste of time. Older adults may view a psychological problem as a sign of weakness, as something to be ashamed of, or as meaning that they are "crazy."[155] For all these reasons, the presentation of depression may be quite different in older adults than in younger persons, discussed at length elsewhere.[156,157]

Some studies indicate that screening for depression may be useful because recognition by the physician leads to attention to the problem and treatment or referral.[5,58,159] German and colleagues,[160] working in a general medical outpatient setting, screened patients of all ages using the General Health Questionnaire (GHQ). Feedback on a randomized group of patients was given to the physicians-in-training consisting of the GHQ score and its interpretation. Patients were examined 6 months later. The screening procedure resulted in a significantly increased rate of detection when compared to major depression only for the patients aged 65 years and older (63% recognition among the patients for whom the doctor received feedback of GHQ score vs 41% for the patients for whom no feedback was given). There was a trend toward greater efforts to manage depression among the group for whom the doctor received feedback.[160] Use of a screening diagnostic questionnaire may increase recognition, but recognition may be less clearly tied to treatment in older persons than in younger persons.[161] These studies add evidence to the argument that screening for depression may be worthwhile among older persons in general medical outpatient settings, and the notion of screening deserves further investigation. However, it seems likely that to improve treatment will require more intensive intervention than use of assessment instruments in screening mode.

The diagnostic features of a major depressive episode are delineated in the fourth edition of the *DSM-IV* of the American Psychiatric Association and are reproduced in Exhibit 3-12.[54] These symptoms of depression should be sought in the complete evaluation, but especially when mental impairment is a consideration, or in the setting of significant life events in which loss is a theme (eg, bereavement or recent diagnosis of cancer). Has the individual felt "blue" or "down in the dumps"? The question, "How are your spirits with everything that is going on with you?" may open a discussion related to depression. Has he or she lost interest in activities that were enjoyed previously? How is his or her "energy level"? How well is the person sleeping? Is he or she eating? Does he or she feel useless or like life is not worth living? Does the family give the history that their loved one has withdrawn from usual activities? Is he or she using alcohol, sedatives, or tranquilizers to excess?

Anxious, somatic, or hypochondriacal complaints without sadness in older adults felt to be clinically depressed have been observed by experienced clinicians.[162,163] Feelings of helplessness[164] and hopelessness[165] may play a more central role in depression among older persons than among younger persons. Other aspects of depression that may be characteristic for older adults are not included in the standard criteria (eg, perceived cognitive deficit[166] or irritability[167]). Anxiety symptoms may accompany depression, persisting even after depres-

Exhibit 3–12 Diagnostic Criteria for a Major Depressive Episode

A. Five (or more) of the following symptoms have been present during the same
2-week period and represent a change from previous functioning; at least one
of the symptoms is either (1) depressed mood or (2) loss of interest or pleasure.
Note: Do not include symptoms that are clearly due to a general medical
condition, or mood-incongruent delusions or hallucinations.

(1) depressed mood most of the day, nearly every day, as indicated by either subjective report (e.g., feels sad or empty) or observation made by others (e.g.,
appears tearful). Note: In children and adolescents, can be irritable mood.

(2) markedly diminished interest or pleasure in all, or almost all, activities
most of the day, nearly every day (as indicated by either subjective account
or observation made by others).

(3) significant weight loss when not dieting or weight gain (e.g., a change of
more than 5% of body weight in a month), or decrease or increase in appetite nearly every day. Note: In children, consider failure to make expected weight gains.

(4) insomnia or hypersomnia nearly every day

(5) psychomotor agitation or retardation nearly every day (observable by others, not merely subjective feelings of restlessness or being slowed down)

(6) fatigue or loss of energy nearly every day

(7) feelings of worthlessness or excessive or inappropriate guilt (which may be
delusional) nearly every day (not merely self-reproach or guilt about being
sick)

(8) diminished ability to think or concentrate, or indecisiveness, nearly every
day (either by subjective account or as observed by others)

(9) recurrent thoughts of death (not just fear of dying), recurrent suicidal
ideation without a specific plan, or a suicide attempt or a specific plan for
committing suicide

B. The symptoms do not meet criteria for a Mixed Episode.

C. The symptoms cause clinically significant distress or impairment in social, occupational, or other important areas of functioning.

D. The symptoms are not due to the direct physiological effects of a substance
(e.g., a drug of abuse, a medication) or a general medical condition (e.g., hypothyroidism).

E. The symptoms are not better accounted for by Bereavement, i.e., after the loss
of a loved one, the symptoms persist for longer than 2 months or are characterized by marked functional impairment, morbid preoccupation with worthlessness, suicidal ideation, psychotic symptoms, or psychomotor retardation.

Source: Reprinted with permission from the *Diagnostic and Statistical Manual of Mental
Disorders,* Fourth Edition. Copyright 1994 American Psychiatric Association.

sion has improved.[168] Fogel and Fretwell[162] observed that since many
depressed older adults do not complain of depression, a diagnosis of
depression emphasizes a symptom that does not speak to the illness
experience of the older person.

An older adult with numerous somatic complaints may be depressed but denies feeling "blue." It may then be hard to convince him or her and the family that depression is the diagnosis since mood disturbance is denied by the individual. The family may misinterpret depressive symptoms as grouchiness, hostility, laziness, or merely complaining.[155,169] Hypochondriasis may serve as a plea for help, to displace anxiety, as a manifestation of unresolved guilt, and as a way to manipulate the environment.[170] In community samples, the dysphoria/anhedonia criterion for major depression was *less likely* to be endorsed by persons 65 years of age and older for the 1 month prior to interview, even adjusting for differences due to level of the symptoms of depression and for characteristics thought to influence the reporting of symptoms, such as gender and level of educational attainment.[171] This raises the possibility that the criteria in use for major depression may not be uniformly valid across all age-groups.[172] The person who denies sadness may yet have significant depression.[157,173]

While depression seems to decrease with age in some studies, hopelessness seems to increase with age. This is important because hopelessness, rather than dysphoria, seems to be an important concomitant of suicidal ideation and suicide.[174,175] Community surveys that permit direct age comparisons of the level of hopelessness are uncommon, but employing the Beck Hopelessness Scale, Greene found a clear and statistically significant trend to increasing levels of hopelessness with advancing age in Dublin among 396 community residents.[176] This dovetails with the work showing that dysphoria is less likely to be endorsed by persons aged 65 and older[171] because it means that to identify older persons at risk for depression and suicide, the physician must consider cognitions related to hopelessness and subsyndromal distress. In other words, the older person must be asked about feelings of helplessness and hopelessness in the context of physical illness, paying close attention to depression and thoughts of death in these circumstances. Suicide risk may be increased among older persons who live alone, are male, are recently bereaved, or have a history of psychiatric disorders including drug or alcohol abuse.

Depression can affect performance on mental status tests. When cognitive impairment is suspected, depression should be considered. The person with the appearance of cognitive impairment secondary to depression remains oriented and with coaxing can perform cognitive tests. Clues that dementia may be secondary to depression include recent onset and rapid progression, a family history of depressive disorders, a personal history of affective disorders, and onset of the disorder after the age of 60 years.[99] A more valuable concept regards depression as frequently coexisting with dementia: patients can be diagnosed with both Alzheimer's dementia and depression. An observer-rated scale specifically for depression in dementia, the National Institute of Mental Health (NIMH) Dementia Mood Assessment Scale, is available.[177] Persons found to have some cognitive impairment with accompanying depression may be at risk for developing dementia.[178,179] A plausible estimate is that 20% of individuals with Alzheimer's disease suffer from a major depressive syndrome.[180,181] Treatment with antidepressants may be the only way to prove that a concomitant depression exists.[33,182,183] Treatment of depression could improve cognitive deficits that are mistakenly ascribed to a primary degenerative dementia, and improve overall functioning.[184]

The relationship of physical illness and medication effects to depression is particularly important for older adults since physical illness and medication use are more common with advancing age. Depression may be a direct manifestation of a physical disorder or medication, may be a reaction to the diagnosis of a chronic illness, or may coexist in a person with physical illness. For example, stroke is especially likely to result in depression if certain brain regions are injured.[185] Depression in persons with cardiovascular disease, on the other hand, may arise as a reaction to functional limitations or to anxiety over sexual issues. The classic lesion associated with depression is carcinoma of the pancreas. Other conditions are pernicious anemia (even without megaloblastic changes or anemia); hypothyroidism; hyperthyroidism; parathyroid and adrenal disease; chronic subdural hematoma; untreated congestive heart failure; systemic vasculitis; infections such as hepatitis, influenza, and encephalitis; drug toxicity from drugs like propranolol and diazepam; and alcoholism.[19,63,103,186]

An argument can be made that some standardized instrument be used to screen older persons for affective disorder (especially in relation to stressful life events such as institutionalization) in the same way that tests can be used to assess cognitive impairment.[187] The instrument might be used to assess the mood of caregivers who themselves are older.[188] When older adults express hopelessness, anxiety, unexplained somatic complaints, or the score on a brief measure indicates possible depression, the criteria of the depression syndrome should be sought (Exhibit 3–12). At the same time, significant depression may occur in persons who do not fulfill these criteria.[157,173] The following sections discuss several brief instruments that can be used to uncover depression or psychological distress.

DEPRESSION SCALES

Symptom scales can be useful to screen for depression or general psychological distress. Consideration must be given to two dimensions when trying to define depression: symptom patterns and severity. Symptom pattern refers to the type of symptoms that form the items of the scale (eg, somatic complaints, hopelessness, or irritability). When items in a scale are summed to obtain a score, the implicit assumption is that the symptoms are given equal weight. Persons with higher scores are assumed to be more depressed, but this does not necessarily account for the severity of symptoms being experienced. While clinical judgment remains paramount, the scales can assist in determining whether the person is making satisfactory progress or needs further assessment or referral. Finally, when scales are used, the time frame for the assessment, such as "in the past 2 weeks," should be specified.

Geriatric Depression Scale

The Geriatric Depression Scale (GDS) has been recommended for clinical use by the Institute of Medicine[148] and is included as a routine part of comprehensive geriatric assessment in *A Core Curriculum in Geriatric Medicine.*[189] Introduced almost 2 decades ago,[190] the GDS is finding increasing use in research on depression in older adults.

The GDS is a questionnaire consisting of 30 items to be answered "yes" or "no," a considerable simplification over scales that use a five-category response set (Exhibit 3–13). The questionnaire is scored by assigning one point for each answer that matches the "yes" or "no" in the parentheses following the written question. A score of 10 or 11 is usually used as the threshold to separate patients into depressed and non-depressed groups.

The GDS was devised by choosing from 100 statements felt by the investigators to relate to 7 common characteristics of depression in later life.[190,191] In particular, the 100 items could be grouped a priori into several domains: (1) somatic concern, (2) lowered affect, (3) cognitive impairment, (4) feelings of discrimination, (5) impaired motivation, (6) lack of future orientation, and (7) lack of self-esteem.[190] Based on administration of the items to 46 depressed and normal elders, the best 30 items were selected by noting their correlation to the total score (the total number of the 100 items present). Somatic symptoms such as anorexia and insomnia did not correlate highly with the

Exhibit 3–13 Geriatric Depression Scale

---

1. Are you basically satisfied with your life? (no)
2. Have you dropped many of your activities and interests? (yes)
3. Do you feel that your life is empty? (yes)
4. Do you often get bored? (yes)
5. Are you hopeful about the future? (no)
6. Are you bothered by thoughts that you just cannot get out of your head? (yes)
7. Are you in good spirits most of the time? (no)
8. Are you afraid that something bad is going to happen to you? (yes)
9. Do you feel happy most of the time? (no)
10. Do you often feel helpless? (yes)
11. Do you often get restless and fidgety? (yes)
12. Do you prefer to stay home at night, rather than go out and do new things? (yes)
13. Do you frequently worry about the future? (yes)
14. Do you feel that you have more problems with memory than most? (yes)
15. Do you think it is wonderful to be alive now? (no)
16. Do you often feel downhearted and blue? (yes)
17. Do you feel pretty worthless the way you are now? (yes)
18. Do you worry a lot about the past? (yes)
19. Do you find life very exciting? (no)
20. Is it hard for you to get started on new projects? (yes)
21. Do you feel full of energy? (no)
22. Do you feel that your situation is hopeless? (yes)
23. Do you think that most persons are better off than you are? (yes)
24. Do you frequently get upset over little things? (yes)
25. Do you frequently feel like crying? (yes)
26. Do you have trouble concentrating? (yes)
27. Do you enjoy getting up in the morning? (no)
28. Do you prefer to avoid social gatherings? (yes)
29. Is it easy for you to make decisions? (no)
30. Is your mind as clear as it used to be? (no)

Score one point for each response that matches the yes or no answer after the question.

Source: Adapted from *Journal of Psychiatric Research,* Vol. 17, J.A. Yesavage and T.L. Brink, Development and Validation of a Geriatric Depression Screening Scale: A Preliminary Report. © 1983, with permission from Elsevier Science.

---

total score, and were dropped from the final instrument. The GDS was then administered to 20 normal elders and 51 elders who were in treatment for depression to evaluate the performance of the new 30-item instrument. Using a cutoff score of 11 or above to designate depressed individuals, the test was 84% sensitive and 95% specific for the diagnosis of depression.[190] Subsequent studies have demonstrated the value of the GDS.[192–198]

Persons with dementia were excluded from formative studies of the GDS, yet Brink was the first to suggest that the GDS may have uncertain validity in the presence of dementia.[199] Insensitivity of the GDS to dementia was suggested by a study of older adults from a comprehensive evaluation clinic.[200] A total of 72 persons with Alzheimer's disease were compared to 70 cognitively intact persons. Overall, the GDS was found to be useful in the detection of depression, but for a demented group the GDS performance was no better than chance. For those with dementia there was no cutoff that yielded a sensitivity and specificity greater than 65%. Another study by Burke and colleagues did not show any difference in performance with cognitive impairment.[201] In this study, the diagnoses were obtained prospectively (ie, after the GDS was administered). The authors explain the discrepancy between the studies as due to differences in the case ascertainment. Despite memory impairment, demented persons in this particular study often were consistent in their responses to questions about depression; however, persons with dementia may deny symptoms of depression in the same way they deny memory difficulties.[202]

Kafonek and associates[203] studied the GDS at an academic nursing home. Of 169 eligible admissions, 134 gave consent for the study, and 70 completed the examination. Residents were classified with regard to depression by a psychiatrist using the criteria of the third edition of the *Diagnostic and Statistical Manual (DSM-III)* and blinded to the results of the GDS. By clinical examination, 59% of the residents were demented, 19% were delirious, and 21% were depressed. Using a cutoff of 13/14, the GDS was 47% sensitive and 75% specific for the diagnosis of depression for the residents as a group. Importantly, the investigators found that GDS sensitivity was markedly diminished in the subset that scored less than 24 on the MMSE. In the current study, sensitivity dropped from 75% in the resident subset scoring normally on the MMSE to 25% in the subset scoring in the abnormal range. In other words, the GDS may not be suitable for detecting depression in the presence of dementia, which is a common type of impairment in nursing homes.

Finally, Parmelee and coworkers[204] examined 708 persons of mean age 84 years and found that 43% had symptoms of depression, 12% meeting criteria for major depression, even in the face of cognitive impairment. The paper sets forth very clearly the thorough attempts made at verifying diagnostic accuracy and reasons for nonparticipation. The GDS showed good agreement with observer ratings of depression whether or not there was dementia. The investigators felt that the GDS gave reliable data as long as cognitive deficits were not so severe as to preclude comprehension of the questions.

A short version of the GDS has been published.[205] The 15 questions of the shorter version are 1–4, 7–9, 10, 12, 14, 15, 17, and 21–23. Scores of 5 or more may indicate depression, according to the authors. Eighty-one volunteers from a continuing care community and a foster grandparent program were randomized to receive either the long GDS form or the short GDS form, and 2 weeks later, the alternative instrument.[206] The correlation coefficient for the scores on the two instruments was 0.66, indicating very high agreement. Using the GDS short form, Cwikel and Ritchie[207] interviewed 285 community respondents aged 65 and older, and a subset of 71 were examined by a clinician. A preliminary study of 20 cases and 20 controls showed that the threshold of 6/7 had the best sensitivity and specificity. Using a threshold of 6/7, the sensitivity was 72% and specificity was 57% for a *DSM-III* diagnosis of major depression. Persons without formal education were more likely to score in the depressed range on the GDS short form. It remains to be seen how specific the GDS is to geriatric depression and how specific to depression as opposed to general psychological distress; however, the GDS can be usefully applied in general medical settings. In using the GDS, it must be remembered that potentially important signals of depression in older people are not included in the GDS, such as sleep disturbance, somatic symptoms, and appetite disturbance with weight loss.

Zung Self-Rating Depression Scale

The Zung Self-Rating Depression Scale comprises 10 positive and 10 negative statements (Exhibit 3–14).[208] The statements are answered with the following phrases: "a little of the time," "some of the time," "a good part of the time," or "most of the time." The responses are scored from 1 to 4, in such a way that a higher score indicates greater depression. The score may be expressed as a percentage of 80, which is the maximum score attainable.

The Zung Self-Rating Depression Scale has been validated for a university outpatient psychiatric population.[209,210] Older persons apparently score higher than other groups.[211] In one study, community-dwelling older adults without psychiatric impairment had a score similar to that which would be considered borderline for the population as a whole.[212] Eighty-eight percent of patients with the diagnosis of depression by psychiatric examination had a score of 50 or greater, and 88% of patients who were not depressed had a score less than 50.[211,213] In a study that compared the Zung Self-Rating Depression Scale with psychiatric examination, the sensitivity was 77%, and the specificity was

Exhibit 3–14 The Zung Self-Rating Depression Scale

1. (−) I feel downhearted and blue.
2. (+) Morning is when I feel the best.
3. (−) I have crying spells or feel like it.
4. (−) I have trouble sleeping at night.
5. (+) I eat as much as I used to.
6. (+) I still enjoy sex.
7. (−) I notice that I am losing weight.
8. (−) I have trouble with constipation.
9. (−) My heart beats faster than usual.
10. (−) I get tired for no reason.
11. (+) My mind is as clear as it used to be.
12. (+) I find it easy to do the things I used to.
13. (−) I am restless and can't keep still.
14. (+) I feel hopeful about the future.
15. (−) I am more irritable than usual.
16. (+) I find it easy to make decisions.
17. (+) I feel that I am useful and needed.
18. (+) My life is pretty full.
19. (−) I feel that others would be better off if I were dead.
20. (+) I still enjoy the things I used to do.

Statements are answered "a little of the time," "some of the time," "a good part of the time," or "most of the time." The responses are given a score of 1 to 4, arranged so that the higher the score, the greater the depression: the statements designated with (+) are given "1" for response "most of the time," while those with (−) are given a "4" for "most of the time"

Source: Reprinted with permission from WWK Zung, A Self-Rating Scale, *Archives of General Psychiatry* Vol. 12, p.65. Copyright © 1965, American Medical Association.

82%. The predictive value of a positive test (for this study, a cutoff of 60 was used) was 65%; for a negative test, it was 89%.[214] The Zung scale contains more physical symptoms than other scales, and older adults, even when not depressed, tend to score higher than younger adults.[211]

General Health Questionnaire

The GHQ is a 60-item self-administered instrument whose purpose is to detect the presence of a psychiatric disorder.[215] A scaled version has been devised consisting of 28 items testing 4 general categories (7 questions each) that include somatic symptoms, anxiety and insomnia, social dysfunction, and depression (Exhibit 3–15). The GHQ is unusual among assessment questionnaires in that it was developed specifically for use in the primary care setting and has been used throughout the world.

Using the GHQ, respondents rate the presence of anxious and depressive symptoms over the past few weeks into one of four categories: "not at all" (coded 1), "no more than usual" (coded 2), "more than usual" (coded 3), or "much more than usual" (coded 4). Goodchild and Duncan-Jones[216] recommended a modified scoring method in which certain symptoms rated "no more than usual" are considered positive responses, reasoning that the GHQ may otherwise fail to detect chronic distress in persons screened for psychological distress in general medical settings.

In a British general practice, using a score of 4 or 5 as a cutoff, with higher scores indicating psychiatric illness, the scale has an 88% sensitivity (ie, 88% of respondents with a psychiatric disorder are correctly classified) and an 84% specificity (ie, 84% of the normal respondents are correctly classified).[217] Similar results were obtained in an American practice; when compared with the examination of a psychiatrist who did not know the result of the GHQ, the sensitivity was 86% with a specificity of 77%.[218]

As mentioned previously, the use of a screening instrument to detect depression in primary medicine can be valuable to increase awareness of depression in primary care practices.[219] Contrary to expectations, older persons as a group did not have any more somatic symptoms on the scale than did the younger subjects. Despite the use of idioms such as "strung up" and "keyed up," the GHQ appears to be sensitive to both anxiety and depression in outpatients, has been used all over the world, and is very well-studied.[158,220-229]

Beck Depression Inventory

The Beck Depression Inventory (BDI) is an instrument that addresses 21 characteristics of depression: mood, pessimism, sense of failure, satisfaction, guilt, sense of punishment, disappointment in oneself, self accusations, self-punitive wishes, crying spells, irritability, social withdrawal, indecisiveness, body image, function at work, sleep disturbance, fatigue, appetite disturbance, weight loss, preoccupation with health, and loss of libido.[230,231] Graber[232] and Gallo and associates[233] illustrate versions of the instrument. The BDI is administered by an interviewer, although it has been adapted for use as a self-administered instrument. Individual items are scored as 0, 1, 2, or 3. As reported in a study by Beck and associates, a score greater than 21 was indicative of severe depression, with about 75% sensitivity and 92% specificity; the value of a positive test in that sample (only 5% of subjects were over 55 years of age) was 75%, and that of a negative test was 92%.[234]

Exhibit 3–15 Items from the Scaled US Version of the General Health Questionnaire (GHQ)

A. *Somatic symptoms*
   A1. Been feeling in need of some medicine to pick you up?
   A2. Been feeling in need of a good tonic?
   A3. Been feeling run down and out of sorts?
   A4. Felt that you are ill?
   A5. Been getting any pains in your head?
   A6. Been getting a feeling of tightness or pressure in your head?
   A7. Been having hot or cold spells?

B. *Anxiety and insomnia*
   B1. Lost much sleep over worry?
   B2. Had difficulty staying asleep?
   B3. Felt constantly under strain?
   B4. Been getting edgy and bad-tempered?
   B5. Been getting scared or panicky for no reason?
   B6. Found everything getting on top of you?
   B7. Been feeling nervous and uptight all the time?

C. *Social dysfunction*
   C1. Been managing to keep yourself busy and occupied?
   C2. Been taking longer over the things you do?
   C3. Felt on the whole you were doing things well?
   C4. Been satisfied with the way you have carried out your tasks?
   C5. Felt that you are playing a useful part in things?
   C6. Felt capable of making decisions about things?
   C7. Been able to enjoy your normal day-to-day activities?

D. *Depression*
   D1. Been thinking of yourself as a worthless person?
   D2. Felt that life is entirely hopeless?
   D3. Felt that life isn't worth living?
   D4. Thought of the possibility that you might do away with yourself?
   D5. Found at times you couldn't do anything because your nerves were too bad?
   D6. Found yourself wishing you were dead and away from it all?
   D7. Found that the idea of taking your own life kept coming into your mind?

There are four responses for each question: score 1 for either of the two answers consistent with depression and 0 for the other two.

Source: Adapted with permission from DP Goldberg and VF Hiller, A Scaled Version of the General Health Questionnaire *Psychological Medicine*, Vol. 9, No. 1, pp. 139–145, © 1979, Cambridge University Press.

Compared with the *DSM-III* criteria for depression, the instrument was 100% sensitive (no missed cases) and 90% specific when a cutoff score of 10 was used to indicate depression in an adult sample with a mean age of about 40 years.[235]

Older adults participating in a psychiatric inpatient program were administered the BDI with good results. Using a score of 11 or greater as indicative of depression, the instrument had 93% sensitivity and 81% specificity. The predictive value of a positive test was 93%.[236] Medically ill older adults over the age of 60 years were administered the BDI on referral to a geriatric clinic. At a cutoff point of 10, the BDI was 89% sensitive and 82% specific when compared with a standardized diagnostic interview.[195]

In a study involving 526 patients in a primary care medical setting, a threshold score of 13 was used as indicative of depression; with this cutoff score, the sensitivity was 79%, and the specificity was 77% for all age groups.[237] The authors suggested using a cutoff score of 10 despite the greater number of false-positive results in order to avoid missing any cases of depression. In another study, a cutoff score of 10 was used for a group of 31 elderly medical outpatients; the BDI proved to be 89% sensitive and 82% specific as regarded the detection of depression.[195] In a study sample with a prevalence of depression estimated at about 12%, using 10 as a cutoff score was found to miss few depressed patients.[187]

A short version of the BDI (ie, the 21 items are reduced to 13) was shown to identify cases of depression as well as the longer instrument. The self-administered 13-item BDI takes 5 minutes to complete. The questions are identical to those in the larger instrument except that the order of the responses is reversed—the patient reads the most negative statements first. Scores of 5 to 7 are consistent with mild depression; scores of 8 to 15 indicate a moderate depression; and scores of 16 or greater show severe depression.[231]

The number of responses for each item in the Beck instruments is a source of potential confusion to the older patient, especially when some degree of mental impairment is present. As is the case with other instruments, older persons with numerous somatic complaints and difficulties may answer the items in such a way as to reflect these multiple physical complaints, rather than depression. The value of a positive test could be considerably lower in a primary care population where the prevalence of major depression would presumably be lower than in a psychiatric practice.[187] This is not necessarily a disadvantage as long as the examiner is prepared to confirm results by clinical interview. A short version of the BDI was recommended for use in primary care by the Depression Guidelines Panel.[147]

Center for Epidemiologic Studies Depression Scale

The Center for Epidemiologic Studies Depression Scale (CES-D; Exhibit 3–16) was developed by the Center for Epidemiologic Studies at the

Exhibit 3–16 Center for Epidemiologic Studies Depression Scale

---

Instructions for questions: Below is a list of the ways you might have felt or behaved. Please tell me how often you have felt this way during the past week.

Rarely or none of the time (less than 1 d)
Some or a little of the time (1–2 d)
Occasionally or a moderate amount of the time (3–4 d)
Most or all of the time (5–7 d)

During the past week:
1. I was bothered by things that usually don't bother me.
2. I did not feel like eating; my appetite was poor.
3. I felt that I could not shake off the blues even with help from my family or friends.
4. I felt that I was just as good as other people.
5. I had trouble keeping my mind on what I was doing.
6. I felt depressed.
7. I felt that everything I did was an effort.
8. I felt hopeful about the future.
9. I thought my life had been a failure.
10. I felt fearful.
11. My sleep was restless.
12. I was happy.
13. I talked less than usual.
14. I felt lonely.
15. People were unfriendly.
16. I enjoyed life.
17. I had crying spells.
18. I felt sad.
19. I felt that people dislike me.
20. I could not get "going."

Source: Reprinted from the Center for Epidemiologic Studies, National Institute of Mental Health.

NIMH for use in studies of depression in community samples.[238–240] The CES-D contains 20 items. Respondents are asked to report the amount of time they have experienced symptoms during the past week by choosing one of the following phrases: "rarely or none of the time"—less than 1 day—score 0; "some or a little of the time"—1 to 2 days—score 1; "occasionally or a moderate amount of time"—3 to 4 days—score 2; "most or all of the time"—5 to 7 days—score 3. Typically, a threshold of 17 and above is taken as defining "caseness,"[241] although higher cutoff points (eg, 24 and above) have been suggested.[242] Among patients in a medical setting, an inordinate number of false positives was generated with higher thresholds on the CES-D, but a higher threshold of 27 was associated with greater specificity.[243] The CES-D did not seem to be biased by somatic complaints in a large community survey of persons aged 55 years and older.[244] Zimmerman and Coryell called attention to the lack of correlation to *DSM-IV* criteria and proposed a revision that would include criteria such as suicidal ideation and psychomotor agitation or retardation,[245] and modifications of the CES-D are in development.[157]

ALCOHOL AND OTHER SUBSTANCE MISUSE

Alcohol consumption is common among older adults although the proportion meeting criteria for alcohol abuse or dependence is much smaller. For example, 10% to 20% of older persons report daily use of alcohol,[246] but the 1-month prevalence of alcohol abuse or dependence was only 1% to 3% for men and less than 0.5% for women aged 65 years and older.[247,248] Of 5,065 adults aged 60 years and older screened in primary care practices in Wisconsin, 10.5% of the men and 3.9% of the women reported problem alcohol use.[249] Numerous factors, including stereotypes of alcoholics and the aged, conspire to make alcoholism difficult to detect in older persons.[250–252] Screening for alcohol use problems should accompany evaluation of older persons with functional impairment, seizures, falls, cognitive impairment, depression, anxiety, insomnia, and adverse reaction to prescribed medications.[106,250] Comorbid psychiatric conditions such as depression and alcoholism may identify older adults at increased risk for suicide.[253,254]

Among the brief measures of alcohol abuse are the 4-item CAGE,[255,256] the 10-item AUDIT,[257–259] and the 24-item MAST-G.[103,260] The CAGE is advantageous as the entire instrument can be committed to memory because each letter in CAGE is associated with a question:

1. Ever felt the need to *cut down* on your drinking? (C)
2. Ever felt *annoyed by* criticism of your drinking? (A)
3. Ever felt *guilty* about drinking? (G)
4. Ever take a morning drink *(eye-opener)*? (E)

Two affirmative answers are said to be suggestive of alcoholism.[255,256,261] The CAGE is widely recommended as a screening instrument for alcohol use problems in primary care settings.[262,263] Two affirmative answers to the four CAGE questions are said to be suggestive of problem drinking.[255,256] When using the CAGE, the examiner should ask about the amount and pattern of drinking to be sure not to miss heavy drinkers in older primary care patients[249] and to permit assessment of change in alcohol consumption.

The AUDIT was developed under the auspices of the World Health Organization and is an acronym for the Alcohol Use Disorder Identification Test (Exhibit 3–17). Each item is rated on 4-point scale; using a cutoff point of 8 was 92% sensitive and 93% specific.[258] Unlike the CAGE, the AUDIT includes items about amount consumed and problems directly related to alcohol consumption.

ANXIETY DISORDERS

Anxiety and worries are important symptoms in the care of older persons. Studies reveal that among long-term users of anxiolytic medicines in primary care, older adults figure prominently.[264–267] For example, compared to adults aged 18 to 44 years, adults aged 65 years and older were almost twice as likely to continue daily benzodiazepine use for more than 60 days even accounting for a number of potential confounders, based on analysis of a pharmacy database.[268] Comorbid anxiety and depression increase recognition of depression[158,269] but also appear to be associated with increased prescription of benzodiazepines,[158,270,271] suggesting that physicians have not appropriately assessed the patients.[270] Despite the importance of anxiety symptoms and the availability of a number of instruments to tap anxiety symptoms,[272–274] an NIMH workshop that focused on anxiety in older persons concluded that the topic has not been well-studied and is not well understood. Further discussion of the mental disorders of late life can be found in other sources.[152,275,276]

CONCLUSION

The instruments discussed in this chapter are valuable in clinical settings to improve the recognition and evaluation of dementia, delirium, depression, and other mental disturbances. It must be emphasized that the screening instruments are tools to supplement clinical assessment. An abnormal score on a short mental status test may be due to something other than dementia, such as an acute confusional state (delirium), vision or hearing impairment, or low educational level. The patient must be examined carefully and appropriate historical data sought before a diagnosis of dementia is made. If dementia is diagnosed, an appropriate attempt should be made to characterize the etiology. The examiner must remember to consider alternative conditions when persons with dementia who have had stable deficits show a decline.

Exhibit 3–17 Alcohol Use Disorder Identification Test (AUDIT)

AUDIT is a brief structured interview, developed by the World Health Organization, which can be incorporated into a medical history. It contains questions about recent alcohol consumption, dependence symptoms, and alcohol-related problems.

Begin the AUDIT by saying: "Now I am going to ask you some questions about your use of alcoholic beverages *during the past year.*" Explain what is meant by alcoholic beverages (ie, beer, wine, liquor [vodka, whiskey, brandy, etc.]).

Record the score for each question in the box on the right side of the question [ ].

1. How often do you have a drink containing alcohol?
   ☐ Never   (0)   [ ]
   ☐ Monthly or less   (1)
   ☐ 2 to 4 times a month   (2)
   ☐ 2 to 3 times a week   (3)
   ☐ 4 or more times a week   (4)

2. How many drinks containing alcohol do you have on a typical day when you are drinking?
   ☐ None   (0)   [ ]
   ☐ 1 or 2   (1)
   ☐ 3 or 4   (2)
   ☐ 5 or 6   (3)
   ☐ 7 or 9   (4)
   ☐ 10 or more (5)

3. How often do you have six or more drinks on one occasion?
   ☐ Never   (0)   [ ]
   ☐ Less than monthly (1)
   ☐ Monthly   (2)
   ☐ Weekly   (3)
   ☐ Daily or almost daily (4)

4. How often during the last year have you found that you were unable to stop drinking once you had started?
   ☐ Never   (0)   [ ]
   ☐ Less than monthly (1)
   ☐ Monthly   (2)
   ☐ Weekly   (3)
   ☐ Daily or almost daily (4)

5. How often during the last year have you failed to do what was normally expected from you because of drinking?
   ☐ Never   (0)   [ ]
   ☐ Less than monthly (1)
   ☐ Monthly   (2)
   ☐ Weekly   (3)
   ☐ Daily or almost daily (4)

continues

Exhibit 3–17 continued

---

6. How often during the last year have you needed a first drink in the morning to get yourself going after a heavy drinking session?
   ☐ Never   (0)   [ ]
   ☐ Less than monthly   (1)
   ☐ Monthly   (2)
   ☐ Weekly   (3)
   ☐ Daily or almost daily   (4)

7. How often during the last year have you had a feeling of guilt or remorse after drinking?
   ☐ Never   (0)   [ ]
   ☐ Less than monthly   (1)
   ☐ Monthly   (2)
   ☐ Weekly   (3)
   ☐ Daily or almost daily   (4)

8. How often during the last year have you been unable to remember what happened the night before because you had been drinking?
   ☐ Never   (0)   [ ]
   ☐ Less than monthly   (1)
   ☐ Monthly   (2)
   ☐ Weekly   (3)
   ☐ Daily or almost daily   (4)

9. Have you or someone else been injured as the result of your drinking?
   ☐ Never   (0)   [ ]
   ☐ Less than monthly   (1)
   ☐ Monthly   (2)
   ☐ Weekly   (3)
   ☐ Daily or almost daily   (4)

10. Has a relative, friend, or a doctor or other health worker been concerned about your drinking or suggested you cut down?
   ☐ Never   (0)   [ ]
   ☐ Less than monthly   (1)
   ☐ Monthly   (2)
   ☐ Weekly   (3)
   ☐ Daily or almost daily   (4)

Record the total of the specific items.   [ ]

A score of 8 or greater may indicate the need for a more in-depth assessment.

Source: Reprinted with permission from T.F. Babor et al., AUDIT--the Alcohol Use Disorders Identification Test: Guidelines for Use in Primary Health Care, World Health Organization/PSA/92.4.

Regardless of the specific properties of the instrument used, the important point is to use some standardized method of mental status testing when assessing older persons. The assessment instruments make data collection uniform, and many have been well studied. In addition, many are brief enough to administer at intervals to assess changes in the individual's condition. Such examinations may be invaluable as a baseline assessment, particularly at the time of nursing home placement or hospitalization. Despite stability or deterioration in scores on cognitive tests, individuals may improve in other ways such as diminished behavioral or psychotic symptoms. For example, despite achieving the same score on the MMSE as was achieved a year ago, a demented older person might rest better at night, cause less worry to caregivers, and enjoy socializing when enrolled in a day-care.[277] Mental status testing must be viewed as one of several integrated facets in the assessment of older adults.

REFERENCES

1. Shepherd M, Cooper B, Brown AC, Kalton GW. *Psychiatric Illness in General Practice*. London: Oxford University Press; 1966.

2. Regier DA, Narrow WE, Rae DS, Manderscheid RW, Locke BZ, Goodwin FK. The de facto US mental and addictive disorders system: Epidemiologic Catchment Area prospective 1-year prevalence rates of disorders and services. *Arch Gen Psychiatry.* 1993;50:85–94.

3. Gallo JJ, Marino S, Ford D, Anthony JC. Filters on the pathway to mental health care: II. Sociodemographic factors. *Psychol Med.* 1995;25:1149–1160.

4. Miranda J, Hohmann AA, Attkisson CC, Larson DB. *Mental Disorders in Primary Care*. San Francisco: Jossey-Bass Publishers; 1994.

5. Higgins ES. A review of unrecognized mental illness in primary care: Prevalence, natural history, and efforts to change the course. *Arch Fam Med.* 1994;3:908–917.

6. Sager MA, Dunham NC, Schwantes A, Mecum L, Halverson K, Harlowe D. Measurement of activities of daily living in hospitalized elderly: A comparison of self-report and performance-based methods. *J Am Geriatr Soc.* 1992;40:457–462.

7. Jacobs J, Bernhard MR, Delgado A, et al. Screening for organic mental syndromes in the medically ill. *Ann Intern Med.* 1977;86:40–46.

8. McCartney JR, Palmatee LM. Assessment of cognitive deficit in geriatric patients: A study of physician behavior. *J Am Geriatr Soc.* 1985;33:467–471.

9. Callahan CM, Hendrie HC, Tierney WM. Documentation and evaluation of cognitive impairment in elderly primary care patients. *Ann Intern Med.* 1995;122:422–429.

10. Larson EB. Recognition of dementia: Discovering the silent epidemic. *J Am Geriatr Soc.* 1998;46:1576–1577.

11. Iliffe S, Booroff A, Gallivan S, Goldenberg E, Morgan P, Haines A. Screening for cognitive impairment in the elderly using the mini-mental state examination. *Br J Gen Pract.* 1990;40:277–279.

12. Cooper B, Eastwood R. *Primary Health Care and Psychiatric Epidemiology.* New York: Tavistock/Routledge; 1992.

13. Cooper B, Bickel H. Population screening and the early detection of dementing disorders in old age: A review. *Psychol Med.* 1984;14:81–95.

14. Ross GW, Abbott RD, Petrovitch H. Frequency and characteristics of silent dementia among elderly Japanese-American men. *JAMA.* 1997;277:800–805.

15. Schneider LS, Reynolds CF, Lebowitz BD, Friedhoff AJ. *Diagnosis and Treatment of Depression in Late Life: Results of the NIH Consensus Development Conference.* Washington, DC: American Psychiatric Association; 1994.

16. Francis J, Kapoor WN. Prognosis after hospital discharge of older medical patients with delirium. *J Am Geriatr Soc.* 1992;40:601–606.

17. Marcantonio ER, Goldman L, Mangione CM, et al. A clinical prediction rule for delirium after elective noncardiac surgery. *JAMA.* 1994;271:134–139.

18. Fields SD, MacKenzie R, Charlson ME, et al. Cognitive impairment: Can it predict the course of hospitalized patients? *J Am Geriatr Soc.* 1986;34:579–585.

19. Murray AM, Levkoff SE, Wetle TT, et al. Acute delirium and functional decline in the hospitalized elderly patient. *J Gerontol.* 1993;48:M181–186.

20. O'Keeffe ST, Lavan JN. Predicting delirium in elderly patients: Development and validation of a risk-stratification model. *Age Ageing.* 1996;25:317–321.

21. Inouye SK, Charpentier PA. Precipitating factors for delirium in hospitalized elderly persons: Predictive model and interrelationship with baseline vulnerability. *JAMA.* 1996;275:852–857.

22. Cooper JK, Mungas D, Weiler PG. Relation of cognitive status and abnormal behaviors in Alzheimer's disease. *J Am Geriatr Soc.* 1990;38:867–870.

23. Henderson AS, Huppert FA. The problem of mild dementia. *Psychol Med.* 1984;14:5–11.

24. Warshaw G. Are mental status questionnaires of clinical value in everyday office practice? An affirmative view. *J Fam Pract.* 1990;30:194–197.

25. Costa PT, Williams TF, Somerfield M, et al. *Early Identification of Alzheimer's Disease and Related Dementias, Clinical Practice Guidelines, No 19.* Rockville, MD: US Dept of Health and Human Services, Public Health Service, Agency for Health Care Policy and Research; 1996. AHCPR Publication Number 97–0703.

26. Kapp MB, Bigot A. *Geriatrics and the Law.* New York: Springer Publishing Co; 1985.

27. Broadhead WE, Blazer DG, George LK, Tse CK. Depression, disability days, and days lost from work in a prospective epidemiologic survey. *JAMA.* 1990;264: 2524–2528.

28. Horwath E, Johnson J, Klerman GL, Weissman MM. Depressive symptoms as relative and attributable risk factors for first-onset major depression. *Arch Gen Psychiatry.* 1992;49:817–823.

29. Johnson J, Weissman MM, Klerman GL. Service utilization and social morbidity associated with depressive symptoms in the community. *JAMA.* 1992;267:1478–1483.

30. Pearson JL, Teri L, Reifler BV, Raskind MA. Functional status and cognitive impairment in Alzheimer's patients with and without depression. *J Am Geriatr Soc.* 1989; 37:1117–1121.

31. Wells KB, Stewart A, Hays RD, et al. The functioning and well-being of depressed patients: Results from the medical outcomes study. *JAMA.* 1989;262:914–919.

32. NIH Consensus Development Panel on Depression in Late Life. Diagnosis and treatment of depression in late life. *JAMA.* 1992;268:1018–1024.

33. Reynolds CF, Schneider LS, Lebowitz BD, Kupfer DJ. Treatment of depression in elderly patients: Guidelines for primary care. In: Schneider LS, Reynolds CF, Lebowitz BD, Friedhoff AJ, eds. *Diagnosis and Treatment of Depression in Late Life: Results of the NIH Consensus Development Conference.* Washington, DC: American Psychiatric Association; 1994:463–490.

34. Auerbach SH, Cicerone KD, Levin HS, Tranel D. What you can learn from neuropsychologic testing. *Patient Care.* 1994;28(July 15):97–116.

35. Strub RL, Black FW. *The Mental Status Examination in Neurology.* 2nd ed. Philadelphia: FA Davis Co; 1985.

36. Jones TV, Williams ME. Rethinking the approach to evaluating mental functioning of older persons: The value of careful observations. *J Am Geriatr Soc.* 1988;36: 1128–1134.

37. Fry PS. *Depression, Stress, and Adaptations in the Elderly: Psychological Assessment and Intervention.* Rockville, MD: Aspen Publishers, Inc; 1986.

38. Feher EP, Doody R, Pirozzolo FJ, Appel SH. Mental status assessment of insight and judgment. *Clin Geriatr Med.* 1989;5:477–498.

39. Kokmen E, Naessens JM, Offord KP. A short test of mental status: Description and preliminary results. *Mayo Clin Proc.* 1987;62:281–288.

40. Mattis S. Mental status examination for organic mental syndrome in the elderly patient. In: Bellak L, Karasu TB, eds. *Geriatric Psychiatry.* New York: Grune & Stratton; 1976:77–121.

41. LaRue A. Memory loss and aging: Distinguishing dementia from benign senescent forgetfulness and depressive pseudodementia. *Psychiatr Clin N Am.* 1982;5:89–103.

42. Blum JE, Jarvik LF, Clark ET. Rate of change on selective tests of intelligence: A twenty-year longitudinal study of aging. *J Gerontol.* 1970;25:171–176.

43. Gallo JJ, Stanley L, Zack N, Reichel W. Multi-dimensional assessment of the older patient. In: Reichel W, ed. *Clinical Aspects of Aging.* 4th ed. Baltimore: Williams & Wilkins; 1995:15–30.

44. Erilsen CW, Hamlin RM, Daye C. Aging adults and rate of memory scan. *Bull Psychono Soc.* 1973;1:259–260.

45. Smith ME. Delayed recall of previously memorized material after fifty years. *J Gen Psychol.* 1963;102:3–4.

46. Grut M, Jorm AF, Fratiglioni L, Forsell Y, Viitanen M, Winblad B. Memory complaints of elderly people in a population survey: Variation according to dementia stage and depression. *J Am Geriatr Soc.* 1993;41:1295–1300.

47. Crook T, Bartus RT, Ferris SH, et al. Age-associated memory impairment: Proposed diagnostic criteria and measures of clinical change: Report of a National Institute of Mental Health work group. *Dev Neuropsychol.* 1986;2:261–276.

48. Kral VA. Senescent forgetfulness: Benign and malignant. *J Can Med Assoc.* 1962; 86:257–260.

49. Rediess S, Caine ED. Aging-associated cognitive changes: How do they relate to the diagnosis of dementia? *Curr Opinion Psychiatry.* 1993;6:531–536.

50. Working Party of the International Psychogeriatric Association in collaboration with the World Health Organization. Aging-associated cognitive decline. *Int Psychogeriatr.* 1994;6:63–68.

51. Blackford RC, La Rue A. Criteria for diagnosing age-associated memory impairment: Proposed improvements from the field. *Dev Neuropsychol.* 1989;5:295–306.

52. Small GW, Okonek A, Mandelkern MA, et al. Age-associated memory loss: Initial neuropsychological and cerebral metabolic findings of a longitudinal study. *Int Psychogeriatr.* 1994;6:23–44.

53. Huppert FA, Brayne C, O'Connor DW. *Dementia and Normal Aging.* Cambridge, England: Cambridge University Press; 1994.

54. American Psychiatric Association: *Diagnostic and Statistical Manual of Mental Disorders, Fourth Edition.* Washington, DC, American Psychiatric Association, 1994.

55. Blazer DG. *Depression in Late Life.* 2nd ed. St Louis, MO: CV Mosby, Co; 1993.

56. Damasio AR. Aphasia. *N Engl J Med.* 1992;326:531–539.

57. Wolf-Klein GP, Silverstone FA, Levy AP, Brod MS. Screening for Alzheimer's disease by clock drawing. *J Am Geriatr Soc.* 1989;37:730–737.

58. Sunderland T, Hill JL, Mellow AM, et al. Clock drawing in Alzheimer's disease: A novel measure of dementia severity. *J Am Geriatr Soc.* 1989;37:725–729.

59. Mendez MF, Ala T, Underwood KL. Development of scoring criteria for the clock drawing task in Alzheimer's disease. *J Am Geriatr Soc.* 1992;40:1095–1099.

60. Tuokko H, Hadjistavropoulos T, Miller JA, Beattie BL. The clock test: A sensitive measure to differentiate normal elderly from those with Alzheimer's disease. *J Am Geriatr Soc.* 1992;40:579–584.

61. Watson YI, Arfken CL, Birge SJ. Clock completion: An objective screening test for dementia. *J Am Geriatr Soc.* 1993;41:1235–1240.

62. Shuttleworth EC. Memory function and the clinical differentiation of dementing disorders. *J Am Geriatr Soc.* 1982;30:363–366.

63. Lipowski ZJ. Delirium (acute confusional states). *JAMA.* 1987;258:1789–1792.

64. Inouye SK, van Dyck CH, Alessi CA, Balkin S, Siegal AP, Horwitz RJ. Clarifying confusion: The confusion assessment method: A new method for detection of delirium. *Ann Intern Med.* 1990;113:941–948.

65. Larson EB, Reifler BV, Featherstone HJ, et al. Dementia in elderly outpatients: A prospective study. *Ann Intern Med.* 1984;100:417–423.

66. Maletta GJ. The concept of "reversible" dementia: How nonreliable terminology may impair effective treatment. *J Am Geriatr Soc.* 1990;38:136–140.

67. Cummings JL, Benson DF. *Dementia: A Clinical Approach.* 2nd ed. Stoneham, MA: Butterworth-Heinemann; 1992.

68. McKhann G, Drachman D, Folstein M, et al. Clinical diagnosis of Alzheimer's disease: Report of the NINCDS-ADRDA work group under the auspices of Department of Health and Human Services Task Force on Alzheimer's Disease. *Neurology.* 1984;34:939–944.

69. Cummings JL, Benson DF. Dementia of the Alzheimer type: An inventory of clinical features. *J Am Geriatr Soc.* 1986;34:12–19.

70. Coen RF, O'Mahoney D, Bruce I, Lawlor BA, Walsh JB, Coakley D. Differential diagnosis of dementia: A prospective evaluation of the DAT inventory. *J Am Geriatr Soc.* 1994;42:16–20.

71. Emery VOB, Gillie EX, Smith JA. Reclassification of the vascular dementias: Comparisons of infarct and noninfarct vascular dementias. *Int Psychogeriatr.* 1996;8:33–61.

72. Larson EB. Illness causing dementia in the very elderly. *N Engl J Med.* 1993;328:203–205.

73. Skoog I. Risk factors for vascular dementia: A review. *Dementia.* 1994;5:137–144.

74. Yao H, Sadoshima S, Ibayashi S. Leukoaraiosis and dementia in hypertensive patients. *Stroke.* 1992;23:1673–1677.

75. Breteler MM, van Swieten JC, Bots ML. Cerebral white matter lesions, vascular risk factors, and cognitive function in a population-based study: The Rotterdam Study. *Neurology.* 1994;44:1246–1252.

76. Breteler MM, van Amerongen NM, van Swieten JC. Cognitive correlates of ventricular enlargement and cerebral white matter lesions on magnetic resonance imaging: The Rotterdam Study. *Stroke.* 1994;25:1109–1115.

77. Manolio TA, Kronmal RA, Burke GL. Magnetic resonance abnormalities and cardiovascular disease in older adults. *Stroke.* 1994;25:318–327.

78. De Reuck J, Crevitz L, De Coster W. Pathogenesis of biswanger chronic progressive subcortical encephalopathy. *Neurology.* 1980;30:920–928.

79. Awad IA, Johnson PC, Spetzler RF, Hodak JA. Incidental subcortical lesions identified on magnetic resonance imaging in the elderly, II: Postmortem pathological correlations. *Stroke.* 1986;17:1090–1097.

80. Chimowitz MI, Estes ML, Furlan AJ, Awad IA. Further observations on the pathology of subcortical lesions identified on magnetic resonance imaging. *Arch Neurol.* 1992;49:747–752.

81. Price TR, Manolio TA, Kronmal RA, et al. Silent brain infarction on magnetic resonance imaging and neurological abnormalities in community-dwelling older adults: The Cardiovascular Health Study, CHS Collaborative Group. *Stroke.* 1997;28:1158–1164.

82. Ferrucci L, Guralnik JM, Salive ME, et al. Cognitive impairment and risk of stroke in the older population. *J Am Geriatr Soc.* 1996;44:237–241.

83. Snowdon DA. Aging and Alzheimer's disease: Lessons from the Nun Study. *Gerontologist.* 1997;37:150–156.

84. Berrios GE. Dementia. In: Berrios GE, Porter R, eds. *A History of Clinical Psychiatry: The Origin and History of Psychiatric Disorders.* Washington Square, NY: New York University Press; 1995:34–51.

85. Dening TR. Stroke and other vascular disorders. In: Berrios GE, Porter R, eds. *A History of Clinical Psychiatry: The Origin and History of Psychiatric Disorders.* Washington Square, NY: New York University Press; 1995:72–85.

86. Devasenapathy A, Hachinski V. Vascular cognitive impairment: A new approach. In: Holmes C, Howard R, eds. *Advances in Old Age Psychiatry: Chromosomes to Community Care.* Bristol, PA: Wrightson Biomedical Publishing, Ltd; 1997:79–95.

87. Steingart A, Hachinski VC, Lau C, et al. Cognitive and neurologic findings in demented patients with diffuse white matter lucencies on computed tomographic scan (leuko-araiosis). *Arch Neurol.* 1987;44:36–39.

88. Hofman A, Ott A, Breteler MMB, et al. Atherosclerosis, apolipoprotein E, and prevalence of dementia and Alzheimer's disease in the Rotterdam Study. *Lancet.* 1997;349:151–154.

89. Snowdon DA, Greiner LH, Mortimer JA, Riley KP, Greiner PA, Markesbery WR. Brain infarction and the clinical expression of Alzheimer's disease: the Nun Study. *JAMA.* 1997;277:813–817.

90. Alexopoulos GS, Meyers BS, Young RC, Campbell S, Silbersweig D, Charlson M. 'Vascular depression' hypothesis. *Arch Gen Psychiatry.* 1997;54:915–922.

91. Emery VOB, Gillie EX, Smith JA. Reclassification of the vascular dementias: Comparisons of infarct and noninfarct vascular dementias. *Int Psychogeriatr.* 1996;8:33–61.

92. Olsen CG, Clasen ME. Senile dementia of the Binswanger's type. *Am Fam Physician.* 1998;58:2068–2074.

93. Bennett DA, Wilson RS, Gilley DW, Fox JH. Clinical diagnosis of Binswanger's disease. *J Neurol Neurosurg Psychiatry.* 1990;53:1–5.

94. Roman GC. Senile dementia of the Binswanger type: A vascular form of dementia in the elderly. *JAMA.* 1987;258:1782–1788.

95. Mahler ME, Cummings JL, Tomiyasu U. Atypical dementia syndrome in an elderly man. *J Am Geriatr Soc.* 1987;35:1116–1126.

96. Meyer JS, Judd BW, Tawakina T, et al. Improved cognition after control of risk factors for multi-infarct dementia. *JAMA.* 1986;256:2203–2209.

97. Hachinski VC, Iliff LD, Zilhka E, et al. Cerebral blood flow in dementia. *Ann Neurol.* 1975;32:632–637.

98. Liston EH, LaRue A. Clinical differentiation of primary degenerative and multi-infarct dementia: A critical review of the evidence: II. Pathological studies. *Biol Psychiatry.* 1983;18:1467–1484.

99. Whitehouse PJ. The concept of subcortical and cortical dementia: Another look. *Ann Neurol.* 1986;19:1–6.

100. McKeith IG. Dementia with Lewy bodies. In: Holmes C, Howard R, eds. *Advances in Old Age Psychiatry: Chromosomes to Community Care.* Bristol, PA: Wrightson Biomedical Publishing, Ltd; 1997:52–63.

101. McKeith LG, Galasko D, Kosaka K. Consensus guidelines for the clinical and pathologic diagnosis of dementia with Lewy bodies (DLB): Report of the Consortium on DLB International Workshop. *Neurology.* 1996;47:1113–1124.

102. Clarfield AM, Larson EB. Should a major imaging procedure (CT or MRI) be required in the workup of dementia? An opposing view. *J Fam Pract.* 1990;31:405–410.

103. Beresford TP. Alcoholism in the elderly. *Int Rev Psychiatry.* 1993;5:477–483.

104. Brody JA. Aging and alcohol abuse. *J Am Geriatr Soc.* 1982;30:123–126.

105. Gottheil E, Druley KA, Skoloda TE. *The Combined Problems of Alcoholism, Drug Addiction, and Aging.* Springfield, IL: Charles C Thomas; 1985.

106. Wattis JP. Alcohol problems in the elderly. *J Am Geriatr Soc.* 1981;29:131–134.

107. Zimberg S. Alcohol abuse among the elderly. In: Carstensen LL, Edelstein BA, eds. *Handbook of Clinical Gerontology.* New York: Pergamon Press; 1987:57–65.

108. Widner S, Zeichner A. Alcohol abuse in the elderly: Review of epidemiology research and treatment. *Clin Gerontologist.* 1991;11:3–18.

109. Moss RJ, Miles SH. AIDS and the geriatrician. *J Am Geriatr Soc.* 1987;35:460–464.

110. Sabin TD. AIDS: The new "great imitator" [editorial]. *J Am Geriatr Soc.* 1987;35:467–468.

111. Larson EB, Reifler BV, Sumi SM, et al. Diagnostic evaluation of 200 elderly outpatients with suspected dementia. *J Gerontol.* 1985;40:536–543.

112. National Center for Cost Containment. *Geropsychology Assessment Resource Guide.* Milwaukee, WI: US Department of Commerce, National Technical Information Service; 1993.

113. McDowell I, Newell C. *Measuring Health: A Guide to Rating Scales and Questionnaires.* 2nd ed. New York: Oxford University Press; 1996.

114. Froehlich TE, Robison JT, Inouye SK. Screening for dementia in the outpatient setting: The time and change test. *J Am Geriatr Soc.* 1998;46:1506–1511.

115. Solomon PR, Pendlebury WW. Recognition of Alzheimer's disease: The 7-minute screen. *Fam Med.* 1998;30:265–271.

116. Keating HJ. "Studying" for the Mini-Mental Status Exam [letter]. *J Am Geriatr Soc.* 1987;35:594–595.

117. Folstein MF, Folstein SE, McHugh PR. "Mini-Mental State": A practical method for grading the cognitive state of patients for the clinician. *J Psychiatr Res*. 1975;12:189–198.

118. Tombaugh TN, McIntyre NJ. The Mini-Mental State Examination: A comprehensive review. *J Am Geriatr Soc*. 1992;40:922–935.

119. Crum RM, Anthony JC, Bassett SS, Folstein MF. Population-based norms for the Mini-Mental State Examination by age and educational level. *JAMA*. 1993;269:2386–2391.

120. Gallo JJ, Anthony JC. Misperception in the scoring of the MMSE [letter]. *Can J Psychiatry*. 1994;39:382.

121. Brandt J, Spencer M, Folstein M. The telephone interview for cognitive status. *Neuropsychiatry Neuropsychol Behav Neurol*. 1988;1:11–17.

122. Tsai L, Tsuang MT. The Mini-Mental State test and computerized tomography. *Am J Psychiatry*. 1979;136:436–439.

123. Fillenbaum G. Comparison of two brief tests of organic brain impairment, the MSQ and the short portable MSQ. *J Am Geriatr Soc*. 1980;28:381–384.

124. Roth M, Tym E, Mountjoy CQ, et al. CAMDEX: A standardised instrument for the diagnosis of mental disorder in the elderly with special reference to the early detection of dementia. *Br J Psychiatry*. 1986;149:698–709.

125. Anthony JC, LeResche L, Niaz U, von Korff M, Folstein MF. Limits of the 'Mini-Mental State' as a screening test for dementia and delirium among hospital patients. *Psychol Med*. 1982;12:397–408.

126. Dick JPR, Guiloff RJ, Stewart A, et al. Mini-Mental State Examination in neurological patients. *J Neurol Neurosurg Psychiatry*. 1984;47:496–499.

127. Webster JS, Scott RR, Nunn B, et al. A brief neuropsychological screening procedure that assesses left and right hemispheric function. *J Clin Psychol*. 1984;40:237–240.

128. Kittner SJ, White LR, Farmer ME, et al. Methodological issues in screening for dementia: The problem of education adjustment. *J Chronic Dis*. 1986;39:163–170.

129. Uhlmann RF, Larson EB. Effect of education on the Mini-Mental State Examination as a screening test for dementia. *J Am Geriatr Soc*. 1991;39:876–880.

130. Pfeiffer E. A short portable mental status questionnaire for the assessment of organic brain deficit in elderly patients. *J Am Geriatr Soc*. 1975;23:433–441.

131. Kahn RL, Goldfarb AI, Pollack M. Brief objective measures for the determination of mental status in the aged. *Am J Psychiatry*. 1960;117:326–328.

132. Erkinjuntt T, Sulkava R, Wikstrom J, et al. Short Portable Mental Status Questionnaire as a screening test for dementia and delirium among the elderly. *J Am Geriatr Soc*. 1987;35:412–416.

133. Smyer MA, Hofland BF, Jonas EA. Validity study of the Short Portable Mental Status Questionnaire for the elderly. *J Am Geriatr Soc*. 1979;27:263–269.

134. Dalton JE, Pederson SL, Blom BE, et al. Diagnostic errors using the Short Portable Mental Status Questionnaire with a mixed clinical population. *J Gerontol*. 1987;42:512–514.

135. Wolber G, Romaniuk M, Eastman E, et al. Validity of the Short Portable Mental Status Questionnaire with elderly psychiatric patients. *J Consult Clin Psychol*. 1984;52:712–713.

136. Fillenbaum GG, Landerman LR, Simonsick EM. Equivalence of two screens of cognitive functioning: The Short Portable Mental Status Questionnaire and the Orientation-Memory-Concentration Test. *J Am Geriatr Soc*. 1998;46:1512–1518.

92   HANDBOOK OF GERIATRIC ASSESSMENT

137. Klein LE, Roca RP, McArthur J, et al. Univariate and multivariate analyses of the mental state examination. *J Am Geriatr Soc.* 1985;33:483–488.

138. Kaufman DM, Weinberger M, Strain JJ, et al. Detection of cognitive deficits by a brief mental status examination: The Cognitive Capacity Screening Examination. *Gen Hosp Psychiatry.* 1979;1:247–254.

139. Omer H, Foldes J, Toby M, et al. Screening for cognitive deficits in a sample of hospitalized geriatric patients: A re-evaluation of a brief mental status questionnaire. *J Am Geriatr Soc.* 1983;31:266–268.

140. Katzman R, Brown T, Fuld P,. Peck A, Schechter R, Schimmel H Validation of a Short Orientation-Memory-Concentration test of cognitive impairment. *Am J Psychiatry.* 1983;140:734–739.

141. Issacs B, Kennie AT. The set test as an aid to the detection of dementia in old people. *Br J Psychiatry.* 1973;123:467–470.

142. Eslinger PJ, Damasio AR, Benson AL, et al. Neuropsychologic detection of abnormal mental decline in older persons. *JAMA.* 1985;253:670–674.

143. Ainslie NK, Murden RA. Effect of education on the clock-drawing dementia screen in non-demented elderly persons. *J Am Geriatr Soc.* 1993;41:249–252.

144. Rook KS, Catano R, Dooley D. The timing of major life events: Effects of departing from the social clock. *Am J Community Psychol.* 1989;17:233–258.

145. Stahelin HB, Monsch AU, Spiegel R. Early diagnosis of dementia via a two-step screening and diagnostic procedure. *Int Psychogeriatr.* 1997;9(suppl 1):123–130.

146. Lebowitz BD, Pearson JL, Schneider LS, et al. Diagnosis and treatment of depression in late life: Consensus statement update. *JAMA.* 1997;278:1186–1190.

147. Depression Guideline Panel. *Depression in Primary Care: Volume 1. Detection and Diagnosis: Clinical Practice Guideline, No 5.* Rockville, MD: US Dept of Health and Human Services, Public Health Service, Agency for Health Care Policy and Research; 1993. AHCPR Publication Number 93–0550.

148. Institute of Medicine. *The Second Fifty Years: Promoting Health and Preventing Disability.* Washington, DC: National Academy Press; 1992.

149. Department of Health and Human Services. *Healthy People 2000: National Health Promotion and Disease Prevention Objectives.* Washington, DC: US Government Printing Office; 1991. DHHS Publication No. PHS 91–50213.

150. Rabins PV. Prevention of mental disorders in the elderly: Current perspectives and future prospects. *J Am Geriatr Soc.* 1992;40:727–733.

151. Conwell Y. Suicide in elderly patients. In: Schneider LS, Reynolds CF, Lebowitz BD, Friedhoff AJ, eds. *Diagnosis and Treatment of Depression in Late Life: Results of the NIH Consensus Development Conference.* Washington, DC: American Psychiatric Association; 1994:397–418.

152. Gallo JJ, Rabins PV, Iliffe S. The 'research magnificent' in late life: Psychiatric epidemiology and the primary health care of older adults. *Int J Psychiatry Med.* 1997;27:185 –204.

153. Newmann JP. Aging and depression. *Psychol Aging.* 1989;4:150–165.

154. National Center for Health Statistics. *Vital Statistics of the United States. 1988, Vol. II: Mortality, Part A.* Washington, DC: US Public Health Service; 1991.

155. Chaisson-Stewart GM. The diagnostic dilemma. In: Chaisson-Stewart GM, ed. *Depression in the Elderly: An Interdisciplinary Approach.* New York: John Wiley & Sons; 1985:18–43.

156. Gallo JJ, Rabins PV. Depression without sadness: Alternative presentations of depression in late life. *Am Fam Physician.* In press.

157. Gallo JJ, Gonzales J. Depression and other mood disorders. In: Adelman A, Daly M, eds. *Twenty Common Problems in Geriatrics.* New York: McGraw-Hill. In press.

158. Ormel J, Van den Brink W, Koeter MWJ, et al. Recognition, management and outcome of psychological disorders in primary care: A naturalistic follow-up study. *Psychol Med.* 1990;20:909–923.

159. Gonzales JJ, Norquist G. Mental health consultation-liaison interventions in primary care. In: Miranda J, Hohmann AA, Attkisson CC, Larson DB, eds. *Mental Disorders in Primary Care.* San Francisco: Jossey-Bass Publishers; 1994:347–373.

160. German PS, Shapiro S, Skinner EA, et al. Detection and management of mental health problems of older patients by primary care providers. *JAMA.* 1987;257:489–493.

161. Valenstein M, Kales H, Mellow A, et al. Psychiatric diagnosis and intervention in older and younger patients in a primary care clinic: Effect of a screening and diagnostic instrument. *J Am Geriatr Soc.* 1998;46:1499–1505.

162. Fogel BS, Fretwell M. Reclassification of depression in the medically ill elderly. *J Am Geriatr Soc.* 1985;33:446–448.

163. Salzman C, Shader RI. Depression in the elderly: I. Relationship between depression, psychologic defense mechanisms and physical illness. *J Am Geriatr Soc.* 1978; 26:253–260.

164. Depure RA, Monroe SM. Learned helplessness in the perspective of the depressive disorders: Concepts and definitional issues. *Abnorm Psychol.* 1978;87:3–20.

165. Abramson LY, Metalsky GI, Alloy LB. Hopelessness depression: A theory based subtype of depression. *Psychol Rev.* 1989;96:358–372.

166. Weiss IK, Nagel CL, Aronson MK. Applicability of depression scales to the old person. *J Am Geriatr Soc.* 1986;34:215–218.

167. Rohrbaugh RM, Siegal AP, Giller EL. Irritability as a symptom of depression in the elderly. *J Am Geriatr Soc.* 1988;36:736–738.

168. Blazer D, Hughes DC, Fowler N. Anxiety as an outcome symptom of depression in the elderly and middle-aged adults. *Int J Geriatr Psychiatry.* 1989;4:273–278.

169. Roth M. Differential diagnosis of psychiatric disorders in old age. *Hosp Pract.* July 1986:111–138.

170. Blazer D, Siegler IC. *A Family Approach to Health Care of the Elderly.* Menlo Park, CA: Addison-Wesley Publishing Co; 1984.

171. Gallo JJ, Anthony JC, Muthen BO. Age differences in the symptoms of depression: A latent trait analysis. *J Gerontol: Psychol Sci.* 1994;49:P251–264.

172. Henderson AS. Does ageing protect against depression? *Soc Psychiatry Psychiatr Epidemiol.* 1994;29:107–109.

173. Gallo JJ, Rabins PV, Lyketsos CG, Tien AY, Anthony JC. Depression without sadness: Functional outcomes of nondysphoric depression in later life. *J Am Geriatr Soc.* 1997;45:570–578.

174. Beck AT, Steer RA, Beck JS, Newman CF. Hopelessness, depression, suicidal ideation, and clinical diagnosis of depression. Suicide and Life Threat Behav. 1993;23: 139–145.

175. Beck AT, Steer RA, Kovacs M. Hopelessness and eventual suicide: A 10-year prospective study of patients hospitalized with suicidal ideation. *Am J Psychiatry.* 1985; 142:559–563.

176. Greene SM. Levels of measured hopelessness in the general population. *Br J Clin Psychol.* 1981;20:11–14.

177. Sunderland T, Alterman IS, Yount D, et al. A new scale for the assessment of depressed mood in demented patients. *Am J Psychiatry.* 1988;145:955–959.

178. Rabins PV, Merchant A, Nestadt G. Criteria for diagnosing reversible dementia caused by depression: Validation by 2-year follow-up. *Br J Psychiatry.* 1984;144:488–492.

179. Devanand DP, Sano M, Tang MX, et al. Depressed mood and the incidence of Alzheimer's disease in the elderly living in the community. *Arch Gen Psychiatry.* 1996; 53:175–182.

180. Rovner B, Broadhead J, Spencer M. Depression in Alzheimer's disease. *Am J Psychiatry.* 1989;146:350–353.

181. Wragg RE, Jeste DV. Overview of depression and psychosis in Alzheimer's disease. *Am J Psychiatry.* 1989;146:577–589.

182. Reynolds CF, Kupfer DJ, Hoch CC, et al. Two-year follow-up of elderly patients with mixed depression and dementia: Clinical and electroencephalographic sleep findings. *J Am Geriatr Soc.* 1986;34:793–799.

183. Caine ED. Pseudodementia. *Arch Gen Psychiatry.* 1981;38:1359–1364.

184. Reifler BV, Larson E, Hanley R. Coexistence of cognitive impairment and depression in geriatric outpatients. *Am J Psychiatry.* 1982;139:623–626.

185. Morris PLP, Robinson RG, Raphael B. Prevalence and course of post-stroke depression in hospitalized patients. *Int J Psychiatry Med.* 1990;20:327–342.

186. Lehmann HE. Affective disorders in the aged. *Psychiatr Clin North Am.* 1982; 5:27–48.

187. Kamerow DB, Campbell TL. Is screening for mental health problems worthwhile in family practice? *J Fam Pract.* 1987;25:181–187.

188. Gallo JJ. The effect of social support on depression in caregivers of the elderly. *J Fam Pract.* 1990;30:430–436.

189. Cobbs EL, Duthie EH, Murphy JB, eds. *Geriatric Review Syllabus. A Core Curriculum in Geriatric Medicine.* 4th ed. New York: American Geriatrics Society; 1999.

190. Brink TL, Yesavage JA, Lum O, et al. Screening tests for geriatric depression. *Clin Gerontol.* 1982;1:37–43.

191. Yesavage JA, Brink TL. Development and validation of a geriatric depression screening scale: A preliminary report. *J Psychiatr Res.* 1983;17:37–49.

192. O'Riordan TG, Hayes JP, O'Neill D. The effect of mild to moderate dementia on the Geriatric Depression Scale and on the General Health Questionnaire. *Age and Ageing.* 1990;19:57–61.

193. Hyer L, Blount J. Concurrent and discriminant validities of the Geriatric Depression Scale with older psychiatric patients. *Psychol Rep.* 1984;54:611–616.

194. Magni G, Shifano F, de Leo D. Assessment of depression in an elderly medical population. *J Affective Disord.* 1986;11:121–124.

195. Norris JT, Gallagher D, Wilson A, Winograd CH. Assessment of depression in geriatric medical outpatients: The validity of two screening measures. *J Am Geriatr Soc.* 1987; 35:989–995.

196. Koenig HG, Meador KG, Cohen HJ. Self-rated depression scales and screening for major depression in the older hospitalized patient with medical illness. *J Am Geriatr Soc.* 1988;36:699–706.

197. Rapp SR, Parial SA, Walsh DA. Detecting depression in elderly medical inpatients. *J Consult Clin Psychol.* 1988;56:509–513.

198. Harper RG, Kotik-Harper D, Kirby H. Psychometric assessment of depression in an elderly general medical population: Over- or underassessment? *J Nerv Ment Dis.* 1990;178:113–119.

199. Brink TL. Limitations of the GDS in cases of pseudodementia. *Clin Gerontol.* 1984;2:60–61.

200. Burke WJ, Houston MJ, Boust SJ. Use of the Geriatric Depression Scale in dementia of the Alzheimer type. *J Am Geriatr Soc.* 1989;37:856–860.

201. Burke WJ, Nitcher RL, Roccaforte WH, Wengel SP. A prospective evaluation of the Geriatric Depression Scale in an outpatient geriatric assessment center. *J Am Geriatr Soc.* 1992;40:1227–1230.

202. Feher EP, Larrabee GJ, Crook TH. Factors attenuating the validity of the Geriatric Depression Scale in a dementia population. *J Am Geriatr Soc.* 1992;40:906–909.

203. Kafonek S, Ettinger WH, Roca R. Instruments for screening for depression and dementia in a long-term care facility. *J Am Geriatr Soc.* 1989;37:29–34.

204. Parmelee PA, Katz IR, Lawton MP. Depression among institutionalized aged: Assessment and prevalence estimation. *J Gerontol.* 1989;44:M22–29.

205. Yesavage JA. The use of self-rating depression scales in the elderly. In: Poon LW, ed. *Clinical Memory Assessment of Older Adults.* Washington, DC: American Psychological Association; 1986.

206. Alden D, Austin C, Sturgeon R. A correlation between the Geriatric Depression Scale long and short forms. *J Gerontol.* 1989;4:P124–125.

207. Cwikel J, Ritchie K. Screening for depression among the elderly in Israel: An assessment of the short Geriatric Depression Scale (S-GDS). *Isr J Med Sci.* 1989;25: 131–137.

208. Zung WWK. A self-rating depression scale. *Arch Gen Psychiatry.* 1965;12:63–70.

209. Zung WWK, Richards DB, Short MF. Self-rating depression scale in an outpatient clinic: Further validation of the SDS. *Arch Gen Psychiatry.* 1965;13:508–515.

210. Zung WWK. Factors influencing the self-rating depression scale. *Arch Gen Psychiatry.* 1967;16:543–547.

211. Zung WWK. Depression in the normal aged. *Psychosomatics.* 1967;8:287–292.

212. Freedman N, Bucci W, Elkowitz E. Depression in a family practice elderly population. *J Am Geriatr Soc.* 1982;30:372–377.

213. Moore JT, Silimperi DR, Bobula JA. Recognition of depression by family medicine residents: The impact of screening. *J Fam Pract.* 1978;7:509–513.

214. Okimoto JT, Barnes RF, Veith RC, et al. Screening for depression in geriatric medical patients. *Am J Psychiatry.* 1982;139:799–802.

215. Goldberg DP. *The Detection of Psychiatric Illness by Questionnaire.* London: Oxford University Press; 1972.

216. Goodchild ME, Duncan-Jones P. Chronicity and the General Health Questionnaire. *Br J Psychiatry.* 1985;146:55–61.

217. Goldberg DP, Hillier VF. A scaled version of the General Health Questionnaire. *Psychol Med.* 1979;9:139–145.

218. Goldberg DP, Rickels K, Downing R, Hesbacher P. A comparison of two psychiatric screening tests. *Br J Psychiatry.* 1976;129:61–67.

219. German PS, Shapiro S, Skinner EA. Mental health of the elderly: Use of health and mental health services. *J Am Geriatr Soc.* 1985;33:246–252.

220. Clarke DM, Smith GC, Herrman HE. A comparative study of screening instruments for mental disorders in general hospital patients. *Int J Psychiatry Med.* 1993;23:323–337.

221. Cleary PD, Goldberg ID, Kessler LG, Nycz GR. Screening for mental disorder among primary care patients. *Arch Gen Psychiatry.* 1982;39:837–840.

222. Ford DE, Anthony JC, Nestadt GR, Romanoski AJ. The General Health Questionnaire by interview: Performance in relation to recent use of health services. *Med Care.* 1989;27:367–375.

223. Lindsay J. Validity of the General Health Questionnaire (GHQ) in detecting psychiatric disturbance in amputees with phantom pain. *J Psychosom Res.* 1986;30:277–281.

224. Lobo A, Perez-Echeverria M, Jimenez-Aznarez A, et al. Emotional disturbances in endocrine patients: Validity of the scaled version of the General Health Questionnaire (GHQ-28). *Br J Psychiatry.* 1990;152:807–812.

225. Marino S, Bellantuono C, Tansella M. Psychiatric morbidity in general practice in Italy: A point-prevalence survey in a defined geographical area. *Soc Psychiatry Psychiatr Epidemiol.* 1990;25:67–72.

226. Rand EH, Badger LW, Coggins DR. Toward a resolution of contradictions: Utility of feedback from the GHQ. *Gen Hosp Psychiatry.* 1988;10:189–196.

227. Samuels JF, Nestadt G, Anthony JC, Romanoski AJ. The detection of mental disorders in the community setting using a 20-item interview version of the General Health Questionnaire. *Acta Psychiatr Scand.* 1994;89:14–20.

228. Simon GE, VonKorff M, Durham ML. Predictors of outpatient mental health utilization by primary care patients in a Health Maintenance Organization. *Am J Psychiatry.* 1994;151:908–913.

229. Von Korff M, Shapiro S, Burke JD, et al. Anxiety and depression in a primary care clinic: Comparison of Diagnostic Interview Schedule, General Health Questionnaire, and practitioner assessments. *Arch Gen Psychiatry.* 1987;44:152–156.

230. Gallagher D. The Beck Depression Inventory and older adults: Review of its development and utility. In: Brink TL, ed. *Clinical Gerontology: A Guide to Assessment and Intervention.* New York: Haworth Press; 1986:149–163.

231. Beck AT, Beck RW. Screening depressed patients in family practice: A rapid technique. *Postgrad Med.* 1972;52:81–85.

232. Graber MA, Toth PP. *The University of Iowa Family Practice Handbook.* St. Louis, MO: Mosby; 1997.

233. Gallo JJ, Reichel W, Andersen LM. *Handbook of Geriatric Assessment.* Gaithersburg, MD: Aspen Publishers; 1988.

234. Beck AT, Ward CH, Mendelson M, et al. An inventory for measuring depression. *Arch Gen Psychiatry.* 1961;4:53–63.

235. Oliver JM, Simmons ME. Depression as measured by the DSM-III and the Beck Depression Inventory in an unselected adult population. *J Consult Clin Psychol.* 1984;52:892–898.

236. Gallagher D, Breckenridge J, Steinmetz J, et al. The Beck Depression Inventory and Research Diagnostic Criteria: Congruence in an older population. *J Consult Clin Psychol.* 1983;51:945–946.

237. Nielsen AC, Williams TA. Depression in ambulatory medical patients: Prevalence by self-report questionnaire and recognition by nonpsychiatric physicians. *Arch Gen Psychiatry.* 1980;37:999–1004.

238. Radloff LS. The CES-D Scale: A self-report depression scale for research in the general population. *Appl Psychol Meas.* 1977;1:385–401.

239. Comstock GW, Helsing KJ. Symptoms of depression in two communities. *Psychol Med.* 1976;6:551–563.

240. Eaton WW, Kessler LG. Rates of symptoms of depression in a national sample. *Am J Epidemiol.* 1981;114:528–538.

241. Katon W, Schulberg HC. Epidemiology of depression in primary care. *Gen Hosp Psychiatry.* 1992;14:237–247.

242. Husaini BA, Neff JA, Harrington JB, et al. Depression in rural communities: Validating the CES-D Scale. *J Community Psychol.* 1980;8:20–27.

243. Schulberg HC, Saul M, McClelland M, Ganguli M, Christy W, Frank R. Assessing depression in primary medical and psychiatric practices. *Arch Gen Psychiatry.* 1985;42:1164–1170.

244. Foelker GA, Shewchuk RM. Somatic complaints and the CES-D. *J Am Geriatr Soc.* 1992;40:259–262.

245. Zimmerman M, Coryell W. Screening for major depressive disorder in the community: A comparison of measures. *Psychol Assess.* 1994;6:71–74.

246. Beresford T, Gomberg E. *Alcohol and Aging.* New York: Oxford University Press; 1995.

247. Robins LN, Regier DA. *Psychiatric Disorders in America: The Epidemiologic Catchment Area Study.* New York: Free Press; 1991.

248. Grant BF, Harford TC, Chou P, et al. Prevalence of DSM-III-R alcohol abuse and dependence: United States, 1988. *Alcohol Health Res World.* 1991;15:91–96.

249. Adams WL, Barry KL, Fleming MF. Screening for problem drinking in older primary care patients. *JAMA.* 1996;276:1964–1967.

250. Thibault JM, Maly RC. Recognition and treatment of substance abuse in the elderly. *Primary Care.* 1993;20:155–165.

251. Curtis JR, Geller G, Stokes EJ, Levine DM, Moore RD. Characteristics, diagnosis, and treatment of alcoholism in elderly patients. *J Am Geriatr Soc.* 1989;37:310–316.

252. Graham K. Identifying and measuring alcohol abuse among the elderly: Serious problems with existing instrumentation. *J Stud Alcohol.* 1986;47:322–326.

253. Cook BL, Winokur G, Garvey MJ, Beach V. Depression and previous alcoholism in the elderly. *Br J Psychiatry.* 1991;158:72–75.

254. Osgood NJ. The alcohol-suicide connection in late life. *Postgrad Med.* 1987;81:379–384.

255. Mayfield DG, McLeod G, Hall P. The CAGE questionnaire: Validation of a new alcoholism screening instrument. *Am J Psychiatry.* 1974;131:1121–1123.

256. Ewing JA. Detecting alcoholism: The CAGE questionnaire. *JAMA.* 1984;252:1905–1907.

257. US Department of Health and Human Services. *Screening and brief intervention. Eighth Special Report to the US Congress on Alcohol and Health from the Secretary of Health and Human Services, September 1993.* Washington, DC: US Dept of Health and Human Services, Public Health Service, National Institute of Health, National Institute on Alcohol Abuse and Alcoholism; 1993:297–317.

258. Babor TF, Grant M. From clinical research to secondary prevention: International collaboration in the development of the Alcohol Use Disorders Identification Test (AUDIT). *Alcohol Health Res World.* 1989;13:371–374.

259. Fleming MF, Barry KL. The alcohol use disorders identification test (AUDIT) in a college sample. *Int J Addict.* 1991;26:1173–1185.

260. Blow FC, Brower KJ, Schulenberg JE, Demo-Dananberg LM, Young JS, Beresford TP. The Michigan Alcoholism Screening Test-Geriatric Version (MAST-G): A new elderly-specific screening instrument. *Alcohol Clin Exp Res.* 1992;16:372.

261. Sackett DL. A primer on the precision and accuracy of the clinical examination. *JAMA.* 1992;267:2638–2644.

262. American Medical Association. *Alcoholism in the Elderly: Diagnosis, Treatment, Prevention; Guidelines for Primary Care Physicians.* Chicago: American Medical Association; 1995.

263. Jones TV, Lindsey BA, Yount P, Soltys R, Farani-Enayat B. Alcoholism screening questionnaires. *J Gen Intern Med.* 1993;8:674–678.

264. Isacson DGL, Bingefors KAL, Antonov KIM. Long-term use of neuroleptics among elderly in a Swedish community. *Ann Pharmacother.* 1992;26:373–377.

265. Simpson RJ, Power KG, Wallace LA, Butcher MH, Swanson V, Simpson EC. Controlled comparison of the characteristics of long-term benzodiazepine users in general practice. *Br J Gen Pract.* 1990;40:22–26.

266. Simpson RJ, Power KG, Swanson V. Age-band prevalence rates of long-term benzodiazepine users [letter]. *Br J Gen Pract.* 1990;40:168–169.

267. Holm M. One year follow-up of users of benzodiazepines in general practice. *Dan Med Bull.* 1990;37:188–191.

268. Simon GE, Von Korff M, Barlow W, Pabiniak C, Wagner E. Predictors of chronic benzodiazepine use in a health maintenance organization sample. *J Clin Epidemiol.* 1996;49:1067–1073.

269. Coyne JC, Schwenk TL, Fechner-Bates S. Nondetection of depression by primary care physicians reconsidered. *Gen Hosp Psychiatry.* 1995;17:3–12.

270. Tollefson GD, Souetre E, Thomander L, Potvin JH. Comorbid anxious signs and symptoms in major depression: Impact on functional work capacity and comparative treatment outcomes. *Int Clin Psychopharmacol.* 1993;8:281–293.

271. Schulberg HC, McClelland M, Gooding W. Six-month outcomes for medical patients with major depressive disorders. *J Gen Intern Med.* 1987;2:312–317.

272. Knight RG, Waal-Manning HJ, Spears GF. Some norms and reliability data for the State-Trait Anxiety Inventory and the Zung Self-Rating Depression Scale. *Br J Clin Psychology.* 1983;22:245–249.

273. Molina S, Borkovec TD. The Penn State Worry Questionnaire: Psychometric properties and associated characteristics. In: Davey G, Tallis F, eds. *Worrying: Perspectives on Theory, Assessment, and Treatment.* New York: John Wiley & Sons; 1994:265–284.

274. Spielberger CD. *Manual for the State-Trait Anxiety Inventory.* Palo Alto, CA: Consulting Psychologists Press, Inc; 1977.

275. Gallo JJ, Lebowitz BD. The epidemiology of common mental disorders in late life: Themes for a new century. Psychiatric Services, in press.

276. Iliffe S, Gallo JJ, Reichel W. The contribution of family doctors in the care of old people. In: Pathy MSJ, ed. *Principles and Practice of Geriatric Medicine*. 3rd ed. Sussex, England: John Wiley & Sons; 1998:1501–1508.

277. Erickson RC, Howieson D. The clinician's perspective: Measuring change and treatment effectiveness. In: Poon LW, ed. *Clinical Memory Assessment of Older Adults*. Washington, DC: American Psychological Association; 1986:69–80.

4

Functional Assessment

The preservation of function has become a prominent theme in geriatrics.[1] A major goal of the *Healthy People: 2000* initiative concerns increasing the span of healthy life for all Americans.[2] The emphasis has appropriately changed from an exclusive concern with delaying mortality to a focus on avoiding morbidity; that is, to preserving function[3,4] and extending active life expectancy.[5] Functional status captures the concept of quality of life in ways that an emphasis on medical diagnoses does not.[6,7] Functional assessment is the key to understanding the impact of medical illness on the older person and family and is the cornerstone of geriatric rehabilitation.[8,9] The typical catalog of medical problems is not sufficient to answer questions about functional capability, such as ability to dress or to use the toilet. Brief methods are emphasized in this chapter to encourage ongoing functional assessment in the office and in other settings.

FOCUS ON FUNCTION

Functioning in daily life may be examined on several levels. Performance in social and occupational roles composes one level.[10,11] The tasks demanded every day such as driving or using public trans-

101

portation compose another. Activities necessary for persons in a modern society such as using the telephone or automatic-teller machine are commonplace. On another plane are the personal care tasks such as dressing, bathing, and toileting. Older adults and others who have difficulty with these tasks must compensate for the disability.

The capacity to function independently is poorly described by the constellation of medical diseases alone. Performance on mental status testing does not necessarily predict functional status.[12,13] Similarly, the severity of disease as measured by standard laboratory tests does not necessarily imply disability. Functional status should be assessed directly and independently of medical and laboratory abnormalities or cognitive impairment.

A 70-year-old woman with diabetes mellitus, hypertension, and congestive heart failure was hospitalized for urinary incontinence. Urologic studies were normal, and the patient was discharged home in her husband's care. Two weeks later she was again admitted for "mental status changes," since she was noted to be increasingly disoriented and incontinent. Her daughter related slow intellectual impairment over the course of at least 1 year. Mental status testing revealed global intellectual deficits in orientation, memory, calculations, and visuospatial skills. Review of the chart from the previous hospitalization showed no documented mental status examination with which to compare findings. It was believed the patient had Alzheimer's disease with superimposed delirium secondary to medication.

Specific functional loss in the elderly is not determined by the locus of disease—urinary incontinence may not indicate disease confined to the urinary tract. Because of the family's difficulty in caring for this patient, she required nursing home care. In a situation with better functional ability or social support, she may have been able to stay at home. Thus, the problem list alone did not give all the information needed to make recommendations.

Cognitive impairment does not necessarily imply an inability to perform enough activities to maintain independent living. Scores on the Short Portable Mental Status Questionnaire (SPMSQ) were only weakly correlated to the ability of older adults to care for themselves. Of 32 persons with moderate to severe impairment on the SPMSQ, 9 were living completely independently, and another 10 needed assistance only with dressing.[14] This observation is borne out by experience. Severely impaired persons may perform quite well in a familiar home setting.

Functional assessment can help the practitioner focus on the person's capabilities, and when there is a change, appropriate resources can be rallied and a search for medical illness initiated. The sometimes delicate state of homeostasis makes the older adult vulnerable to disability from a variety of sources. Going beyond the medical model is critical since medical or psychiatric illness may present as a nonspecific deterioration in functional status. It is not enough to enumerate the medical problems and treat them in isolation. When a medical illness is diagnosed, how it affects the elder's functional capacity must always be considered. Conversely, the person's functional status must be considered in formulating the treatment plan.

Consider an 83-year-old man who lives alone and has a history of paraplegia since an early age with confinement to a wheelchair, osteoarthritis, scoliosis, atrial fibrillation with controlled ventricular response on digoxin, a suprapubic catheter for a neurogenic bladder, cataracts, and poor dental hygiene with full dentures. This patient's mental status is normal. Despite his physical limitations and medical problems, he lives in his home alone with the periodic visits from his niece and visiting nurses. Suppose one knew that this person was not able to transfer from his wheelchair to the toilet or to the bed or that he was incapable of taking his medication properly. One can see how difficulty in one of these areas might change the situation and temper one's judgment about a person's ability to reside at home. Except for walking, this person's functional status is good.

The multitude of medical, social, and psychological challenges presented by the older adult can overwhelm health care professionals. They should attack small problems with major consequences first. Ameliorating problems that interfere with safe driving and ambulation would be an important focus for intervention. Among the illnesses or complaints presented by the older person, which one or two are presenting the most difficulty in terms of functional capacity? For example, cataracts might present more difficulty with eating, shopping, and meal preparation than osteoarthritis. The physician should look closely at the less serious although treatable conditions that contribute to disability. Correction of minor problems could enhance the person's quality of life. Something as simple as modifying the diuretic drug dosing schedule to obviate the need for evening and nightly trips to the bathroom may enhance the sleep of the older person and his or her caregiver.

Asking about driving habits and accidents is an important inquiry in its own right, but also signals that more basic tasks, such as shopping, dressing, and bathing are probably adequately performed. Driving is given special attention in a separate chapter. Difficulties with the telephone or improper use of medications may signal cognitive impairment[15] or depression.[16]

The information from functional assessment has an important, practical role in advising and counseling clients and their families, and in following clients after significant medical events.[10] A functional scale has been used to predict the need for institutionalization (at least on a temporary basis) after hip fracture.[17] This scale consists of components assessing physical health (eg, vision, hearing, and mental status), ambulatory ability, daily activities, social situation (eg, lives alone, with spouse, or in nursing home), and disabilities (eg, incontinence, paralysis, amputation, decubitus, and contracture). The Functional Rating Scale for the Symptoms of Dementia, discussed below, is also an example of a functional assessment questionnaire that evaluates the need for nursing home placement in the patient with dementia.[18] The Determination of Need Functional Assessment is an example of a rating scale that has been specifically developed to evaluate the risk for nursing home placement and to assist with care planning for community-based services.[19,20]

Functional ability is prognostic of mortality. For example, a retrospective study compared persons who died within 1 year of placement in a nursing home with those who "survived." The latter group was found to be more independent, especially in bathing and dressing.[21] Mortality was also associated with poor functioning following hospitalization.[22] The inability to perform tasks such as traveling, shopping, meal preparation, housework, and handling money predicts mortality as well.[23,24] Inability to perform simple tasks such as carrying a bag of groceries predicts further functional decline[25] and institutionalization.[26]

A person's home can speak volumes about the performance of activities of daily living (ADL). How well arranged is the home for bathing and toileting? Are there obvious safety hazards (eg, frayed wires, ashtrays near the bed, slippery floors or rugs, and firearms stored in the home of a person with dementia)? How well does the older person maneuver about the home (ie, transfer and ambulation)? How well are nutritional needs met (ie, food in the refrigerator, shopping, and cooking)? How well is the home maintained (ie, shelter, cleanliness, clutter)? In addition to the other benefits of home visits, such as the assessment of social support available to the patient, there is also less need for second-hand information about the functional ability of the older adult.[27,28]

Functional impairment can be listed independently of the problem list in the problem-oriented medical record. For example, two persons with rheumatoid arthritis may differ in their abilities to eat. The physician would then list "difficulty with feeding" independently of the medical diagnosis of rheumatoid arthritis. This helps quantify functional impairment and alerts other clinicians to the implications of the functional impairment (in this case, a problem with nutrition).

A complete problem-oriented medical record, listing functional as well as undefined problems, organizes them and helps establish priorities for solution. Seen as "building blocks," efforts to assist the patient are cumulative because some problems are selected for immediate attention whereas others are worked on gradually. Medical diagnosis remains important, but functional assessment keeps the problems in perspective and provides a complementary viewpoint. Functional impairment should prompt a timely and thorough search for cognitive impairment, depression, substance abuse, adverse medication effects, and sensory impairment.[7]

Functional assessment can be a positive force in caring for older adults. Since so much professional training focuses on the negative aspects of age and its losses, taking care to determine functional capacity compels health professionals to see evaluation in a positive light. Despite multiple diseases, the patient functions well. How well does he or she function in his or her own environment? What adaptations and concessions have been made to make up for deficiencies? Lastly, how can professionals and other caregivers promote and initiate adaptations to allow the most independent, fulfilling life possible? This is a taste of the kinds of issues facing clinicians, who may use some of the instruments discussed later in this chapter to facilitate thinking along these lines.

THE COMPONENTS OF FUNCTIONAL STATUS

A systematic approach to each domain of geriatric assessment, including functional assessment, is desirable. The items generally agreed on as composing functional assessment are the ADL and the instrumental ADL or IADL, although other categorizations are possible.[29] The ADL are the functions that are fundamental to independent living, such as dressing and bathing. The IADL include more complex daily activities, such as using the telephone, housekeeping, and managing money. Statistical methods applied to self-report data on difficulty with activities resulted in similar groupings consisting of: (1) activities related to mobility and exercise such as walking, (2) complex tasks such as paying bills and shopping, (3) self-care activities such as toileting, and (4) upper extremity tasks such as grasping and reaching.[30] Driving and sexual functioning are other important arenas to consider in functional assessment, and are discussed in other chapters.

Evaluation of functional status is not limited to the assessment of specific activities and tasks, although that is the emphasis here. Assessment may also include significant happenings in a person's life or family that have a bearing on the health status or situation (events of daily living); demands placed on the person from within or from the family and society (demands of daily living); the nature of the physical environment (environment of daily living); and the person's values and beliefs that determine decisions and responses regarding health care (values and beliefs in daily living).[31,32]

Activities of Daily Living

Just as is true for mental status testing instruments, ADL scales may have ceiling or threshold effects.[33] In other words, if the activities chosen for assessment are too easy, many persons will do well on the scale; thus, a prominent ceiling effect occurs. Such an ADL scale may be useful for assessing or defining the frail elderly, but most community-dwelling older adults would be able to perform the activities on the list without much trouble.[34] Asking about driving and instrumental ADL is apt to be more fruitful in functional assessment of ambulatory older persons.

The term "frailty" has been used to describe older adults whose management of day-to-day tasks is tenuous. The definition of frail has been couched in functional terms to describe those persons who need help performing ADL,[35,36] with effects on behavior and quality of life.[37] A dynamic model assumes that it is the balance between assets and deficits that determines frailty; the assets and deficits are components of geriatric assessment, such as caregiver burden, resources, attitudes, and health status.[38] A change in status on one domain may tip the balance into frailty. Frail older adults may rely heavily on neighbors or family to perform routine jobs that fully independent persons do for themselves. Frailty implies health conditions that require frequent hospitalizations, medication, and visits to physicians' offices.

Ideally, practitioners need a set of questions that are quick and easy to administer periodically to detect older adults who are beginning to experience difficulty in the activities usually associated with independent living. Something similar to the Apgar score used to evaluate newborns might be desirable for this purpose. Details regarding the use of indexes of function and measurement theory can be found elsewhere.[1,33,39-43] Further theoretical considerations can be found in the Institute of Medicine Report, *Disability in America*.[44] In the next section, specific instruments used to assess ADL and IADL are discussed.

Katz Index of Activities of Daily Living

A basic schedule to assess ADL, published in 1963, is the Katz Index of ADL, which includes bathing, dressing, toileting, transfer, continence, and feeding (Exhibit 4–1).[45] It provides a framework for assessing the ability to live independently, or, if deficiencies are found, it is the focal point for remediation. A person dependent in a single activity might need assistance at isolated times of the day, such as for bathing, but more help might be needed by persons dependent on assistance in many activities.

A three-tiered scale for the ADL is found to be more reliable and is reproducible even when scored by personnel with minimal training. The three-point scale might consist of the ratings "independent," "semi-independent" (needs a part-time assistant), and "dependent," rather than a checklist with four or five gradations defining how much assistance is required.[46]

Considering the basic ADL items in evaluation of an older person has several important advantages. For one, focusing on functional abilities allows matching of services to needs. For example, someone requiring only assistance in bathing may be maintained independently with an aide to perform the task once a week. In addition, keying in on specific tasks allows interventions to be more focused. In dealing with difficulty in dressing, a caregiver might try putting picture labels on drawers, grouping items that belong together, and taking the individual by the hand and starting the desired action as a cue. In other cases, multiple areas of dependence would make it clear that it is not possible to provide the necessary help to continue the multiple ADL that keep the person at home.[45,47,48]

Subjective estimates of disease severity or mere use of a diagnostic label may not be as helpful as an emphasis on functional assessment. An individual with rheumatoid arthritis may have major functional deficits that could be improved with physical therapy, appliances, or the provision of help with key ADL such as bathing. In the care of a patient after a stroke, following his or her progress on ADL is useful.[49] In addition to matching services to needs, persons unable to perform one or more of these ADL may be at risk for hospitalization or nursing home placement.

Barthel Index

The Barthel Index has also been used to assess ability for self-care, but the items are weighted to account for the amount of physical assistance that would be required if the individual is unable to carry out the function. In one study in a rehabilitative setting for patients with neuromuscular disorders, the Barthel Index was used to document im-

Exhibit 4–1 Katz Index of Activities of Daily Living (ADL)

---

1. *Bathing* (sponge, shower, or tub)
   I: receives no assistance (gets in and out of tub if tub is the usual means of bathing)
   A: receives assistance in bathing only one part of the body (such as the back or a leg)
   D: receives assistance in bathing more than one part of the body (or not bathed)

2. *Dressing*
   I: gets clothes and gets completely dressed without assistance
   A: gets clothes and gets dressed without assistance except in tying shoes
   D: receives assistance in getting clothes or in getting dressed or stays partly or completely undressed

3. *Toileting*
   I: goes to "toilet room," cleans self, and arranges clothes without assistance (may use object for support such as cane, walker, or wheelchair and may manage night bedpan or commode, emptying it in the morning)
   A: receives assistance in going to "toilet room" or in cleansing self or in arranging clothes after elimination or in use of night bedpan or commode
   D: doesn't go to room termed "toilet" for the elimination process

4. *Transfer*
   I: moves in and out of bed as well as in and out of chair without assistance (may be using object for support such as cane or walker)
   A: moves in and out of bed or chair with assistance
   D: doesn't get out of bed

5. *Continence*
   I: controls urination and bowel movement completely by self
   A: has occasional "accidents"
   D: supervision helps keep urine or bowel control; catheter is used, or is incontinent

6. *Feeding*
   I: feeds self without assistance
   A: feeds self except for getting assistance in cutting meat or buttering bread
   D: receives assistance in feeding or is fed partly or completely by using tubes or intravenous fluids

   Abbreviations: I, independent; A, assistance; D, dependent

   Source: Adapted with permission from S. Katz et al., *Studies of Illness in the Aged: The Index of ADL, Activities of Daily Living Scale,* Vol. 185, p. 915. Copyright © 1963, American Medical Association.

---

provement. Patients who did not improve their score during rehabilitation were believed to have poor potential for recovery.[50]

A modified Barthel Index has been devised and, when used to assess the need for home health services, correlated to the number of activities the person was able to do independently.[42,51] Persons scoring less than 60 on the modified Barthel Index (Table 4–1) were able to perform no more than 10 of the defined ADL and IADL tasks. A score of less than 60 was especially associated with the need for help in feeding, bathing, grooming, dressing, toileting, transferring, doing housework, and preparing meals.[51] The modified Barthel Index may be a good indicator of the need for support in ADL.

Instrumental Activities of Daily Living

In addition to the ADL, another set of activities required for independent living are the IADL.[52,53] These activities are the more complex and demanding skills of using the telephone, traveling, shopping, preparing meals, doing housework, taking medicine properly, and managing money (Exhibit 4–2). The IADL may emphasize tasks traditionally performed by women, especially for the current cohort of older persons.[54] This bias notwithstanding, these chores are required daily activities for most persons, and if someone is unable to perform them, the tasks must be performed by a caregiver.

The IADL have been distilled into five items, which form a simple screening test to determine who may require a more comprehensive

Table 4–1 Modified Barthel Index

	Independent		Dependent	
	Intact	Limited	Helper	Null
Drink from cup/feed from dish	10	5	0	0
Dress upper body	5	5	3	0
Dress lower body	5	5	2	0
Don brace or prosthesis	0	0	-2	0
Grooming	5	5	0	0
Wash or bathe	4	4	0	0
Bladder incontinence	10	10	5	0
Bowel incontinence	10	10	5	0
Care of perineum/clothing at toilet	4	4	2	0
Transfer, chair	15	15	7	0
Transfer, toilet	6	5	3	0
Transfer, tub or shower	1	1	0	0
Walk on level 50 yd or more	15	15	10	0
Up and down stairs for one flight or more	10	10	5	0
Wheelchair 50 yd (only if not walking)	15	5	0	0

Source: Adapted with permission from RH Fortinsky et al., The Use of Functional Assessment in Understanding Home Care Needs, *Medical Care* Vol. 19, No.5, p. 491, © 1981, JB Lippincott Company.

Exhibit 4–2 Instrumental Activities of Daily Living (IADL)

1. *Telephone*
   I: able to look up numbers, dial, receive, and make calls without help
   A: able to answer phone or dial operator in an emergency, but needs special phone or help in getting number or dialing
   D: unable to use the telephone

2. *Traveling*
   I: able to drive own car or travel alone on bus or taxi
   A: able to travel, but not alone
   D: unable to travel

3. *Shopping*
   I: able to take care of all shopping with transportation provided
   A: able to shop, but not alone
   D: unable to shop

4. *Preparing meals*
   I: able to plan and cook full meals
   A: able to prepare light foods, but unable to cook full meals alone
   D: unable to prepare any meals

5. *Housework*
   I: able to do heavy housework (like scrub floors)
   A: able to do light housework, but needs help with heavy tasks
   D: unable to do any housework

6. *Medication*
   I: able to take medications in the right dose at the right time
   A: able to take medications, but needs reminding or someone to prepare it
   D: unable to take medications

7. *Money*
   I: able to manage buying needs, write checks, pay bills
   A: able to manage daily buying needs, but needs help managing checkbook, and paying bills
   D: unable to manage money

Abbreviations: I, independent; A, assistance; D, dependent

Source: Adapted with permission from Duke University Center for the Study of Aging and Human Development, *The Multidimensional Functional Assessment Questionnaire,* Ed 2, pp 169–170, 154–156, and 157–162, © 1978, Duke University at Durham, North Carolina.

assessment.[23] The five items concern travel, shopping, meal preparation, housework, and handling money (Exhibit 4–3). The five-item IADL scale has some interesting features.

First, as mentioned previously, the inability to perform these tasks is correlated to mortality. Second, when the items are arranged vertically, knowing a person can pass or perform one item indicates that person can pass or perform all items below it on the scale but none of the items listed above it. For example, when rated from the most difficult to the least difficult, the five items are ordered: housework, travel, shopping, finances, and cooking.[23,55]

This five-item scale can demonstrate change as well, which may identify who needs help, and might be administered on a scheduled basis for all older patients in a primary care practice. For example, con-

---

Exhibit 4–3 The Five-Item Instrumental Activities of Daily Living (IADL) Screening Questionnaire

---

1. Can you *get to places* out of walking distance:
   1 Without help (can travel alone on bus, taxi, or drive your own car)
   0 With some help (need someone to help you or go with you when traveling) or are you unable to travel unless emergency arrangements are made for a specialized vehicle such as an ambulance?
   – Not answered

2. Can you *go shopping* for groceries or clothes (assuming you have transportation):
   1 Without help (taking care of all your shopping needs yourself, assuming you have transportation)
   0 With some help (need someone to go with you on all shopping trips), or are you completely unable to do any shopping?
   – Not answered

3. Can you *prepare your own meals:*
   1 Without help (plan and cook meals yourself)
   0 With some help (can prepare some things but unable to cook full meals yourself), or are you completely unable to prepare any meals?
   – Not answered

4. Can you do your *housework:*
   1 Without help (can scrub floors, etc.)
   0 With some help (can do light housework but need help with heavy work), or are you unable to do any housework?
   – Not answered

5. Can you *handle your own money:*
   1 Without help (write checks, pay bills, etc.)
   0 With some help (manage day-to-day buying but need help with managing your checkbook and paying your bills), or are you completely unable to handle money?
   – Not answered

Source: Adapted with permission from G Fillenbaum, Screening the Elderly: A Brief Instrumental Activities of Daily Living Measure, *Journal of the American Geriatric Society,* Vol. 33, pp. 683–706, © 1985, Lippincott Williams & Wilkins.

sider a 63-year-old woman presenting for routine examination and re-newal of blood pressure medications. Last year she had no difficulties getting places, shopping, preparing meals, doing housework, or han-dling money. Today she admits some recent trouble managing her checkbook and reluctantly relates her worries about declining memory and lack of concentration. The Folstein Mini-Mental State score is nor-mal. On further questioning, vegetative symptoms of depression are found. The items of ADL and IADL translate readily into services. Knowledge of the ability of clients to perform various tasks becomes an indicator of what services might be needed. For example, nursing care, personal care, continuous supervision, meal preparation, or homemaker assistance may be required because of recent hospitaliza-tion or illness.[56]

Combined IADL and ADL Assessments

Several instruments have been developed that combine both ADL and IADL domains. Although combined ADL and IADL instruments have generally been developed for specific purposes, they may have broader utility because the combined spectrum of behaviors is ad-dressed. An instrument that combines both ADL and IADL in a single evaluation was developed by Paveza and colleagues[19,20] for use by per-sons working in community care settings. It has features that permit the practitioner to separate impairment on a behavior from the need for assistance with that same behavior. The developers of this instru-ment argue that not unlike the relationship of diagnosis to level of need for functional assistance, impairment in and of itself does not necessarily suggest the level of other personal assistance that an im-paired older person may require. Need for assistance is based not only on impairment, but also on what assistive devices may be in use and what support systems may already be providing help.[19,20] The practi-tioner needs to consider help already in place when determining what additional assistance to request. Moreover, by focusing on the broad spectrum of behaviors, the evaluator can more easily place the older adult on a continuum of care and can even estimate the likelihood that he or she is at risk for institutionalization.[19,20]

Determination of Need Assessment

The Determination of Need Assessment (DONA) is an ADL and IADL combined assessment designed by Paveza and his collaborators[57] as part of a Medicaid waiver project (Exhibit 4–4). As such, this instrument was designed with the needs of the community-based practitioner in mind and approaches the assessment of functional status from a unique perspective. The DONA separates functional incapacity or impairment from the need for assistance. The authors argue that these are really separate phenomena, one dictated by the inability to perform a behavior based on some physical, emotional, or cognitive problem, and the other by what assistance may already be in place or adaptations that the older adult may have already made to accommodate for the specific disability.

Furthermore, the scale defines levels of impairment on a multiple-point scale in which impairment can range from none to mild, moderate, or severe. The DONA also distinguishes these levels of impairment from the behaviors that the ratings are to evaluate. The need for assistance is placed on a similar four-point scale that primarily asks the evaluator to consider the degree to which the person is at health risk if no additional help above the current level of functioning is provided.[19,20] The diversity in the construction of this scale allows the person doing the evaluation to discuss both function and assistance on various levels from the behavior specific to a global combined assessment. Another important aspect of this instrument is that it was normed against a Medicaid-supported institutional population. Thus, the authors note in their discussion of this instrument that if a person scores 15 or above on the impairment section of this instrument that he or she is similar in level of functional impairment to the most disabled two thirds of an institutional sample. Such a result suggests that the person is at high risk for institutionalization and should definitely be considered for community-based services.[19,20] Because it was specifically developed for use in community-based, long-term care programs, its qualities can be particularly useful when thinking about community care for the older adult.

Medical Outcomes Study Short Form 36

The Short Form 36 (SF-36) represents eight health concepts: physical functioning, role disability due to physical health problems, bodily pain, general health perceptions, vitality, social functioning, role disability due to emotional problems, and general mental health (Exhibit 4–5).[58] The scientific literature pertaining to the use of the SF-36 in studies of older adults was recently reviewed by McHorney,[59] who concluded that, generally speaking, the SF-36 scales were predictive of mortality and hospitalization over the course of a 2-year follow-up. Correlation between SF-36 subscales was similar in cognitively im-

Exhibit 4-4 Determination of Need Functional Assessment

Function	Level of Impairment	Unmet Need for Care	Case Comments: Identify resources, and describe special needs and circumstances that should be taken into account when developing a care plan.
1. Eating	0 1 2 3	0 1 2 3	
2. Bathing	0 1 2 3	0 1 2 3	
3. Grooming	0 1 2 3	0 1 2 3	
4. Dressing	0 1 2 3	0 1 2 3	
5. Transfering	0 1 2 3	0 1 2 3	
6. Incontinence	0 1 2 3	0 1 2 3	
7. Managing money	0 1 2 3	0 1 2 3	
8. Telephoning	0 1 2 3	0 1 2 3	
9. Preparing meals	0 1 2 3	0 1 2 3	
10. Laundry	0 1 2 3	0 1 2 3	

11. Housework	0 1 2 3	0 1 2 3
12. Outside home	0 1 2 3	0 1 2 3
13. Routine health	0 1 2 3	0 1 2 3
14. Special health	0 1 2 3	0 1 2 3
15. Being alone	0 1 2 3	0 1 2 3
Box A: subtotal column A, items 1–6	Box A	Box B: subtotal column B, items 1–6	Box B
Box C: subtotal column A, items 7–15	Box C	Box D: subtotal column B, items 7–15	Box D
Box E: subtotal box A and box C	Box E	Box F: subtotal box B and box D	Box F
		Box G: subtotal box E and box F	Box G

Source: G. Pavesa et al., A Brief Assessment Tool for Determining Eligibility and Need for Community-Based Long-Term Care Services, *Behavior Health and Aging*, Vol. 1, pp. 121–132, © 1990, Springer Publishing Company, Inc., New York 10012. Used by permission.

paired older subjects as in cognitively intact subjects. The SF-36 has been employed in studies of outcome of patient care[58-62] and appears to be reliable and valid even in frail older adults.[63]

PERFORMANCE ASSESSMENT OF FUNCTION

Consider the source of information about functional impairment.[64] Persons may perceive their level of functioning to be at a higher level than the evaluation of nurses familiar with them would suggest. Assuming the nurses' evaluations were the most accurate, clients overrated their functional status, whereas families underrated it.[65] Self-ratings were found to most closely reflect the direct observations of research staff.[66] Pincus and colleagues found that self-reports on a simple questionnaire of functional status was significantly correlated to objective measures of physical impairment in rheumatoid arthritis.[67] In the Framingham follow-up, older residents did not seem reluctant to assent to functional limitations when compared to limitations noted on observation.[68] In clinical settings, physicians should use information from both the client and the caregiver. Is the activity performed? Could the activity be performed if necessary? Since data from self-report of function predict mortality, it is obvious that self-report information is very valuable.

Because direct observation of the client is desirable to confirm information given by the client or caregiver about functional status, a number of instruments have been developed.[69-71] Measures that appear to be adequate for primary care practice, however, are few.[72] One early performance test used props much as does the Denver Developmental Screening Examination for children. Example items included drinking from a cup, lifting food on a spoon to the mouth (props: spoon and candy), making a telephone call, brushing teeth (prop: toothbrush), and telling the time.[73] Performance tests focusing on manual dexterity predict the need for formal support services and appear to be unaffected by age or educational level,[74-77] but require specialized equipment.

Simple tests are sometimes used to assess functional status. In the "get up and go," the older person is timed while he or she rises from a chair, walks a given distance, turns, and sits down.[78,79] Impaired performance may identify older persons at risk of falling.[80] In functional reach, the distance that the person can extend the arm is measured.[81] The observation of performance may produce a more accurate assessment of capability than relying on report of function from the clients or caregivers. At the same time, the addition of performance measures

Exhibit 4–5 Medical Outcomes Study Short Form 36 (SF 36)

Instructions: This survey asks for your views about your health. This information will help keep track of how you feel and how well you are able to do your usual activities. Answer every question by marking the answer as indicated. If you are unsure about how to answer a question, please give the best answer you can.

1. In general, would you say your health is:

   (Circle one)

   Excellent 1
   Very good 2
   Good 3
   Fair 4
   Poor 5

2. *Compared to 1 year ago,* how would you rate your health in general now?

   (Circle one)

   Much better now than 1 year ago 1
   Somewhat better now than 1 year ago 2
   About the same now as 1 year ago 3
   Somewhat worse now than 1 year ago 4
   Much worse now than 1 year ago 5

3. The following items are about activities you might do during a typical day. Does *your health* now limit you in these activities? If so, how much?

   (Circle one number on each line)

Activities	Yes, Limited a Lot	Yes, Limited a Little	No, Not Limited at All
a. Vigorous activities, such as running, lifting heavy objects, or participating in strenuous sports	1	2	3
b. Moderate activities, such as moving a table, pushing a vacuum cleaner, bowling, or playing golf	1	2	3
c. Lifting or carrying groceries	1	2	3
d. Climbing several flights of stairs	1	2	3
e. Climbing one flight of stairs	1	2	3
f. Bending, kneeling, or stooping	1	2	3
g. Walking more than a mile	1	2	3
h. Walking several blocks	1	2	3
i. Walking one block	1	2	3
j. Bathing or dressing yourself	1	2	3

continues

Exhibit 4–5 continued

4. During the *past 4 weeks,* have you had any of the following problems with your work or other regular daily activities *as a result of your physical health?*

(Circle one number on each line)

	Yes	No
a. Cut down on the amount of time you spent on work or other activities	1	2
b. Accomplished less than you would like	1	2
c. Were limited in the kind of work or other activities	1	2
d. Had difficulty performing the work or other activities (for example, it took extra effort)	1	2

5. During the *past 4 weeks,* have you had any of the following problems with your work or other regular activities *as a result of any emotional problems* (such as feeling depressed or anxious)?

(Circle one number on each line)

	Yes	No
a. Cut down on the amount of time you spent on work or other activities	1	2
b. Accomplished less than you would like	1	2
c. Didn't do work or other activities as carefully as usual	1	2

6. During the *past 4 weeks,* to what extent has your physical health or emotional problems interfered with your normal social activities with family, friends, neighbors, or groups?

(Circle one)

Not at all 1
Slightly 2
Moderately 3
Quite a bit 4
Extremely 5

7. How much *bodily* pain have you had during the *past 4 weeks?*

(Circle one)

None 1
Very mild 2
Mild 3
Moderate 4
Severe 5
Very severe 6

continues

Exhibit 4–5 continued

8. During the *past 4 weeks,* how much did *pain* interfere with your normal work (including both work outside the home and housework)?

(Circle one)

Not at all 1
A little bit 2
Moderately 3
Quite a bit 4
Extremely 5

9. These questions are about how you feel and how things have been with you during the *past 4 weeks.* For each question, please give the one answer that comes closest to the way you have been feeling. How much of the time during the *past 4 weeks*

(Circle one number on each line)

	All of the Time	Most of the Time	A Good Bit of the Time	Some of the Time	A Little of the Time	None of the Time
a. Did you feel full of pep?	1	2	3	4	5	6
b. Have you been a very nervous person?	1	2	3	4	5	6
c. Have you felt so down in the dumps that nothing could cheer you up?	1	2	3	4	5	6
d. Have you felt calm and peaceful?	1	2	3	4	5	6
e. Did you have a lot of energy?	1	2	3	4	5	6
f. Have you felt downhearted and blue?	1	2	3	4	5	6
g. Did you feel worn out?	1	2	3	4	5	6
h. Have you been a happy person?	1	2	3	4	5	6
i. Did you feel tired?	1	2	3	4	5	6

10. During the *past 4 weeks,* how much of the time had your *physical health or emotional problems* interfered with your social activities (like visiting with friends, relatives, etc)?

(Circle one)

All of the time 1
Most of the time 2
Some of the time 3
A little of the time 4
None of the time 5

continues

Exhibit 4–5 continued

11. How TRUE or FALSE is *each* of the following statements for you?
(Circle one number on each line)

	Definitely True	Mostly True	Don't Know	Mostly False	Definitely False
a. I seem to get sick a little easier than other people	1	2	3	4	5
b. I am as healthy as anybody I know	1	2	3	4	5
c. I expect my health to get worse	1	2	3	4	5
d. My health is excellent	1	2	3	4	5

Source: Courtesy of Quality Metric, Inc., Lincoln, Rhode Island.

increases the time required for assessment and may not tap all pertinent domains.[82]

Physical Performance Test

The Physical Performance Test permits direct assessment of performance on a set of basic tasks that simulate the ADL.[83,84] The Physical Performance Test consists of:

1. writing a sentence
2. simulated eating
3. lifting a book and putting it on a shelf
4. putting on and removing a jacket
5. picking up a penny from the floor
6. turning 360 degrees
7. walking
8. climbing stairs.

Explicit instructions for administrating and scoring are provided. Bed mobility, transfer skills, standing up from a chair, standing balance, stepping up one step with a handrail, and walking are the activities rated in another performance measure suitable for hospitalized older patients.[85]

Direct Assessment of Functioning Scale

The utility of the Direct Assessment of Functioning Scale (DAFS)[69] is that it was developed specifically for use in working with persons who are demented. As such, it can assist with understanding what areas of behavior are affected by the dementia. Moreover, given the findings by Freels and colleagues,[86] that for many demented persons the ADL are not lost until well into the later stages of the disease, an instrument that is sensitive to early stages of dementia can help practitioners target interventions.

The DAFS was developed by Lowenstein and colleagues[69] out of concern that many of the functional assessment instruments rely on self-report rather than direct observation. As noted previously, there is some tendency when using self report data for an impaired person to overestimate his or her functional abilities, but when the report is obtained from an informant, particularly a family member, functional status is underestimated. The DAFS, as its name implies, requires the direct measurement and observation of a number of behaviors, including ADL and IADL, as well as some measure of cognitive functioning.

Because this instrument requires both the use of props and observation by the examiner, the DAFS is best suited for an office environment. However, its unique aspects make it particularly suited for use with demented persons, particularly those with Alzheimer's disease. Indeed, it is the strong relationship to both the Blessed Dementia Rating Scale and the Mini Blessed Dementia Rating Scale that makes the DAFS a useful instrument when working with persons who have already been diagnosed or are currently undergoing evaluation for dementia. Moreover, the ability to distinguish nondepressed and nondemented older adults from depressed or demented ones makes the DAFS a practical assessment for inclusion in a diagnostic workup.[69] Furthermore, the demonstrated ability to adequately track changes in functioning over time suggests that, unlike some instruments, the DAFS does not have an appreciable ceiling or floor effect and can, therefore, assist the practitioner with monitoring changes in older persons' functioning over time.

Case Study: Assessment of ADL

History

Mrs. Jones was a 72-year-old white woman who was recently widowed. She had a history of hypertension, treated with an angiotensin-converting enzyme inhibitor and a mild diuretic, and osteoarthritis, especially of the lower back, treated intermittently with a nonsteroidal anti-inflammatory drug. She lived alone in her own home. A 48-year-old working, married daughter lived in the same town and visited on the weekends to run errands and do some light housekeeping. An unmarried son lived in a larger city some 400 miles away.

Since her bereavement some 4 months ago, the woman, who did not drive, had been socially isolated, especially since she was unable to attend her usual functions, such as church meetings and bridge club. Her daughter was quite concerned because of her mother's lack of appetite and neglect of personal care. On questioning, Mrs. Jones admitted to early morning awakening, lack of appetite, weight loss, and crying spells. There was no prior history of depression, but the woman was thought to be depressed as part of her grief reaction.

The daughter was able to rearrange her schedule in order to provide transportation to the bridge club and to church. Counseling was arranged to help her cope with the grieving process. Participating in Meals on Wheels was suggested as a means to increase her social contact, but Mrs. Jones refused. Overall, these efforts mitigated some of her feelings of depression, and she improved considerably over the next several months.

Follow-Up

She remained at the same functional level, receiving assistance from her daughter, with her son keeping in touch by phone and helping out financially, until, at age 77, Mrs. Jones sustained a hip fracture after slipping on the ice on the way to her mailbox. She was hospitalized with a fracture of the left femoral neck and made a good recovery after insertion of a pin to stabilize her hip. She spent 2 months in a nursing home receiving physical therapy and rehabilitation and kept her spirits up with the thought of returning home. She was discharged home where she ambulated with a walker.

To accommodate her, the bedroom was moved downstairs, a commode was placed at her bedside, nightlights were obtained, and a ramp to eliminate the need for stairs to the outside was installed. Her movement, however, was more severely limited. Her daughter continued to provide help with shopping and housework and was able to enlist the help of the postal carrier as a daily check on Mrs. Jones' well-being.

Present Condition

Three years later, Mrs. Jones is now 80 years old. Her daughter, at age 56, is hospitalized for a myocardial infarction and will not be able to keep up the same level of help. At least temporarily, she will no longer be available to assist her mother in shopping, housekeeping, laundry, meal planning and preparation, and bathing, or to provide emotional support. Mrs. Jones does not wish to leave her home, but some of these activities are not getting done.

When her son visits, he is surprised and a little angry at the "condition Mom is in," although he keeps it to himself, considering his sister's recent heart attack. He believes Mrs. Jones should be immediately placed in a protective environment. Since Mrs. Jones is adamant about staying home, her son makes a compromise agreement with her to allow a live-in housekeeper. Although he tries to find a satisfactory live-in helper, he cannot find one who is satisfactory both to Mrs. Jones and him.

Resolution

Since her son must return to work, and the daughter is unable to care for her mother, Mrs. Jones reluctantly agrees to nursing home placement in an intermediate care facility, at least on a trial basis. The risk factors for nursing home placement in this case included living alone, old age, lack of a caregiver, and impaired mobility.

DEMENTIA RATING SCALES

A combination of mental status questions, ADL, and IADL items are sometimes blended into a score used to quantify the severity of dementia, a common clinical problem in geriatric practice. The dementia rating scales may be considered a hybrid type of instrument. Dementia rating scales have been used not only to identify dementia but also to quantify it, that is, to assign a stage or degree of severity. One example is the Blessed Dementia Score (Exhibit 4–6), which can be correlated to pathologic changes seen in brains of demented older persons at autopsy.[87] Many of these scales might be used in clinical practice, particularly if the practice includes a significant number of demented patients. The ideal dementia rating scale should be short and easy to score, just like the mental status screening instruments, to facilitate its use in clinical practice. The rating instrument should allow some quantification of dementia with a few differentiating points to categorize the severity of dementia. It would also be helpful if the practitioner could use it to follow the progression of the dementing illness. Several of these instruments are discussed in this section.

Exhibit 4–6 Blessed Dementia Score

---

1. Inability to perform household tasks
2. Inability to cope with small sums of money
3. Inability to remember short lists of items
4. Inability to find way outdoors
5. Inability to find way about familiar streets
6. Inability to interpret surroundings
7. Inability to recall recent events
8. Tendency to dwell in the past
9. Eating:
    Messily, with spoon only
    Simple solids, such as biscuits (2 points)
    Has to be fed (3 points)
10. Dressing:
    Occasionally misplaced buttons, etc
    Wrong sequence, forgets items (2 points)
    Unable to dress (3 points)
11. Sphincter control:
    Occasional wet beds
    Frequent wet beds (2 points)
    Doubly incontinent (3 points)
12. Increased rigidity
13. Increased egocentricity
14. Impairment of regard for feelings of others
15. Coarsening of affect
16. Impairment of emotional control
17. Hilarity in inappropriate situations
18. Diminished emotional responsiveness
19. Sexual misdemeanor (de novo in old age)
20. Hobbies relinquished
21. Diminished initiative or growing apathy
22. Purposeless hyperactivity

Total score _____

Scores range from 0 to 27; the higher the score, the greater the degree of dementia. Each item scores 1 except the items noted. A second part, the Information Score, contains items testing orientation and memory.

Source: Adapted with permission from G Blessed et al., The Association Between Quantitative Measures of Dementia and Senile Changes in the Cerebral Grey Mater of Elder Subjects, *British Journal of Psychiatry* Vol. 114, pp. 797–811, © 1968, The Royal College of Psychiatrists.

Functional Dementia Scale

A brief instrument to assess the severity of dementia is the Moore Functional Dementia Scale.[88] This questionnaire (Exhibit 4–7) can be given to family members in either written or oral form. The questionnaire gives results that quantify the dementia as well as provide a "review of systems" (or more accurately "review of symptoms") concerning the problems of dementia. No published guidelines on whether the scale shows change with time are available. It would be of interest to know if, beyond a certain score, more persons require nursing home placement. Perhaps one would then give certain undesirable or difficult characteristics higher weight, such as incontinence, which is often an especially troublesome problem.

Revised Memory and Behavior Problems Checklist

The Revised Memory and Behavior Problems Checklist assesses the frequency of observable problem behaviors and, on a separate dimension, the caregiver's response (Exhibit 4–8).[89–91] The frequency of the

---

Exhibit 4–7 Functional Dementia Scale

1. Has difficulty in completing simple tasks on own, such as dressing, bathing, doing arithmetic
2. Spends time either sitting or in apparently purposeless activity
3. Wanders at night or needs to be restrained to prevent wandering
4. Hears things that are not there
5. Requires supervision or assistance in eating
6. Loses things
7. Appearance is disorderly if left to own devices
8. Moans
9. Cannot control bowel function
10. Threatens to harm others
11. Cannot control bladder function
12. Needs to be watched so does not injure self, such as by careless smoking, leaving the stove on, or falling
13. Destructive of materials within reach, such as breaks furniture, throws food trays, or tears up magazines
14. Shouts or yells
15. Accuses others of doing him or her bodily harm or stealing his or her possessions when you are sure the accusations are not true
16. Is unaware of limitations imposed by illness
17. Becomes confused and does not know where he or she is
18. Has trouble remembering
19. Has sudden changes of mood, such as gets upset, angered, or cries easily
20. If left alone, wanders aimlessly during the day or needs to be restrained to prevent wandering

Each item is rated by the caregiver as follows: none or little of the time, some of the time, a good part of the time, or most or all of the time.

Source: J. Moore et al., A Functional Dementia Scale, Vol. 16, p. 503, © 1983, Dowden Publishing Company, Inc. Reproduced with permission from *The Journal of Family Practice*.

Exhibit 4-8 Revised Memory and Behavior Problems Checklist

The following is a list of problems patients sometimes have. Please indicate if any of these problems have occurred *during the past week*. If so, how much has this bothered or upset you when it happened? Use the following scales for the frequency of the problem and your reaction to it. Please read the description of the ratings carefully.

FREQUENCY RATINGS:
0 = never occurred
1 = not in the past week
2 = 1 to 2 times in the past week
3 = 3 to 6 times in the past week
4 = daily or more often
9 = don't know/not applicable

REACTION RATINGS:
0 = not at all
1 = a little
2 = moderately
3 = very much
4 = extremely
9 = don't know/not applicable

Please answer all the questions below. Please circle a number from 0–9 for both *frequency* and *reaction*.

	Frequency	Reaction
1. Asking the same question over and over.	0 1 2 3 4 9	0 1 2 3 4 9
2. Trouble remembering recent events (e.g., items in the newspaper or on TV).	0 1 2 3 4 9	0 1 2 3 4 9
3. Trouble remembering significant past events.	0 1 2 3 4 9	0 1 2 3 4 9
4. Losing or misplacing things.	0 1 2 3 4 9	0 1 2 3 4 9
5. Forgetting what day it is.	0 1 2 3 4 9	0 1 2 3 4 9
6. Starting, but not finishing, things.	0 1 2 3 4 9	0 1 2 3 4 9
7. Difficulty concentrating on a task.	0 1 2 3 4 9	0 1 2 3 4 9
8. Destroying property.	0 1 2 3 4 9	0 1 2 3 4 9
9. Doing things that embarrass you.	0 1 2 3 4 9	0 1 2 3 4 9

10. Waking you or other family members up at night.	0 1 2 3 4 9	0 1 2 3 4 9
11. Talking loudly and rapidly.	0 1 2 3 4 9	0 1 2 3 4 9
12. Appears anxious or worried.	0 1 2 3 4 9	0 1 2 3 4 9
13. Engaging in behavior that is potentially dangerous to self or others.	0 1 2 3 4 9	0 1 2 3 4 9
14. Threats to hurt oneself.	0 1 2 3 4 9	0 1 2 3 4 9
15. Threats to hurt others.	0 1 2 3 4 9	0 1 2 3 4 9
16. Aggressive to others verbally.	0 1 2 3 4 9	0 1 2 3 4 9
17. Appears sad or depressed.	0 1 2 3 4 9	0 1 2 3 4 9
18. Expressing feelings of hopelessness or sadness about the future (eg, "Nothing worthwhile ever happens," "I never do anything right").	0 1 2 3 4 9	0 1 2 3 4 9
19. Crying and tearfulness.	0 1 2 3 4 9	0 1 2 3 4 9
20. Commenting about death of self or others (eg, "Life isn't worth living," "I'd be better off dead").	0 1 2 3 4 9	0 1 2 3 4 9
21. Talking about feeling lonely.	0 1 2 3 4 9	0 1 2 3 4 9
22. Comments about feeling worthless or being a burden to others.	0 1 2 3 4 9	0 1 2 3 4 9
23. Comments about feeling like a failure or about not having any worthwhile accomplishments in life.	0 1 2 3 4 9	0 1 2 3 4 9
24. Arguing, irritability, and/or complaining.	0 1 2 3 4 9	0 1 2 3 4 9

Source: Courtesy of Dr. L. Teri, © 1992, Seattle, Washington.

behavior is rated using the following phrases: (1) "never," (2) "not in the past week," (3) "one to two times in the past week," (4) "three to six times in the past week," or (5) "daily." The degree to which each behavior upsets the caregiver is rated by the caregiver on a five-point scale: (1) "not at all," (2) "a little," (3) "moderately," (4) "very much," and (5) "extremely." The assessment of caregiver distress is an advantage when considering disturbing behaviors sometimes associated with dementia. The development of depression in caregivers is predicted primarily by their subjective evaluations of circumstances rather than objective measures of function of the elder.[92]

Functional Rating Scale for the Symptoms of Dementia

The Texas Tech Functional Rating Scale for the Symptoms of Dementia is a questionnaire devised to predict who may require nursing home placement.[18] According to the investigators, this is a brief dementia scale that measures severity, shows change, and may be valuable in predicting when nursing home placement is necessary (Exhibit 4–9). The concept that persons reaching a certain level of functional disability require nursing home placement is attractive because such objective measures are generally lacking in assessment for long-term care.

Scores on the Functional Rating Scale for the Symptoms of Dementia range from 0 (not demented) to 42. Persons were tested over a 2-year period every few months and were divided at the start of the study into two groups: (1) those with scores above 21 and (2) those with scores below 21. Persons with a score greater than 21 had an average of 7 months until nursing home placement occurred, and those with scores of 21 or less did not require nursing home placement for an average of 18 months. Scores at the time of admission to the nursing home were about the same for both groups (ie, about 32).[18]

Three items on the Functional Rating Scale for the Symptoms of Dementia were especially predictive of nursing home placement. If two of the three were present, 83% of these patients were in a nursing home before the next evaluation. The items were incontinence of bowel and bladder, inability to speak coherently, and inability to bathe and groom oneself. The investigators who developed this instrument suggested that scores above 30 may indicate a need for nursing home placement.[18] If the physician can say that most persons reaching a certain level of disability require nursing home placement, it may help alleviate family guilt. Of course, such a scale should be used only in the context of other relevant medical, social, psychological, and economic data.

Exhibit 4–9 Functional Rating Scale for the Symptoms of Dementia

Instructions
1. The scale must be administered to the most knowledgeable informant available. This usually is a spouse or close relative.
2. The scale should be read to the informant one category at a time. The informant is presented the description for behavior in each category. The informant is read each of the responses beginning with zero response. All responses should be read before the informant endorses the highest number response that best describes the behavior of the patient.
3. When responses have been obtained for each category, the circled numbers from each category are summed to give an overall score for functional rating of symptoms of dementia.

Circle the highest number of each category that best describes behavior during the past 3 months.

Eating
0 Eats neatly using appropriate utensils
1 Eats messily, has some difficulty with utensils
2 Able to eat solid foods (eg, fruits, crackers, and cookies) with hands only
3 Has to be fed

Dressing
0 Able to dress appropriately without help
1 Able to dress self with occasionally mismatched socks, disarranged buttons or laces
2 Dresses out of sequence, forgets items, or wears sleeping garments with street clothes, needs supervision
3 Unable to dress alone, appears undressed in inappropriate situations

Continence
0 Complete sphincter control
1 Occasional bed wetting
2 Frequent bed wetting or daytime urinary incontinence
3 Incontinent of both bladder and bowel

Verbal communication
0 Speaks normally
1 Minor difficulties with speech or word-finding difficulties
2 Able to carry out only simple, uncomplicated conversations
3 Unable to speak coherently

Memory for names
0 Usually remembers names of meaningful acquaintances
1 Cannot recall names of acquaintances or distant relatives
2 Cannot recall names of close friends of relatives
3 Cannot recall name of spouse or other living partner

Memory for events
0 Can recall details and sequences of recent experiences
1 Cannot recall details or sequences of recent events
2 Cannot recall entire events (eg, recent outings or visits of relatives or friends) without prompting
3 Cannot recall entire events even with prompting

continues

Exhibit 4–9 continued

Mental alertness
0 Usually alert, attentive to environment
1 Easily distractible, mind wanders
2 Frequently asks the same questions over and over
3 Cannot maintain attention while watching television

Global confusion
0 Appropriately responsive to environment
1 Nocturnal confusion on awakening
2 Periodic confusion during daytime
3 Nearly always quite confused

Spatial orientation
0 Oriented, able to find and keep his or her bearings
1 Spatial confusion when driving or riding in local community
2 Gets lost when walking in neighborhood
3 Gets lost in own home or in hospital ward

Facial recognition
0 Can recognize faces of recent acquaintances
1 Cannot recognize faces of recent acquaintances
2 Cannot recognize faces of relatives or close friends
3 Cannot recognize spouse or other constant living companion

Hygiene and grooming
0 Generally neat and clean
1 Ignores grooming (eg, does not brush teeth and hair, shave)
2 Does not bathe regularly
3 Has to be bathed and groomed

Emotionality
0 Unchanged from normal
1 Mild change in emotional responsiveness—slightly more irritable or more passive, diminished sense of humor, mild depression
2 Moderate change in emotional responsiveness—growing apathy, increased
  rigidity, despondent, angry outbursts, cries easily
3 Impaired emotional control—unstable, rapid cycling or laughing or crying in
  inappropriate situations, violent outbursts

Social responsiveness
0 Unchanged from previous, "normal"
1 Tendency to dwell in the past, lack of proper association for present situation
2 Lack of regard for feelings of others, quarrelsome, irritable
3 Inappropriate sexual acting out or antisocial behavior

Sleep patterns
0 Unchanged from previous, "normal"
1 Sleeps, noticeably more or less than normal
2 Restless, nightmares, disturbed sleep, increased awakenings
3 Up wandering for all or most of the night, inability to sleep

Source: Reprinted with permission of JT Hutton et al., Predictors of Nursing Home Placement of Patients with Alzheimer's Disease, *Texas Medicine,* Vol. 7, No. 81, p. 41, © 1985 Texas Medical Association.

Global Deterioration Scale

Another approach to the problem of assessing the severity of cognitive impairment uses a clinical staging system. In Alzheimer's disease three stages have been commonly recognized. First, a forgetfulness stage occurs, in which memory problems and impaired visuospatial skills predominate. Then a confusional stage ensues, in which language and calculations are affected, with some changes in personality. Finally, a dementia stage develops in which intellectual functions are severely deteriorated.[93]

The Global Deterioration Scale (GDS) for Primary Degenerative Dementia is one such staging system (Exhibit 4–10).[93] The person's stage is related to prognosis, and, as expected, the more advanced the stage, the worse is the prognosis. For example, in the older adult with mild cognitive decline (stage 3), the prognosis is primarily benign, at least over a 4-year period. Persons in early stages may actually have aging-associated cognitive decline. On the other hand, when cognitive decline is severe (stage 6), one third of the persons have died after 4 years, and most have been placed in institutions.

The stages of the GDS correlate with results of the Mini-Mental State Examination (MMSE). Patients with GDS stage 4, indicating mild Alzheimer's disease, scored from 16 to 23 on the MMSE.[94] Independent validation of the MMSE set a cutoff score of 24 to detect dementia.[95–97] Persons at more impaired stages of the GDS had correspondingly lower scores on the MMSE.[94] Several recent articles have questioned the utility of this scale. These articles have noted that the functional deterioration proposed in the GDS is actually much more heterogeneous in the population than the scale suggests.[98,99] Some investigators contend that both families and practitioners may be better served by staying with the broader concepts of mild, moderate, and severe dementia based on neuropsychological testing and then describing the actual levels of functional impairment and behavioral disturbance rather than trying to place a single value on the level of deterioration.[98,99]

Functional Assessment Staging of Alzheimer's Disease

The GDS has been expanded into a more elaborate staging system called the Functional Assessment Staging of Alzheimer's Disease (FAST).[100,101] Stages 1 through 5 of the FAST correspond exactly to stages 1 through 5 of the GDS. Stages 6 and 7 of the GDS have been subdivided into five and six substages, respectively, in the FAST (Exhibit 4–11).

Exhibit 4–10 Global Deterioration Scale for Primary Degenerative Dementia with 4-Year Prognosis Data

---

Stage 1: No cognitive decline

Stage 2: Very mild cognitive decline

The patient complains of memory loss, especially forgetting where objects were placed or familiar names. There is no objective evidence of memory deficit in the clinical interview and no deficits in employment or social situations.

Prognosis: Benign in 95% over a 4-year period.*

Stage 3: Mild cognitive decline (early confusion)

Memory loss is evident on testing. Decreased ability to remember names of new acquaintances. Coworkers are aware of memory problems. Gets lost in travel. Associated anxiety or denial.

Prognosis: >80% show no further decline in 4 years.*

Stage 4: Moderate cognitive decline (late confusion)

Trouble concentrating on a task. Lessened knowledge of personal history, current events, and recent events. Trouble with travel and finances. Remains oriented to time and place. Denial is a prominent defense mechanism.

Prognosis: In 4 years, one fourth show no change, one fourth are worse but at home, one fourth are in institutions, and one fourth are dead.*

Stage 5: Moderately severe cognitive decline

The phase of dementia. Unable to recall major events of current life. Disoriented to time and place. Occasionally dresses improperly but feeds and toilets independently.

Prognosis: After 4 years, most are worse.*

Stage 6: Severe cognitive decline

Incontinent. Sleep-wake cycle disturbances. Personality changes. Forgets even the names of close relatives and spouse.

Prognosis: One third are dead in 4 years; two thirds are in institutions.*

Stage 7: Very severe cognitive decline

Late dementia, with no speech or psychomotor skills.

*The 4-year prognosis data are from *Psychiatric Annals* (1985;15:319–322), Copyright © 1985, Charles B Slack Inc.

Source: American Journal of Psychiatry, Vol. 139, pp. 1136–1139, 1982. Copyright © 1982, American Psychiatric Association. Reprinted by permission. *Psychiatric Annals,* Vol. 15, pp. 319–322, © 1985, Charles B. Slack Inc.

This hierarchical arrangement accomplishes several objectives. First, when cognitive deficit yields only baseline or zero scores on a mental status examination, further delineation of severity is possible when stages are employed. Second, and more important clinically, when the patient experiences difficulty that seems to vary with the expected se-

Exhibit 4–11 Functional Assessment Staging of Alzheimer's Disease Symptomatology and Differential Diagnostic Considerations

FAST Characteristic	FAST Stage	Differential Diagnosis If FAST Stage Is Early
No functional decrement subjectively or objectively	1	
Complains of forgetting location of objects Subjective work difficulties	2	Anxiety neurosis Depression
Decreased functioning in demanding work settings evident to coworkers Difficulty traveling to new locations	3	Depression Subtle manifestations of medical pathology
Decreased ability to perform complex tasks (eg, planning dinner, shopping, or personal finances)	4	Depression Psychosis Focal process (eg, Gerstmann)
Requires assistance selecting attire May require coaxing to bathe properly	5	Depression
Difficulty dressing properly	6a	Arthritis Sensory deficit Stroke Depression
Requires assistance bathing (fear of bathing)	b	Same as 6a
Difficulty with mechanics of toileting	c	Same as 6a
Urinary incontinence	d	Urinary tract infection Other causes
Fecal incontinence	e	Infection Malabsorption syndrome Other causes
Vocabulary limited to one to five words	7a	Stroke Other dementing disorder (eg, space-occupying lesion)
Intelligible vocabulary lost	b	Same as 7a
Ambulatory ability lost	c	Parkinsonism Neuroleptic-induced or other secondary extrapyramidal syndrome Creutzfeldt-Jakob disease Normal pressure hydrocephalus Hyponatremic dementia Stroke Hip fracture

continues

Exhibit 4–11 continued

		Arthritis
		Overmedication
Ability to sit lost	d	Arthritis
		Contractures
Ability to smile lost	e	Stroke
Ability to hold up head lost	f	Head trauma
Ultimately, stupor or coma		Metabolic abnormality
		Overmedication
		Other causes

Source: Reprinted with permission from *Geriatrics,* Vol. 41, No. 4, © 1986, p. 34. Copyright by Advanstar Communications Inc. Advanstar Communications Inc. retains all rights to this material.

quence for Alzheimer's disease, the clinician can consider a treatable condition in the differential diagnosis, rather than ascribing a new change to a progression of Alzheimer's disease.

Consider a 75-year-old man whose wife relates that he has trouble dressing, but still picks out his clothes. Since picking the appropriate items should be lost before difficulty dressing (stage 5 versus stage 6a), the clinician might consider superimposed depression or stroke as precipitating the trouble, rather than a worsening of the underlying dementia. Similarly, a 60-year-old woman who complains of inability to handle personal finances, but is able to function well in a demanding job may be depressed rather than have Alzheimer's disease. Here stage 4 (personal finances) appearing before stage 3 (working) is the clue to the diagnosis of depression. Another example of the clinical utility of FAST is premature development of urinary incontinence, suggesting the presence of a urinary tract infection. Finally, premature loss of speech in an otherwise uncomplicated setting of Alzheimer's disease may suggest focal cerebral pathology such as an infarction.[100,101]

Clinical Dementia Rating Scale

The Clinical Dementia Rating Scale (CDR) was found to correlate to results of the SPMSQ and to the Blessed Dementia Score, but the CDR was able to differentiate a greater number of degrees of severity over the range of dementia (Exhibit 4–12). For example, persons in CDR 2 scored 8.4 on the SPMSQ, and in CDR 3, an indistinguishable 8.7.[102] The CDR correlates with screening tests of cognitive function such as the SPMSQ[103] and has good reliability.[104] The CDR correlates more strongly than do tests of mental status with functional impairment.[12,105]

The clinical stage assigned depends on the pattern of the answers to the questions on the rating scale form (Figure 4–1). The best description of the patient in each of six domains is checked off or circled on the rating scale form. The six areas to be evaluated are memory, orientation, judgment and problem solving, community affairs, home and hobbies, and personal care. The CDR scale can be employed for the assessment of elderly demented patients in primary care practice to have a standard form to use to assess severity of dementia.

Shaded areas in Figure 4–1 show the defined range into which the scores must fall in order to be assigned a specific CDR stage. Memory is considered the primary category, and if at least three other categories are given the same score as memory, then the rating is the same as the rating that describes the memory function. Otherwise, if three or more secondary categories are given a score greater or less than the memory score, the rating is the score of the majority of the secondary categories. If the secondary assessments lie to either side of the memory score, the rating is the same as the memory score.[102] Alternative algorithms for scoring the CDR have been devised to diminish the influence that the memory assessment has on the final CDR score.[106]

ASSESSMENT FOR LONG-TERM CARE

Various facets of assessment and instruments whose use helps maintain consistency and a systematic approach are reviewed in this book. It is hoped that assessment of areas such as performance of ADL helps achieve some congruity between needs and resources. An algorithm that provides an overview of long-term care assessment has been suggested by Williams and Williams (Exhibit 4–13).[107]

Levels of care to be provided depend on the amount of medical, ADL, or social help required. There is a continuum from acute hospitalization to the skilled nursing facility to the intermediate care facility to domiciliary care to the person's own home. The algorithm essentially is a hierarchy based on mental state and the ability to perform ADL and IADL, as well as the need for special medical interventions, such as provision of oxygen.

If the issue is nursing home placement, precipitating factors should be kept in mind.[108,109] Why is nursing home placement being considered at this time? If a precipitating factor is relieved, can the person be cared

Exhibit 4–12 Clinical Dementia Rating Scale (CDR)

	Healthy CDR 0	Questionable Dementia CDR 0.5	Mild Dementia CDR 1	Moderate Dementia CDR 2	Severe Dementia CDR 3
Memory	No memory loss or slight inconstant forgetfulness	Mild consistent forgetfulness; partial recollection of events; "benign" forgetfulness	Moderate memory loss, more marked for recent events; defect interferes with everyday activities	Severe memory loss; only highly learned material retained; new material rapidly lost	Severe memory loss; only fragments remain
Orientation	Fully oriented		Some difficulty with time relationships, oriented for place and person at examination, but may have geographic disorientation	Usually disoriented in time, often to place	Orientation to person only
Judgment, problem solving	Solves everyday problems well, judgment good in relation to past performance	Only doubtful impairment in solving problems, similarities, differences	Moderate difficulty in handling complex problems; social judgment usually maintained	Severely impaired in handling problems, similarities, differences; social judgment usually impaired	Unable to make judgments or solve problems

continues

Community affairs	Independent function at usual level in job, shopping, business and financial affairs, volunteer and social groups	Only doubtful or mild impairment, if any, in these activities	Unable to function independently at these activities though may still be engaged in some; may still appear normal to casual inspection	No pretense of independent function outside home
Home, hobbies	Life at home, hobbies, intellectual interests well maintained	Life at home, hobbies, intellectual interests well maintained or only slightly impaired	Mild, but definite impairment of function at home; more difficult chores abandoned; more complicated hobbies and interests abandoned	Only simple chores preserved; very restricted interests, poorly sustained	No significant function in home outside of own room
Personal care	Fully capable of self-care		Needs occasional prompting	Requires assistance in dressing, hygiene, keeping of personal effects	Requires much help with personal care; often incontinent

Note: Score each item as 0.5, 1, 2, or 3 only if impairment is due to cognitive loss.

Source: Adapted with permission from *The British Journal of Psychiatry*, Vol. 140, pp. 566–572, © 1982, The Royal College of Psychiatrists.

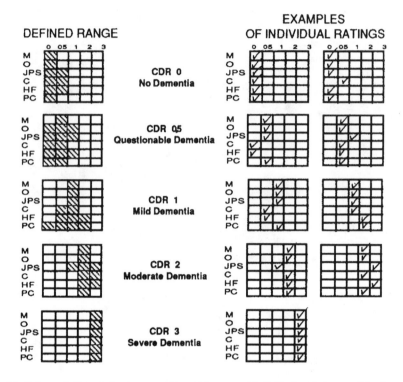

Shaded areas indicate defined range within which scores of individual subjects must fall to be assigned a given CDR.

M = Memory; O = Orientation; JPS = Judgment and problem solving; CA = Community affairs; HH = Home, hobbies ; PC = Personal care.

Instructions for assigning the CDR are as follows:

Use all information and make the best judgment. Score each category (M, O, JPS, CA, HH, PC) as independently as possible. Mark in only one box, rating each according to subject's cognitive function. For determining the CDR, memory is considered the primary category; all others are secondary. If at least three secondary categories are given the same numerical score as memory, then CDR = M. If three or more secondary categories are given a score greater or less than the memory score, CDR = score of majority of secondary categories, unless three secondary categories are scored on one side of M and two secondary categories are scored on the other side of M. In this last circumstance, CDR = M.

When M = 0.5, CDR = 1 if at least three of certain others (O, JPS, CA, HH) are scored 1 or greater (PC not influential here). If M = 0.5, CDR cannot be 0; CDR can only be 0.5 or 1. If M = 0, CDR = 0 unless there is slight impairment in two or more secondary categories, in which case CDR = 0.5.

Figure 4–1 How to determine level of dementia using the CDR scale. *Source:* Adapted with permission from *The British Journal of Psychiatry,* Vol. 140, pp. 566–572, © 1982, The Royal College of Psychiatrists.

Exhibit 4-13 Algorithm for Deciding Need for Long-Term Care

I. 1. Is the patient medically unstable?
    2. Is the patient mentally unstable to the extent of being a danger to himself or herself or others?

    NO (continue below)   YES → ACUTE HOSPITAL

II. 1. Is the patient totally disoriented chronically?
    2. Is the patient immobile (ie, always requires human assistance in locomotion)?
    3. Does the patient have need of special therapy (eg, intravenous line, tracheostomy, oxygen, or ostomy)?
    4. Does the patient require total supervision?
    5. Does the patient require total ADL care?

    NO (continue below)   YES → SKILLED NURSING
                                                    FACILITY
                                                or
                                          HOME IF SUPPORT
                                          AVAILABLE

III. 1. Does the patient have intermittent disorientation or wandering?
     2. Does the patient fluctuate in ADL ability?
     3. Does the patient require a structured environment—some supervision?
     4. Does the patient require special therapeutics (eg, complex diet, complex medication schedule, close monitoring)?

    NO (continue below)   YES → INTERMEDIATE LEVEL
                                                    FACILITY
                                                or
                                          HOME IF SUPPORT
                                          AVAILABLE

IV. Can the patient do all of the following:

1. Feed self	7. Plan meals
2. Bathe	8. Use transportation
3. Dress	9. Use telephone
4. Use the toilet without help	10. Handle finances
5. Change position	11. Manage medications
6. Shop	

    NO (continue below)   YES → HOME

V. Are resources available to meet these needs?

    NO → DOMICILIARY CARE   YES → HOME WITH SUPPORT

Source: Reprinted with permission from the *Journal of the American Geriatric Society,* Vol. 30, No. 7, p. 73, Lippincott Williams & Wilkins.

---

for at home? Is the precipitating factor a change in the person's functioning in a specific ADL? Has the coping ability of a key caregiver become diminished? Thorough physical assessment and documentation of mental status are essential. Issues of guilt and the restructuring of family roles should not be neglected if the decision is finally made that nursing home placement is the most appropriate course of action.[109]

The primary care practitioner is in an excellent position to assess the older person's mental status and ability to perform ADL and IADL. When decline is noted, it alerts the practitioner to search for a cause. Perhaps, help is no longer available to perform some necessary function. Recommendations about resources prescribed or changes in routine can be made to accommodate the loss. The line may be crossed when it is no longer possible to provide enough assistance to keep the person functioning adequately at home, and then alternative arrangements such as nursing home placement can be recommended.

Case Study: Assessment for Long-Term Care

History

Mr. Smith was a fit 78-year-old white man who lived with his 67-year-old wife in their own home. He exhibited considerable memory impairment thought to be Alzheimer's disease, scoring 5 of 10 on the SPMSQ. He had no major physical problems. He performed ADL with some coaxing from his wife (eg, bathing, dressing when she lays out his clothes, and feeding himself). He had occasional lapses in judgment, such as wandering and urinating at inappropriate places or times. The couple had no children. The man's sister-in-law lived several blocks away. A next-door neighbor provided assistance with shopping and transportation to the physician's office for years. In addition, the neighbor had been a source of social interaction for the man's wife. Mr. Smith's behavior made it difficult for Mrs. Smith to do some of the things she used to do for relaxation. She found a woman in the neighborhood to sit with Mr. Smith so she could run errands and obtain some time for herself for respite.

Follow-Up

Over the years Mr. Smith's memory worsened and catastrophic reactions increased in frequency and intensity. He hallucinated and talked to himself in the mirror. He frequently did not recognize his wife, which of course disturbed her. Mr. Smith's physician helped Mrs. Smith realize that she had become socially isolated, depressed, and even more preoccupied with her husband's care than in years past. Interviewing Mrs. Smith, the physician rates Mr. Smith's behavior according to the Texas Tech Functional Rating Scale for the Symptoms of Dementia. His score was 30. On occasion, the physician in similar circumstances has used the Moore Functional Dementia Scale as a questionnaire for the family member while the patient was being examined.

Resolution

Because of Mr. Smith's deteriorating ability to perform ADL, increasing confusion, and catastrophic reactions, including wandering, the physician recommends nursing home placement. The physician anticipates guilt and depression in Mrs. Smith and plans to counsel her to deal with the loss of the husband she knew.

CONCLUSION

The use of instruments to assess the functional status of older persons is an area frequently neglected by physicians. For the older adults, however, functional assessment is critical because the ability to remain independent may hinge on the ability to perform ADL.[1,9] The focus on functional needs puts the emphasis on what is important to the person. How can the person maximize functioning at home and in the community? The functional status directs attention to the health and support services required and the possible alternative settings or levels of care.[110]

A systematic approach to functional assessment is helpful because it provides a task-specific framework to check that the person can perform (or has help performing) the tasks that are required to live independently, such as toileting or preparing meals. In fact, problems found in these areas should be listed alongside the patient's medical problems, thereby yielding a clear picture of his or her difficulties, which can then be organized to find a solution. As Weed suggested, creating such a problem list may help the clinician find hitherto unrecognized correlations among physical, mental, and functional spheres.[111] The comprehensive problem-oriented medical record keeps the constellation of medical diagnoses, undiagnosed conditions, and problems of daily living to the fore.

REFERENCES

1. Applegate WB, Blass JP, Williams TF. Instruments for the functional assessment of older patients. *N Engl J Med.* 1990;322:1207–1214.

2. Department of Health and Human Services. *Healthy People 2000: National Health Promotion and Disease Prevention Objectives.* Washington, DC: US Government Printing Office; 1991. DHHS Publication No. PHS 91–50213.

142   HANDBOOK OF GERIATRIC ASSESSMENT

3. Fried LP, Bush TL. Morbidity as a focus of preventive health care in the elderly. *Epidemiol Rev.* 1988;10:48–64.

4. Hadley EC, Ory MG, Suzman R, Weindruch R, Fried L. Physical frailty: A treatable cause of dependence in old age. *J Gerontol.* 1993;48:1–88.

5. Katz S, Branch LG, Branson MH, et al. Active life expectancy. *N Engl J Med.* 1983; 309:1218–1224.

6. George LK, Bearon LB. *Quality of Life in Older Persons: Meaning and Measurement.* New York: Human Sciences Press; 1980.

7. Rubenstein LV, Calkins DR, Greenfield S, et al. Health status assessment for elderly patients: Report of the Society of General Internal Medicine Task Force on Health Assessment. *J Am Geriatr Soc.* 1988;37:562–569.

8. Granger CV, Gresham GE. *Functional Assessment in Rehabilitation Medicine.* Baltimore: Williams & Wilkins; 1984.

9. Mosqueda LA. Assessment of rehabilitation potential. *Clin Geriatr Med.* 1993;9: 689–703.

10. Heath JM. Comprehensive functional assessment of the elderly. *Primary Care.* 1989;16:305–327.

11. Guralnik JM, Simonsick EM. Physical disability in older Americans. *J Gerontol.* 1993;48:3–10.

12. Skurla E, Rogers JC, Sunderland T. Direct assessment of activities of daily living in Alzheimer's disease: A controlled study. *J Am Geriatr Soc.* 1988;36:97–103.

13. Reed BR, Jagust WJ, Seab J. Mental status as a predictor of daily function in progressive dementia. *Gerontologist.* 1989;29:804–807.

14. Brink TL, Capri D, DeNeeve V, et al. Senile confusion: Limitations of assessment by the Face-Hand Test, Mental Status Questionnaire, and staff ratings. *J Am Geriatr Soc.* 1978;26:380–382.

15. Barberger-Gateau P, Commenges D, Gagnon M, Letenneur L, Sauvel C, Dartigues JF. Instrumental activities of daily living as a screening tool for cognitive impairment and dementia in elderly community dwellers. *J Am Geriatr Soc.* 1992;40:1129–1134.

16. Iliffe S, Tai SS, Haines A, et al. Assessment of elderly people in general practice: 4. Depression, functional ability and contact with services. *Br J Gen Pract.* 1993;43:371–374.

17. Keene JS, Anderson CA. Hip fractures in the elderly. *JAMA.* 1982;248:564–567.

18. Hutton JT, Dippel RL, Loewenson RB, et al. Predictors of nursing home placement of patients with Alzheimer's disease. *Tex Med.* 1985;81:40–43.

19. Paveza GJ, Cohen D, Hagopian M, Prohaska T, Blaser CJ, Brauner D. A brief assessment tool for determining eligibility and need for community-based long-term care services. *Behav, Health Aging.* 1990;1:121–132.

20. Paveza GJ, Cohen D, Blaser CJ, Hagopian M. A brief form of the Mini-Mental State Examination for use in community care settings. *Behav, Health Aging.* 1990;1:133–139.

21. Lichtenstein MJ, Federspiel CF, Shaffner W. Factors associated with early demise in nursing home residents: a case control study. *J Am Geriatr Soc.* 1985;33:315–319.

22. Incalzi AR, Capparella O, Gemmo A, Porcedda P, Raccis G. A simple method of recognizing geriatric patients at risk for death and disability. *J Am Geriatr Soc.* 1992;40: 34–38.

23. Fillenbaum G. Screening the elderly: A brief instrumental activities of daily living measure. *J Am Geriatr Soc.* 1985;33:698–706.

24. Koyano W, Shibata H, Nakazato K, Haga H, Suyama Y, Matsuzaki T. Mortality in relation to instrumental activities of daily living: One year follow-up in a Japanese urban community. *J Gerontol.* 1989;44:S107–109.

25. Mor V, Murphy J, Masterson-Allen S, Willey C, Razmpour A. Risk of functional decline among frail elders. *J Clin Epidemiol.* 1989;42:895–904.

26. Mor V, Wilcox V, Rakowski W, Hiris J. Functional transitions among the elderly: Patterns, predictors, and related hospital use. *Am J Public Health.* 1994;84:1274–1280.

27. Burton JR. The house call: An important service for the frail elderly. *J Am Geriatr Soc.* 1985;33:291–293.

28. Levy MT. Psychiatric assessment of elderly patients in the home. *J Am Geriatr Soc.* 1985;33:9–12.

29. Reuben DB, Solomon DH. Assessment in geriatrics: Of caveats and names. *J Am Geriatr Soc.* 1989;37:570–572.

30. Fried LP, Ettinger WH, Lind B, Newman AB, Gardin J. Physical disability in older adults: A physiological approach. *J Clin Epidemiol.* 1994;47:747–760.

31. Yurick AG, Spier BE, Robb SS, et al. *The Aged Person and the Nursing Process.* 2nd ed. Norwalk, CT: Appleton-Century-Crofts; 1984.

32. Carnevali DL, Patrick M. *Nursing Management for the Elderly.* 2nd ed. Philadelphia: JB Lippincott Company; 1986.

33. Applegate WB. Use of assessment instruments in clinical settings. *J Am Geriatr Soc.* 1987;35:45–50.

34. Siu AL, Reuben DB, Hays RD. Hierarchical measures of physical function in ambulatory geriatrics. *J Am Geriatr Soc.* 1990;38:1113–1119.

35. Blazer D, Siegler IC. *A Family Approach to Health Care of the Elderly.* Menlo Park, CA: Addison-Wesley Publishing Co; 1984.

36. Woodhouse K, Wynne H, Baillie S, et al. Who are the frail elderly? *Q J Med.* 1988; 28:505–506.

37. Schulz R, Williamson GM. Psychosocial and behavioral dimensions of physical frailty. *J Gerontol.* 1993;48:39–43.

38. Rockwood K, Fox RA, Stolee P, Robertson D, Beattie BL. Frailty in elderly people: An evolving concept. *Can Med Assoc J.* 1994;150:489–495.

39. Feinstein AR. An additional basic science for clinical medicine: IV. The development of clinimetrics. *Ann Intern Med.* 1983;99:843–848.

40. Feinstein AR, Josephy BR, Wells CK. Scientific and clinical problems in indexes of functional disability. *Ann Intern Med.* 1986;105:413–420.

41. Becker PM, Cohen HJ. The functional approach to the care of the elderly: A conceptual framework. *J Am Geriatr Soc.* 1984;32:923–929.

42. Granger CV, Albrecht GL, Hamilton BB. Outcome of comprehensive medical rehabilitation: Measurement by PULSES profile and the Barthel index. *Arch Phys Med Rehabil.* 1979;60:145–154.

43. Kane RA, Kane RL. *Assessing the Elderly: A Practical Guide to Measurement.* Lexington, MA: Lexington Books; 1981.

44. Pope AM, Tarlov AR. *Disability in America: Toward a National Agenda for Prevention.* Washington, DC: National Academy Press; 1991.

45. Katz S, Ford AB, Moskowitz RW, et al. Studies of illness in the aged: The index of ADL. *JAMA.* 1963;185:914–919.

46. Bruett TL, Overs RP. A critical review of 12 ADL scales. *Phys Ther.* 1969;49:857–862.

47. Katz PR, Dube DH, Calkins E. Use of a structured functional assessment format in a geriatric consultative service. *J Am Geriatr Soc.* 1985;33:681–686.

48. Katz S, Downs TD, Cash HR, et al. Progress in development of the index ADL. *Gerontologist.* Spring 1970; part 1:20–30.

49. Kelly JF, Winograd CH. A functional approach to stroke management in elderly patients. *J Am Geriatr Soc.* 1985;33:48–60.

50. Mahoney FI, Barthel DW. Functional evaluation: the Barthel index. *Md State Med J.* 1965;14:61–65.

51. Fortinsky RH, Granger CV, Seltzer GB. The use of functional assessment in understanding home care needs. *Med Care.* 1981;19:489–497.

52. Lawton MP, Brody EM. Assessment of older people: Self-maintaining and instrumental activities of daily living. *Gerontologist.* 1969;9:179–186.

53. The Older American Resources and Services (OARS) Methodology. *Multidimensional Functional Assessment Questionnaire.* 2nd ed. Durham, NC: Duke University Center for the Study of Aging and Human Development; 1978:169–170.

54. Teresi JA, Cross PS, Golden RR. Some applications of latent trait analysis to the measurement of ADL. *J Gerontol.* 1989;44:196–204.

55. Suurmeijer TPBM, Doeglas DM, Moum T, et al. The Groningen Activity Restriction Scale for measuring disability: Its utility in international comparisons. *Am J Public Health.* 1994;84:1270–1273.

56. Gallo JJ, Franch MS, Reichel W. Dementing illness: The patient, caregiver, and community. *Am Fam Phys.* 1991;43:1669–1675.

57. Paveza GJ, Prohaska T, Hagopian M, Cohen D. *Determination of Need Revision: Final Report.* Vol I. Chicago: Gerontology Center, University of Illinois at Chicago; 1989.

58. Stewart AL, Ware JE. *Measuring Functioning and Well-Being.* Durham, NC: Duke University Press; 1993.

59. McHorney CA. Measuring and monitoring general health status in elderly persons: Practical and methodological issues in using the SF-36 health survey. *Gerontologist.* 1996;36:571–583.

60. Wells KB, Stewart A, Hays RD, et al. The functioning and well-being of depressed patients: Results from the Medical Outcomes Study. *JAMA.* 1989;262:914–919.

61. Stewart AL, Greenfield S, Hays RD, et al. Functional status and well-being of patients with chronic conditions: Results from the Medical Outcomes Study. *JAMA.* 1989; 262:907–913.

62. Stewart AL, Hays RD, Ware JE. The MOS Short-form General Health Survey: Reliability and validity in a patient population. *Med Care.* 1988;26:724–735.

63. Stadnyk K, Calder J, Rockwood K. Testing the measurement properties of the Short Form-36 health survey in a frail elderly population. *J Clin Epidemiol.* 1998;51:827–835.

64. Branch LG, Meyers AR. Assessing physical function in the elderly. *Clin Geriatr Med.* 1987;3:29–51.

65. Rubenstein LZ, Schairer C, Willard GD, et al. Systematic biases in functional status assessment of elderly adults. *J Gerontol.* 1984;39:686–691.

66. Dorevitch MI, Cossar RM, Bailey FJ, et al. The accuracy of self and informant ratings of physical functional capacity in the elderly. *J Clin Epidemiol.* 1992;45:791–798.

67. Pincus T, Callahan LF, Brooks RH, Fuchs HA, Olsen NJ, Kaye JJ. Self-report questionnaire scores in rheumatoid arthritis compared with traditional physical, radiographic, and laboratory measures. *Ann Intern Med.* 1989;110:259–266.

68. Kelly-Hayes M, Jette AM, Wolf PA, D'Agostino RB, Odell PM. Functional limitations and disability among elders in the Framingham study. *Am J Public Health.* 1992; 82:841–845.

69. Lowenstein DA, Amigo E, Duara R, et al. A new scale for the assessment of functional status in Alzheimer's disease and related disorders. *J Gerontol: Psychol Sci.* 1989; 44:P114–P121.

70. Marsiske M, Willis SL. Dimensionality of everyday problem solving in older adults. *Psychol Aging.* 1995;10:269–282.

71. Diehl M, Willis SL, Schaie KW. Practical problem solving in older adults: Observational assessment and cognitive correlates. *Psychol Aging.* 1995;10:478–491.

72. Guralnik JM, Branch LG, Cummings SR, Curb JD. Physical performance measures in aging research. *J Gerontol.* 1989;44:M141–146.

73. Kuriansky J, Gurland B. The Performance Test of Activities of Daily Living. *Int J Aging Hum Dev.* 1976;7:343–352.

74. Williams ME, Hadler NM, Earp JAL. Manual ability as a marker of dependency in geriatric women. *J Chronic Dis.* 1982;35:115–122.

75. Williams ME. Identifying the older person likely to require long-term care. *J Am Geriatr Soc.* 1987;35:761–766.

76. Williams ME, Gaylord SA, McGaghie WC. Timed manual performance in a community elderly population. *J Am Geriatr Soc.* 1990;38:1120–1126.

77. Williams ME, Gaylord SA, Gerrity MS. The timed manual performance test as a predictor of hospitalization and death in a community-based elderly population. *J Am Geriatr Soc.* 1994;42:21–27.

78. Tinetti M. Performance-oriented assessment of mobility problems in elderly patients. *J Am Geriatr Soc.* 1986;34:119–126.

79. Mathias S, Nayak USL, Isaacs B. Balance in elderly patients: The "get up and go" test. *Arch Phys Med Rehabil.* 1986;67:387–389.

80. Salgado R, Lord SR, Packer J, Ehrlich F. Factors associated with falling in elderly hospital patients. *Gerontology.* 1994;40:325–331.

81. Duncan PW, Weiner DK, Chandler J, Studentski S. Functional reach: A new clinical measure of balance. *J Gerontol: Med Sci.* 1990;45:192–197.

82. Guralnik JM, Reuben DB, Buchner DM, Ferrucci L. Performance measures of physical function in comprehensive geriatric assessment. In: Rubenstein LZ, Wieland D, Bernabei R, eds. *Geriatric Assessment Technology: The State of the Art.* New York: Springer Publishing Co; 1995:59–74.

83. Reuben DB, Siu AL. An objective measure of physical function of elderly outpatients: The Physical Performance Test. *J Am Geriatr Soc.* 1990;38:1105–1112.

84. Rozzini R, Frisoni GB, Bianchetti A, et al. Physical Performance Test and activities of daily living scales in the assessment of health status in elderly people. *J Am Geriatr Soc.* 1993;41:1109–1113.

85. Winograd CH, Lemsky CM, Nevitt MC, et al. Development of a physical performance and mobility examination. *J Am Geriatr Soc.* 1994;42:743–749.

86. Freels S, Cohen D, Eisdorfer C, et al. Functional status and clinical findings in patients with Alzheimer's disease. *J Gerontol: Med Sci.* 1992;47:M177–M182.

87. Blessed G, Tomlinson BE, Roth M. The association between quantitative measures of dementia and of senile changes in the cerebral grey matter of elderly subjects. *Br J Psychiatry.* 1968;114:797–811.

88. Moore J, Bobula JA, Short TB, et al. A Functional Dementia Scale. *J Fam Pract.* 1983;16:499–503.

89. Teri L, Truax P, Logsdon R, Uomoto J, Zarit S, Vitaliano PP. Assessment of behavioral problems in dementia: The revised Memory and Behavior Problems checklist. *Psychol Aging.* 1992;7:622–631.

90. Zarit SH, Todd PA, Zarit J. Subjective burden of husbands and wives as caregivers: A longitudinal study. *Gerontologist.* 1986;26:260–266.

91. Zarit SH, Anthony CR, Boutselis M. Interventions with care givers of dementia patients: Comparison of two approaches. *Psychol Aging.* 1987;2:225–232.

92. Gallo JJ. The effect of social support on depression in caregivers of the elderly. *J Fam Pract.* 1990;30:430–436.

93. Reisberg B, Ferris SH, DeLeon MJ, et al. The global deterioration scale for assessment of primary degenerative dementia. *Am J Psychiatry.* 1982;139:1136–1139.

94. Reisberg B, Ferris SH, Borenstein J, et al. Assessment of presenting symptoms. In: Poon LW, ed. *Clinical Memory Assessment of Older Adults.* Washington, DC: American Psychological Association; 1986.

95. Smyer MA, Hofland BF, Jonas EA. Validity study of the Short Portable Mental Status Questionnaire for the elderly. *J Am Geriatr Soc.* 1979;27:263–269.

96. Shuttleworth EC. Memory function and the clinical differentiation of dementing disorders. *J Am Geriatr Soc.* 1982;30:363–366.

97. Fillenbaum G. Comparison of two brief tests of organic brain impairment, the MSQ and the Short Portable MSQ. *J Am Geriatr Soc.* 1980;28:381–384.

98. Eisdorfer C, Cohen D, Paveza GJ, et al. An empirical evaluation of the Global Deterioration Scale for staging Alzheimer's disease. *Am J Psychiatry.* 1992;149:190–194.

99. Paveza GJ, Cohen D, Jankowski LM, Freels S. An analysis of the Global Deterioration Scale in older persons applying for community care services. *J Ment Health Aging.* 1995;1:35–45.

100. Reisberg B. Dementia: A systematic approach to identifying reversible causes. *Geriatrics.* 1986;41:30–46.

101. Reisberg B, Ferris SH, Franssen E. An ordinal functional assessment tool for Alzheimer-type dementia. *Hosp Community Psychiatry.* 1985;36:593–595.

102. Hughes CP, Berg L, Danziger WL, et al. A new clinical scale for the staging of dementia. *Br J Psychiatry.* 1982;140:566–572.

103. Davis PB, Morris JC, Grant E. Brief screening tests versus clinical staging in senile dementia of the Alzheimer type. *J Am Geriatr Soc.* 1990;38:129–135.

104. Burke WJ, Miller JP, Rubin EH, et al. Reliability of the Washington University clinical dementia rating. *Arch Neurol.* 1988;45:31–32.

105. Winograd CH. Mental status tests and the capacity for self care. *J Am Geriatr Soc.* 1984;32:49–53.

106. Gelb DJ, St. Laurent RT. Alternative calculation of the Global Clinical Dementia Rating. *Alzheimer Dis Assoc Disord.* 1993;7:202–211.

107. Williams TF, Williams ME. Assessment of the elderly for long-term care. *J Am Geriatr Soc.* 1982;30:71–75.

108. Rabins P, Mace NL, Lucas MJ. The impact of dementia on the family. *JAMA.* 1982;248:333–335.

109. Pace WD, Anstett RE. Placement decisions for the elderly: A family crisis. *J Fam Pract.* 1984;18:31–46.

110. Williams TF. Assessment of the geriatric patient in relation to needs for services and facilities. In: Reichel W, ed. *Clinical Aspects of Aging.* 2nd ed. Baltimore: Williams & Wilkins; 1983:543–548.

111. Weed L. *Medical Records, Medical Education, and Patient Care.* Cleveland, OH: Case Western Reserve Press; 1970.

5

The Older Driver

David Carr and George W. Rebok

INTRODUCTION

The automobile is the most important source of transportation for older adults. The ability to drive or be driven is crucial for older persons to maintain an important link with society. Functional assessment, which can include driving ability, is a key component for clinicians involved in providing geriatric care. Clinicians should determine whether their patients are currently driving, provide information on healthy driving behaviors, assess medical conditions or physiologic variables that place their patients at increased risk for a motor vehicle injury or driving cessation, and intervene and treat medical illnesses that can impair driving skills.

Some clinicians may be reluctant to address driving habits. However, one could argue that impaired driving skills should not be viewed any differently from the prevention, detection, and improvement of impaired walking, which can result in a fall or other injury. Epidemiological studies have just begun to identify risk factors for driving cessation and motor vehicle crash or injury in older adults.[1] There is still a need to validate current risk factors and to determine additional risk factors and study whether interventions are a benefit to the patient or society. While awaiting further investigation in this area, the clinician should not delay in assessing or assisting older adults with their driving skills.

BEHAVIORS AND CHARACTERISTICS OF OLDER DRIVERS

There will be a rapid increase in the number of older drivers on the road in the next few decades. This can be attributed to the aging of our driving population in the United States and especially to an increase in the number of older adult female drivers.[2] It appears that each new cohort of older drivers is increasing their average miles driven per year, but still drive fewer miles per year than other age groups.[3] However, the percentage of the population that is actively driving decreases with each decade.[4] Older drivers report less driving at night or during adverse weather conditions, and avoid rush hour or congested thoroughfares. Most importantly, functionally impaired older adults appear to even further restrict their exposure.[5]

The traffic violation rate per licensed driver is increased for both the younger and older driver.[6] Older adults tend to be ticketed for making left-hand turns, failure to yield, or missing stop or traffic signs. These violations tend to reflect problems with attention and complex traffic situations. Older drivers have been noted to take longer to complete turns in intersections.[7] In contrast, younger people tend to have higher rates of violations for speeding, reckless driving, and driving while intoxicated. Older adult drivers (over age 65 years) account for a very small percentage of the motor vehicle crashes and injuries in comparison to other age groups due to fewer number of licensed drivers and reduced exposure. However, public safety concerns about the driving performance of this group have been raised by many studies that reveal an increased crash rate per mile driven for drivers aged 70 years or more.[8] This crash rate has been attributed to age-related changes in driving skills such as visual search and reaction time,[9] in addition to the presence of medical diseases.[10] The actual contribution of each of these factors to this increase in crash rate is unknown.

Dementia may be one of the major medical illnesses that contributes to the increased crash rate in older adults.[11] This may not be surprising given the prevalence of dementia of the Alzheimer type, which doubles every 5 years over the age of 65 years.[12] One study that administered a mental status screen to older adults during driver license renewal revealed that 20% of drivers over age 80 demonstrated significant cognitive impairment.[13] Studies in tertiary referral centers have revealed an increased crash rate in drivers with dementia of the Alzheimer type in comparison with controls[14-16] although there have been exceptions.[17] Larger population-based studies that are able to identify cognitively impaired drivers by brief cognitive screens have found modest increases in crash rates in older adult drivers.[18] However, it is often difficult to find associations between cognitive and visual impairment and crashes because of the infrequent occurrence of these events, along with the reduction in the number of trips made over time.

OLDER DRIVERS AT RISK FOR A MOTOR VEHICLE CRASH OR DRIVING CESSATION

Risk for a Motor Vehicle Crash

Common diseases in older drivers that have been noted to affect driving ability include, but are not limited to, visual impairment,[19] diabetes mellitus,[20] seizure disorders,[21] Alzheimer's disease,[22] cerebrovascular accidents,[23] depression,[24] cardiovascular disease,[25] sleep disorders,[26] arthritis and related musculoskeletal disorders,[27] and alcohol and drug use.[28]

There are relatively few studies that have focused on older drivers and medical conditions as risk factors for motor vehicle crashes. One study utilizing a case control approach from a health maintenance organization found an increase in the crash and injury rate for older diabetics taking insulin or hypoglycemic agents.[29] A recent population-based study reported an increase in crashes and ticketed violations among older adults with heart disease.[30] Some studies have found greater risk associated with physiologic variables than with medical diagnoses.[31] More studies are needed to examine the effect of multiple illnesses on the driving task.

Diseases should be graded as to their severity and ability to impact on driving errors or the human factors. For instance, diabetes has a potential to affect the three important domains of driving: (1) perception (eg, from retinopathy or cataract), (2) cognition (eg, from hypoglycemia), and (3) motor response (eg, from neuropathy). Thus, a clinician may have to make a determination as to the severity of the disease and weigh this finding with the set of patient characteristics. Doing so becomes more difficult in older drivers when one may be dealing with multiple mild to moderate diseases (eg, visual impairment, mild cognitive impairment, and arthritis).

Another approach to index crash risk in older adults is to perform functional or physiologic measures.[32] With increasing age and the presence of age-related diseases, studies have documented a decline in vision,[33] hearing,[34] and reaction time.[35] A decline in glare recovery time,[36] contrast sensitivity,[37] dynamic visual acuity,[38] visual fields,[39] visuospatial skills,[40] complex reaction time,[41] selective,[42] and divided attention[43] have all been noted to adversely affect driving skills. There has been a decline noted in the functional visual field or "useful field of view" with age, and this measure has also been correlated with crash data in an older driver sample that was screened to be at high risk for a crash.[44] There is a brief computerized version of the useful field of vision that is available to clinicians. However, its utility as an office screen or assessment tool awaits further studies to determine its sensitivity, specificity, and positive predictive value in additional settings such as outpatient medical clinics or other high-risk cohorts of older drivers.

Diseases or syndromes such as angina, arrythmias, diabetes, seizures, syncope, transient ischemic attacks, cerebrovascular accidents, and arthritis should be assessed for disease severity to determine whether the disease can have an impact on driving. Polypharmacy is not uncommon in older adults. There are many common medication classes that have been studied and noted to either increase crash risk or impair driving skills when assessed by simulators or road tests. These include, but are not limited to, narcotics, benzodiazepines, antihistamines, antidepressants, antipsychotics, hypnotics, alcohol, and muscle relaxants. A recent study focused on older drivers noted that long-acting benzodiazepines have been associated with increased crash rates.[45] Another report suggests that there may be a significant number of older adults driving while intoxicated or under the influence of other medications.[46,47]

There is a growing consensus among clinicians and experts in the field that there are many conditions and decrements in physiologic variables that can impact driving and can easily be assessed by clinicians.[48-50] The interested clinician can check static visual acuity with the Snellen chart; hearing with the whisper test or hand held audiometry; attention and reaction time with Trails A or B; visual spatial skills with the clock-drawing task; and judgment, insight, muscle strength, and joint range of motion with a physical exam. Impairments in any of these variables should be assessed for their etiologies, and a treatment plan developed. Referral to a subspecialist may be in order.

Clinicians should also incorporate an injury control approach into their health maintenance practice for older adults. Important driving issues that the clinician should discuss with the older driver include using a seat belt, drinking alcohol, using a cellular phone while driving, obeying the speed limit, and enrolling in refresher courses such as 55 Alive sponsored by the American Association of Retired Persons.

Cessation

There are times when the clinician may have to recommend that his or her patient stop driving, especially when a significant medical condition is involved. Many older drivers have been driving longer than their physicians have been practicing medicine. Hence, it is important for health professionals to discuss these issues in a sensitive manner. The physician can play an important role in enforcing driving cessation by encouraging the patient's acceptance of the situation. The physician should also suggest alternative transportation resources. These discussions should be documented in the patient's chart.

Public transportation systems[51] may have reduced fares for senior citizens. Due to restricted sites and the physical or cognitive limitations in the older driver, these services are typically underutilized. State- or local-sponsored services may provide door-to-door transportation for older adults in large vans, many of which are equipped with lifts. Local communities, societies, retirement centers, or local church groups may use funds or volunteers to provide services to physicians' offices, grocery stores, and meetings.

Patients may refuse to stop driving despite advice from a family member or a clinician. The patient may request a referral for another opinion. This should only be reserved for questionable cases since some evaluations (private or state) may be cursory or superficial. The clinician may consider writing a letter to the state department of motor vehicles (DMV). The ethics and legal ramifications of this letter are discussed in the last section of this chapter.

Special mention is made of the older adult driver who does not have insight into his or her own illness such as when he or she is suffering from Alzheimer's disease. The spouse, family, physician, occupational therapist, and DMV may need to work together to keep those individuals judged to be unsafe from driving. In situations where the patient does not have insight into his or her driving limitations, these efforts may include involving the police or DMV to confiscate the driver's license, or involving family members to remove access to car keys, move the automobile off the premises, change door locks, file down the ignition keys, or disable the battery cable.

ASSESSING DRIVING SKILLS

Referral Sources

There are many health professionals and organizations that may assist in the education, training, or assessment of the older driver. These include, but are not limited to, subspecialists in the field of medicine (eg, neurology and cardiology), neuropsychologists, occupational therapists, physical therapists, courses such as 55 Alive, the medical advisory board of the state or driver improvement office, and insurance companies. A driving simulator may also play a role in assessing driving abilities.

Road performance tests are yet another method for evaluating driving skills. Road tests have some limitations since they are often scored subjectively, the road conditions may vary, and the tests may be performed in a car on a driving course that is unfamiliar to the subject. However, road tests have been advocated by several authors as the preferred method to assess driving competency.[52,53] Occupational therapists, often based at rehabilitation centers, may have specific training and experience in evaluating drivers with medical impairments. The therapist may be able to assist in modifications to the vehicle that could enable its safe and timely operation.

The physical therapist can be an indispensable member of the driving rehabilitation team. Large studies on older adult drivers in the community indicate that back pain, arthritis,[54] and the use of pain medications[55] are associated with increased crash rates. Thus, limitations in muscle strength due to pain or disuse, or restrictions in range of motion of joints such as the hands, feet, and neck may play an important role in driving impairment. Interventions to improve muscle strength and joint function have the potential to improve driving skills.

ETHICAL, LEGAL, AND PUBLIC POLICY ISSUES

Patients and families do not always comply or agree with clinicians' recommendations to stop driving. Physicians may simply decide to document this refusal in the chart, as long as the opinion is given to someone who has decision-making capacity. However, this situation may justify a letter to the state's DMV. This breach of confidentiality may be appropriate when performed in the best interest of the community.[56] Obviously, the state DMV will ultimately have the final decision as to whether someone can remain licensed to drive. Most states will follow the advice of the physician or occupational therapist. There are appeal processes for these situations, however. The decision to report patients to the DMV varies depending on personal practices and state requirements. Since the common law and statutes vary among states, legal counsel should be obtained to help guide the evaluation process and determine the regulations that should apply for practices in each state. Some states such as California require physicians to report specific medical conditions such as dementia of the Alzheimer type.

FUTURE RESEARCH NEEDS AND CONCLUSIONS

Current research and studies on older drivers have focused on methods to identify the medically impaired driver who is at risk for a motor vehicle crash or at risk for driving cessation. A comprehensive, step-by-step approach appears to be the most appropriate method to assess older adult drivers when safety issues or functional impairment have been raised or identified. Physicians should take an active role in assessing risk for injury while driving. Referral to other professionals or organizations may be helpful in the evaluation and treatment process as well as in the maintenance of the driving skills of older adults.

REFERENCES

1. Marottoli RA, Richardson ED, Stowe MH, et al. Development of a test battery to identify older drivers at risk for self-reported adverse driving events. *J Am Geriatr Soc.* 1998;46:562–568.

2. Retchin SM, Anapolle J. An overview of the older driver. *Clin Geriatr Med.* 1993;9:279–296.

3. O'Neil, D. The older driver. *Rev Clin Gerontol.* 1996;6:295–302.

4. Foley DJ, Wallace RB, Eberhard J. Risk factors for motor vehicle crashes among older drivers in a rural community. *J Am Geriatr Soc.* 1995;43:776–781.

5. Ball K, Owsley C, Stalvey B, et al. Driving avoidance and functional impairment in older drivers. *Accident Analysis Prev.* 1998;30:313–322.

6. Graca JL. Driving and aging. *Clin Geriatr Med.* 1986;2:577.

7. Cox AB, Cox DJ. Compensatory driving strategy of older people may increase driving risk. *J Am Geriatr Soc.* 1998;46:1058–1059.

8. Evans L. Older driver involvement in fatal and severe traffic crashes. *J Gerontol.* 1988;43:S189.

9. Reuben D. Assessment of older drivers. *Clin Geriatr Med.* 1993;9:445–459.

10. Waller J. Cardiovascular disease, aging, and traffic accidents. *J Chronic Dis.* 1967;20:615–620.

11. Odenheimer G. Dementia and the older driver. *Clin Geriatr Med.* 1993;9:349–364.

12. Jorm AF, Korten AE, Henderson AS. The prevalence of dementia: A quantitative integration of the literature. *Acta Psychiatr Scand.* 1987;76:465–479.

13. Stutts JC, Stewart JR, Martell CM. Cognitive test performance and crash risk in an older driver population. *Accident Analysis Prev.* 1998;30:337–346.

14. Friedland R, Koss E, Kumar A, et al. Motor vehicle crashes in dementia of the Alzheimer type. *Ann Neurol.* 1988;24:782–786.

15. Drachman D, Swearer J. Driving and Alzheimer's disease: The risk of crashes. *Neurology.* 1993;43:2448–2456.

16. Dubinsky R, Williamson A, Gray C, Glatt S. Driving in Alzheimer's disease. *J Am Geriatr Soc.* 1992;40:1112–1116.

17. Trobe JD, Waller PF, Cook-Flannagan CA, Teshima SM, Bieliauskas LA. Crashes and violations among drivers with Alzheimer's disease. *Arch Neurol.* 1996;53:411–416.

18. Foley DJ, Wallace RB, Eberhard J. Risk factors for motor vehicle crashes among older drivers in a rural community. *J Am Geriatr Soc.* 1995;43:776–781.

19. Shinar D, Schieber F. Visual requirements for safety and mobility of older drivers. *Hum Factors.* 1991;33:505–519.

20. Crancer JA Jr, McMurray L. Accident and violation rates of Washington's medically restricted drivers. *JAMA.* 1968;205:272–276.

21. Hansotia P, Broste SK. The effect of epilepsy or diabetes mellitus on the risk of automobile accidents. *N Engl J Med.* 1991;324:22–26.

22. Drachman DA, Swearer JM. Driving and Alzheimer's disease: The risk of crashes. *Neurology.* 1993;42:2448–2456.

23. Wilson T, Smith T. Driving after stroke. *Int Rehabil Med.* 1983;5:170–177.

24. Doege TC, Engelberg AL, eds. *Medical Conditions Affecting Drivers.* Chicago: American Medical Association; 1986.

25. Waller JA. Chronic medical conditions and traffic safety: Review of the California experience. *N Engl J Med.* 1965;273:1413–1420.

26. Findley LJ, Unverzagt ME, Suratt PM. Automobile accidents involving patients with obstructive sleep apnea. *Am Rev Respir Dis.* 1988;138:337–340.

27. Roberts WN, Roberts P. Evaluation of the elderly driver with arthritis. *Clin Geriatr Med.* 1993;9:311–322.

28. Ray WA, Gurwitz J, Decker MD, Kennedy DL. Medications and the safety of the older driver: Is there a basis for concern? *Hum Factors.* 1992;34:33–47.

29. Koepsell TD, Wolf ME, McCloskey L, Buchner DM, Louie D, Wagner EH, and Thompson RS. Medical conditions and motor vehicle collision injuries in older adults. *J Am Geriatr Soc.* 1994;42:695–700.

30. Gallo JJ, Rebok GW, Lesikar SE. The driving habits of adults aged 60 years and older. *J Am Geriatr Soc.* 1999;47:335–341.

31. Sims RV, Owsley C, Allman RM, et al. A preliminary assessment of the medical and functional factors associated with vehicle crashes by older adults. *J Am Geriatr Soc.* 1998; 46:556–561.

32. Wallace RB, Retchin SM. A geriatric and gerontologic perspective on the effects of medical conditions on older drivers: Discussion of Waller. *Hum Factors.* 1992;34:17–24.

33. Kline DW, Schieber F. Vision and aging. In: Birren JE, Schaie KW, eds. *Handbook of the Psychology of Aging.* 3rd ed. New York: Van Nostrand Reinhold; 1990:296–331.

34. Olsho L, Harkins S, Lenhardt M. Aging and the auditory system. In: Birren JE, Schaie KW, eds. *Handbook of the Psychology of Aging.* 3rd ed. New York: Van Nostrand Reinhold; 1985:332–377.

35. Salthouse T. Speed of behavior and its implications for cognition. In: Birren JE, Schaie KW, eds. *Handbook of the Psychology of Aging.* 2nd ed. New York: Van Nostrand Reinhold; 1985:400–426.

36. Burg A. *The Relationship Between Vision Test Scores and Driving Record: General Findings.* Los Angeles: Department of Engineering, University of California, Los Angeles; 1967. Report 67–24.

37. Shinar D, Schieber F. Visual requirements for safety and mobility of older drivers. *Hum Factors.* 1991;33:511.

38. Burg A. *Vision Test Scores and Driving Record: Additional Findings.* Department of Engineering, University of California, Los Angeles; 1968. Report 68–27.

39. Johnson CA, Keltner JL. Incidence of visual field loss in 20,000 eyes and its relationship to driving performance. *Arch Ophthalmol.* 1983;101:371–375.

40. van Zomeren A, Brouwer W, Minderhound J. Acquired brain damage and driving: A review. *Arch Phys Med Rehabil.* 1987;6:702.

41. Mihal W, Barrett G. Individual differences in perceptual information processing and their relation to automobile involvement. *J Appl Psychol.* 1976;6:229–233.

42. Avolio B, Kroeck K, Panek P. Individual differences in information-processing ability as a predictor of motor vehicle accidents. *Hum Factors.* 1985;27:577–587.

43. Trobe JD. Test of divided visual attention predicts automobile crashes among older adults. *Arch Ophthalmol.* 1998;116:665.

44. Owsley C, Ball K, McGwin G, et al. Visual processing impairment and risk of motor vehicle crash among older adults. *JAMA.* 1998;279:1083–1088.

45. Hemmelgarn B, Suissa S, Huang A, et al. Benzodiazepine use and the risk of motor vehicle crash in the elderly. *JAMA.* 1997;278:27–31.

46. Higgins JP, Wright SW, Wrenn KD. Alcohol, the elderly, and motor vehicle crashes. *Am J Emerg Med.* 1996;14:265–267.

47. Johansson K, Bryding G, Dahl ML, et al. Traffic dangerous drugs are often found in fatally injured older male drivers. *J Am Geriatr Soc.* 1997;45:1029–1031.

48. Underwood M. The older driver. Clinical assessment and injury prevention. *Arch Intern Med.* 1992;152:735–740.

49. Foley KT, Mitchell SJ. The elderly driver: What physicians need to know. *Cleve Clin J Med.* 1997;64:423–428.

50. Marottoli RA, Cooney LM, Wagener DR, Doucette J, Tinetti ME. Predictors of automobile crashes and moving violations among elderly drivers. *Ann Intern Med.* 1994;121:842–846.

51. Roper TA, Mulley GP. Caring for older people: Public transport. *BMJ.* 1996;313:415–418.

52. Donnelly R, Karlinsky H. The impact of Alzheimer's disease on driving ability: A review. *J Geriatr Psychiatry Neurol.* 1990;3:67–72.

53. Kapust L, Weintraub S. To drive or not to drive: Preliminary results from road testing of patients with dementia. *J Geriatr Psychiatry Neurol.* 1992;5:210–216.

54. Foley DJ, Wallace RB, Eberhard J. Risk factors for motor vehicle crashes among older drivers in a rural community. *J Am Geriatr Soc.* 1995;43:776–781.

55. Tuokko H, Beattie BC, Tallman K, et al. Predictors of motor vehicle crashes in a dementia clinic population: The role of gender and arthritis. *J Am Geriatr Soc.* 1995;43:1444–1445.

56. Graca JL. Driving and aging. *Clin Geriatr Med.* 1986;2:577.

6

Social Assessment

Social assessment, medical assessment, including mental status, and functional assessment are the three critical elements of any comprehensive geriatric assessment.[1] Social assessment for older patients has two dimensions: (1) the sources and kinds of help available to the older person from the social network; and (2) the assessment of the primary caregiver or the "hidden patient," who is often the client's spouse.[2]

There are several elements that make up the social assessment. These elements include social support of both the client and the caregiver; caregiver burden; economic well-being, including health coverage; assessment of the client's living environment, including the immediate surrounding external environment; assessment for elder mistreatment; and assessment and assistance with values clarification to help clients prepare advance directives. The last issue is discussed in Chapter 7.

Social assessment is essential to a comprehensive assessment because it provides information vital to understanding the "fabric" of the client's life. This fabric permits either the individual assessor or the geriatric assessment team to develop an effective care plan. Such care plans must take into account who is providing care, how much money the client has available to pay for services, whether the client is at risk for mistreatment and whether that risk can be diminished, and whether the physical environment in which the client lives is conducive to his or her ability to remain in the community.

Social assessment may be the most time-consuming element of a comprehensive assessment. It may easily take the team or independent practitioner as long or longer to complete the social part of the assessment as it does to complete the medical history and functional assessments. Without proper information in this area, however, the capacity to plan for care will be adversely affected.[1]

No special sequence need be followed in conducting a social assessment. Rather, the needs of the client, family, or assessor should dictate how it is conducted. Regardless of the order chosen, all of the information discussed in this chapter should be covered.

ASSESSMENT OF SOCIAL SUPPORT

For many older adults, life is immeasurably enhanced by their relationship with their families. At no other time of life, save perhaps for childhood, does family play such a pivotal role. The benefits of the relationship are reciprocal. Older members of the family may give gifts and financial aid or may assist with domestic chores such as housekeeping or child care. They may assume the major role in raising grandchildren. In addition to these tangible tasks, older family members provide a sense of the life cycle to younger members. On the other hand, younger family members may provide companionship, nursing, transportation, and a source of pride to older members.

Children who find themselves caring for older parents may themselves be of retirement age or older. One fourth of all caregivers are 65 to 74 years of age, and 10% are over age 75.[3] One in ten persons over age 65 has a child who is at least 65 years of age.[4] Not uncommonly, the caregiver is a woman in her 60s caring for her mother in her 90s. Because more persons are living to advanced age, the average woman in 1980 might expect to spend more years caring for an elderly parent than would her counterpart in 1900.[5] Trends toward smaller families and, hence, fewer adult children to serve as caregivers as well as the increasing participation of women in the workplace further strain the support system for the older person.

The assessment of the social situation, particularly of the support available to the person unable to perform independently all the activities of daily living (ADL), is intimately intertwined with the issues surrounding nursing home placement. Numerous studies indicate the presence of a caregiver is the most important factor in the disposition of elderly patients from the hospital.[6-12] For example, a clinic at the University of Wisconsin assessed persons with Alzheimer's disease who were living in the community at the time of assessment. Those who eventually had to be placed in a nursing home did not differ from the others in their ability to perform the ADL or in health status. The major precipitating reason for placement was lack of a willing caregiver.[8] Despite myths to the contrary, families continue to provide help for their older members, sometimes stretching financial and emotional resources to the limit.

The support system of older adults comprises three components: the informal network, the formal support system, and semiformal supports.[13,14] Informal supports are provided by family and friends. Formal supports include Social Security, Medicaid, and the social welfare agencies. Semiformal support refers to the support provided by neighborhood organizations such as churches or senior citizen centers.[13]

Informal supports are generally selected by the older persons themselves, often based on longstanding relationships. The informal network is the constellation of social relationships that provides not only social interaction and discourse, such as daily phone contact, but also services, such as transportation to the physician's office or to the grocery store. A social network is the constellation of a person's social relationships, but social support is the actual help (ie, financial, emotional, or otherwise) that the social network provides.[15] Persons in the social network may or may not be helpful (ie, provide social support). For example, a son who lives nearby does not ensure adequate support for an elderly widow.

Neighbors who deal with the older person on a daily basis may perform chores or errands for him or her. The family may be unaware of the extent of the help provided by this "natural helper" network; indeed, the older person may not fully comprehend it.[16] The postal carrier who sees to it that the mail is picked up, the grocery clerk who helps with bags, and neighbors who bake and share their cooking and company are examples of natural helpers. In rural communities, informal helpers may acquire considerable importance because of geographic isolation and reluctance to participate in formal programs.[17] Some rural older persons are not comfortable receiving even informal assistance unless they have accumulated "social credit," that is, they have helped others.[18]

The *formal support system* consists of social welfare and other social service and health care delivery agencies. These programs play an important role in the social and physical well-being of older persons, especially in a mobile industrialized society, in which children move far from their parents.

Semiformal support such as church groups, neighborhood organizations, and clubs are important sources of social support for older adults. For many kinds of support, the older adult must take the initiative to gain access to services and might require encouragement or assistance to do so from health professionals or family members. Professionals who are providing care for older people should familiarize themselves with the available support and get a sense of what informal, formal, and semiformal help the older persons have employed in the past.

The assessment of social support can be conducted in a structured manner through the use of a variety of instruments that have been tested over time to assess social support, or through a more informal means by asking a series of questions aimed at gathering information about who provides help and support to both the older adult and the caregiver. The most fruitful method for providing the practitioner with the desired information may be a combination of a structured assessment instrument and open-ended questions.

One such formal assessment instrument is the Norbeck Social Support Questionnaire (Exhibit 6–1),[19,20] which has been shown to have strong construct validity. Moreover, it has been demonstrated to have utility for measuring social support not only with caregivers, but also for the clients themselves. This instrument's subscales likewise permit the determination of the areas in which a person perceives adequate social support and those areas in which the person perceives social support is lacking. The scale permits the ascertainment of information about complex social networks, including the actual perceived sources of support. Furthermore, this measure of social support has been linked to life stress indicators, suggesting the low social support scores are likely to be predictive of high stress and high scores with low stress. As has already been noted, it is this stress that puts many older adults at risk for institutionalization. Also, as will be discussed in detail later in this chapter, stress has been linked to elder mistreatment as well.[21]

The administration of this scale is fairly simple, and it can be included in those forms that the caregiver and client are asked to complete in the waiting room. The instrument requires that the person develop a list of supports, informal and semiformal, and then answer a brief set of questions about each of the listed supports. Experience suggests that it takes about 10 minutes for a person to complete the scale.

Exhibit 6–1 Norbeck Social Support Questionnaire

Please read all directions before starting.

Please list each significant person in your life and their relationship to you in the section headed Personal Network. Consider all the persons who provide personal support for you or who are important to you.

Use only first names or initials, and then indicate the person's relationship to you by choosing a corresponding number from the following list:

1 = spouse
2 = family member or relative
3 = friend
4 = work or school associate
5 = neighbor
6 = health care provider
7 = counselor or therapist
8 = minister/priest/rabbi
9 = other

Example:

1.	Mary T.	3
2.	Bob	2
3.	M.T.	6
4.	Sam	5
5.	Mrs. R.	7

You do not have to use all the spaces. Use only as many as you have important persons in your life.

When you have finished your list, please answer questions 1 through 8 for each of the persons on your personal network list.

PERSONAL NETWORK

First Name	Relationship
1. _____	1. _____
2. _____	2. _____
3. _____	3. _____
4. _____	4. _____
5. _____	5. _____
6. _____	6. _____
7. _____	7. _____
8. _____	8. _____
9. _____	9. _____
10. _____	10. _____

continues

Exhibit 6–1 continued

For each person that you listed, please answer the following questions by writing in the number that applies.

1 = not at all
2 = a little
3 = moderately
4 = quite a bit
5 = a great deal

Question 1:

How much does this person make you feel liked or loved?

1. _____
2. _____
3. _____
4. _____
5. _____
6. _____
7. _____
8. _____
9. _____
10. _____

Question 2:

How much does this person make you feel respected or admired?

1. _____
2. _____
3. _____
4. _____
5. _____
6. _____
7. _____
8. _____
9. _____
10. _____

Question 3:

How much can you confide in this person?

1. _____
2. _____
3. _____
4. _____
5. _____
6. _____
7. _____
8. _____
9. _____
10. _____

Question 4:

How much does this person agree with or support your actions or thoughts?

1. _____
2. _____
3. _____
4. _____
5. _____
6. _____
7. _____
8. _____
9. _____
10. _____

Question 5:

If you needed to borrow $10, a ride to the doctor, or some other immediate help, how much could this person usually help?

1. _____
2. _____

Question 6:

If you were confined to bed for several weeks, how much could this person help you?

1. _____
2. _____

continues

Exhibit 6–1 continued

3. _____   3. _____
4. _____   4. _____
5. _____   5. _____
6. _____   6. _____
7. _____   7. _____
8. _____   8. _____
9. _____   9. _____
10. _____   10. _____

Question 7:

How long have you known this person?

1 = less than 6 months
2 = 6 to 12 months
3 = 1 to 2 years
4 = 2 to 5 years
5 = more than 5 years

1. _____
2. _____
3. _____
4. _____
5. _____
6. _____
7. _____
8. _____
9. _____
10. _____

Question 8:

How frequently do you usually have contact with this person? (Phone calls, visits, or letters)

5 = daily
4 = weekly
3 = monthly
2 = a few times a year
1 = once a year or less

1. _____
2. _____
3. _____
4. _____
5. _____
6. _____
7. _____
8. _____
9. _____
10. _____

Question 9:

During the past year, have you lost any important relationship due to moving, a job change, divorce or separation, death, or some other reason?

0 = NO
1 = YES

If yes:
a. Please indicate the number of persons from each category who are no longer available to you.
_____ spouse
_____ family members or relatives
_____ friends
_____ work or school associates

continues

Exhibit 6–1 continued

_____ neighbors
_____ health care providers
_____ counselor or therapist
_____ minister/priest/rabbi
_____ other(specify)

b. Overall, how much of your support was provided by these people who are no longer avaliable to you?

0 = none at all

1 = a little

2 = a moderate amount

3 = quite a bit

4 = a great deal

Source: Adapted with permission from J Norbeck et al., The Development of an Instrument to Measure Social Support, _Nursing Research,_ Vol. 30, No. 5, pp. 264–269, © 1981, and Vol. 32, No. 1, pp. 4–9, © 1983, Lippincott Williams & Wilkins.

Another scale that can be considered for assessment of social support is the Lubben Social Network Scale.[22] This scale, through a series of nine questions, seeks information about the nature of the client's social support system. This instrument, like the Norbeck scale, can be used equally well with the client and the caregiver to provide a broad-based picture about the size of the support network and its availability to assist with care and decision making.

If the practitioner believes that the use of a formal scale would either be too time-consuming or simply not fit into the assessment process, a number of options are available. Kane[23] has recently suggested that the minimum assessment of a person's social network should consist of three questions: (1) whether the person has anyone he or she can contact when the person needs help and who that person is, (2) how many _relatives_ other than children the person feels close to and with whom he or she has contact at least once a month, and (3) how many _friends_ the person feels close to and has contact with at least once a month. While these questions certainly would provide some sense of the size of the network and whether at least one person could be counted on for assistance, social support might more critically be seen as not only the numbers of persons, but also the willingness of those persons to provide assistance when needed.[19,23] As such, additional questions such as those suggested by Seeman and Berkman[24] or as suggested by Kane[23] are essential. Whatever format the practitioner uses, the size of the network and the availability of assistance for the client as well as the caregiver should be understood at the conclusion of the social support assessment.

ASSESSMENT OF CAREGIVER BURDEN

In a similar vein, the assessment of caregiver burden is as critical as the assessment of social support because of the significant risk associated with the caregiving experience. The task of caregiving can be demanding and onerous to the caregiver. Research suggests a clear link between the caregiving experience and the risk of depression among caregivers.[25,26] Furthermore, caregiver depression, particularly among those caring for family members with Alzheimer's disease, has been linked to increased risk of elder abuse.[27] These risks suggest that it is crucial for the practitioner to carefully assess for caregiver burden. Caregiver burden has been conceptualized into three components.[28] The first deals with the impairment of the older adult, including assessing the ability to perform ADL, sociability, disruptive behavior, and mental status. The severity of symptoms or impairment alone, however, may be a poor predictor of the degree of caregiver stress.[29] Second, the tasks that correspond to the older adult's needs are rated as difficult, tiring, or upsetting. Dealing with bowel or bladder incontinence, for example, would probably be considered more difficult, tiring, and upsetting than assisting with meals. Lastly, the impact of the behaviors and associated tasks on the caregiver's life is assessed. For example, having to care for an older family member may result in a change of job (eg, quitting or turning down a promotion) or redefined family relationships.[28] Administration of a short instrument, such as the Zarit Burden Interview, introduces the topic of caregiver stress. Instruments used to detect depression might also be used to screen the older caregiver. The prevalence of depression in caregivers may be very high, and the perceived burden of care may be greater when depression is present.[30,31]

Caregiver burden is often linked with the caregiver's coping capabilities and perception of mechanisms he or she can use to assist in handling the stresses inherent in the caregiving situation.[32] It is useful for the clinician to seek information about coping style, including the use of a variety of techniques that have been described by Pearlin[33,34] and by Stephens and her colleagues.[35] Given the increased physical burden of caregiving, and that many caregivers are over 65 themselves,[4] assessing the physical well-being of the caregiver has practical value as well. The caregiver with cardiovascular problems, arthritis, or chronic back problems cannot be expected to do heavy lifting in the course of caring for an impaired older person. This emphasizes again the need to consider the functional status of older caregivers. In one survey, one third of caregivers rated their health as "fair or poor."[4] Other investigators showed that caregivers had three times as many stress-related symptoms and used more psychoactive drugs than similar control subjects.[26]

In addition to assessing burden and coping styles, the clinician might wish to expand the caregiver assessment into other areas that are likely to affect the caregiver's ability to provide useful care. While this may lengthen the process, if conducted by a coworker or ancillary worker, this part of the assessment may be conducted while the physician is completing other parts of the assessment. Areas of caregiver assessment that should also be considered included a formal assessment for depression as well as one of the caregiver's social support system, mental status, and functional status. While the need for assessing these may appear obvious, clinical experience suggests that these areas are often overlooked. Unaddressed, these issues may affect the ability of the caregiver to provide care, thereby resulting in a more rapid institutionalization of the primary client.

Caregiver depression can increase the caregiver's sense of hopelessness in coping with the caregiving experience. It is also possible that while the primary client may describe a reasonable support system, the caregiver may describe a very different one. When this is the case, the physician needs to view the caregiver as fragile and in need of strengthening through the infusion of external services. Of equal importance is taking the time to check the mental and functional status of the caregiver. Clinical experience with caregivers of persons with Alzheimer's has shown caregivers who are as cognitively impaired as and sometimes more than the family members diagnosed with the disease. Such a caregiver, particularly when a spouse, is often simply better at hiding the problem than the diagnosed family member. This kind of caregiving situation could easily result in both persons suffering from lack of care. A similar possibility exists if the clinician fails to assess the functional ability of the caregiver. Again, clinical experience has demonstrated that it is not unusual to have a caregiver that has equal or greater functional impairment than the primary client. Failure to assess this may result in the primary client's and the caregiver's being hospitalized or placed in a long-term care facility prematurely.

ASSESSMENT OF ELDER MISTREATMENT

Assessment of elder mistreatment for many health providers constitutes a dilemma because state laws require them to report suspected elder mistreatment, but providers are concerned that doing so may damage the doctor-patient bond. While this concern is understandable, failure to assess for elder mistreatment increases the risk of premature institutionalization and in some cases premature death.

Currently all 50 states and most U.S. territories have either adult protection statutes or elder abuse statutes. These laws are specifically designed to assist with providing needed social services to older adults who are the victims of mistreatment. While it is true that in some states these statutes are part of the criminal code in which punishment of the abuser is of equal concern, in almost all states in which there are criminal protective statutes, there are also statutes whose purpose is to help provide needed assistance to the older adult who may be the victim of such mistreatment.

It is critical that the health care provider understand the extent and seriousness of elder mistreatment. The National Elder Abuse Incidence Study (NEAIS)[36] indicated that approximately 450,000 older adults in domestic settings, who are not living in institutions, were abused or neglected in 1996. The study also suggests that if the number of older adults who self-neglect are included, the number increases to over 500,000. While these numbers may seem to suggest that abuse is a rare event, the NEAIS suggests that many older adults who are abused and neglected never come to the attention of sentinels or state investigative agencies.[36] If this is the case, then regardless of whether the health care provider chooses to report, he or she must assess for abuse and neglect or failure to provide an adequate standard of care.

While still in its infancy, research in the field of elder abuse and neglect has provided useful information regarding how to identify those at risk for abuse and neglect. Most often those at risk are among the more physically vulnerable who are often dependent on family members for physical care.[37] Other studies suggest that the most vulnerable are women[36] and that abuse is equally divided between spouse caregivers and child caregivers.[21,38] More recently, several studies have suggested that the prevalence of violence may be greater in families providing care to a member with Alzheimer's disease.[27,39,40] Moreover, these articles also suggest there are some unique factors that place persons suffering from Alzheimer's at greater risk for violence. These included depression, living arrangement, burden, years of care, hours of care per day, and whether the caregiver was the object of violence from the primary client.[27,39,40] It is important to remember that this work focuses on those older adults who are living in the general community. There has been little work on the presence of violence and neglect in institutional settings. Yet many of the older adults that health care providers see are living in just such situations.

As with other aspects of social assessment, assessment of elder mistreatment may be accomplished with the use of formal instruments or modifications of formal instruments. For instance, a modification of the Conflict Tactics Scale can be used to assess for physical abuse targeted toward older adults.[27,37,38,41] Other alternatives include the abuse assessment instrument developed by Fulmer and her colleagues[42] (Exhibit 6–2) for quickly assessing patients presenting in an emergency department setting. This instrument provides the health care provider with the types and range of questions that he or she needs to ask.

In cases of elder mistreatment, the practitioner must ensure that adequate and appropriate referral is made to either adult protective services or another social service agency capable of providing the needed interventions. The health care provider must understand, just like the victim must come to understand, that mistreatment rarely just stops, nor does it stop with some counseling.[43,44] Bringing an end to mistreatment requires consistent and ongoing intervention in almost all cases.

Once the health care provider has completed the social assessment to this stage, he or she must consider branching out into the broader aspects of the client's life including issues related to finances and living environment. Other issues that need to be addressed include the client's sexual functioning, spirituality, risk for suicide, and advance directives.

ECONOMIC ASSESSMENT

On the whole, older persons have come a long way in bettering their economic situations, particularly if money "in kind," meaning goods and services available free or at a cost below market value, is added to income. In addition, older adults receive special tax treatment, such as additional personal exemptions, property tax deductions, and, in some states, deferment of taxes until the homeowner's death.[45] The major economic problems affecting all but the wealthiest of elders remain catastrophic illness and long-term care, particularly nursing home costs.

For individuals, economic factors may have an impact on health, nutrition, and place of residence. Although the physician need not

Exhibit 6–2 Elder Abuse Assessment Form

Patient Stamp

Date: _____ Person completing form: _____

Patient Information

Name:_____ Age: _____ Unit #: _____

Address: _____

       Street   Phone #

    City, State, ZIP

Residence: Home ☐ Nursing home ☐ W10 form attached No ☐ Yes ☐

Accompanied to ED by: _____

                                    Name

    Street Address

    City, State, ZIP

Phone #: _____ Relationship to Patient: _____

Family Contact Person:

Name:_____

Street Address   City, State, ZIP   Phone #

Reason for visit (Please check primary reason.)

Cardiac ☐   Orthopaedic ☐   Fall ☐   GI ☐   Psychiatric ☐

Changed mental status ☐   Other (describe) _____

Current mental status

Oriented ☐   Confused ☐   Unresponsive ☐

Who provides home care?

_____

1. General assessment	*Very Good*	*Good*	*Poor*	*Very Poor*
a. clothing				
b. hygiene				
c. nutrition				
d. skin integrity				

Additional comments:_____

_____

_____

---

continues

Exhibit 6–2 continued

2. Possible abuse indicators	No Evidence	Possible Evidence	Probable Evidence	Definite Evidence
a. bruising				
b. lacerations				
c. fractures				
d. various stages of healing of any bruises or fractures				
e. evidence of sexual abuse				
f. statement by older adult regarding abuse				

Additional comments:_____

_____

_____

3. Possible neglect indicators	No Evidence	Possible Evidence	Probable Evidence	Definite Evidence
a. contractures				
b. decubitus ulcers				
c. dehydration				
d. diarrhea				
e. depression				
f. impaction				
g. malnutrition				
h. urine burns				
i. poor hygiene				
j. repetitive falls				
k. failure to respond to warning of obvious disease				
l. inappropriate medications (under/over)				
m. repetitive hospital admissions due to probable failure of health care surveillance				
n. statement by elder regarding neglect				

Additional comments:_____

_____

_____

continues

Exhibit 6–2 continued

4. Possible exploitation indicators	No Evidence	Possible Evidence	Probable Evidence	Definite Evidence
a. misuse of money				
b. evidence of exploitation				
c. reports of demands for goods in exchange for services				
d. inability to account for money/property				
e. statement by elder regarding exploitation				

Additional comments:_____

_____

5. Possible abandonment indicators	No Evidence	Possible Evidence	Probable Evidence	Definite Evidence
a. evidence that a caretaker has withdrawn care precipitously without alternate arrangements				
b. evidence that elder is left alone in an unsafe environment for extended periods of time without adequate support				
c. statement by elder regarding abandonment				

Additional comments:_____

_____

6. Summary indicators	No Evidence	Possible Evidence	Probable Evidence	Definite Evidence
a. evidence of abuse				
b. evidence of neglect				
c. evidence of exploitation				
d. evidence of abandonment				

continues

Exhibit 6–2 continued

Comments: _____

_____

_____

_____

_____

_____

_____

_____

_____

Examples of High Risk Signs and Symptoms

Abuse	Unexplained bruises, repeated falls, lab values inconsistent with history, fracture or bruises in various stages of healing (any report by patient of being physically abused should be followed up immediately).
Neglect	Listlessness, poor hygiene, evidence of malnourishment, inappropriate dress, decubitus ulcers, urine burns, reports of being left in an unsafe situation, reports of inability to get needed medications.
Exploitation	Unexplained loss of Social Security or pension checks, any evidence that material goods are being taken in exchange for care, any evidence that personal belongings (eg, house, jewelry, and car) are being taken over without consent or approval.
Abandonment	Evidence that the older adult has been dropped off at the emergency room or the family unit with no intention of coming back for him or her.
Other high-risk situations	Drug or alcohol addiction in the family, isolation of the older adult, history of untreated psychiatric problems, evidence of unusual family stress, excessive dependence of elder on caretaker.

Source: Adapted with permission from T Fulmer and T Wetle, Elder Abuse Screening and Intervention, *Nurse Practitioner,* Vol. 11, No. 5, pp. 33–38, © 1986, W.B. Saunders Company.

make detailed economic inquiries, he or she should keep in mind the reality of how older persons cope with their limited incomes. For example, an older person may fail to take prescribed medication or might alter the dosage schedule because of financial considerations.

Complaints that an older adult brings to the primary care practitioner can be a direct result of economic factors. Weight loss may occur when the person cannot afford proper nutrition or dentures that fit. The clinician may or may not use formal screening instruments analogous to those discussed for mental status testing; economic issues are ignored, however, only at the risk of recommending impractical therapies. Most definitions of comprehensive assessment include some evaluation of financial factors.[46-49]

Medicare, the government health insurance program, consists of two parts: part A, dealing with hospital insurance and paid for through payroll deductions of workers, and part B, paying for physician's bills and other costs and financed by voluntary participation of workers with a matching contribution from the government. Because of rising health care costs, a gap developed between the cost of health care and the amount of protection afforded by Medicare. Acute care costs, for example, for the last year of life are estimated to amount to 30% of all Medicare dollars, or 1% of the gross national product.[50] Medicare pays an average of 48% of the older adult's medical costs, at a time when more is spent on health care than before Medicare legislation in 1965.[45,51]

Medicare pays about 75% of hospital bills, 55% of physicians' bills, and, contrary to what many older persons think, just 2% of nursing home bills.[52] Some older persons think, incorrectly, that Medicare will cover their nursing home expenses. Part A of Medicare pays for 90 days of hospitalization and the first 20 days of skilled nursing facility care. The next 80 days of rehabilitative care are partially covered. After that, the resident uses personal resources, which, at current nursing home costs, would rapidly deplete all but the most wealthy person's resources.

Part B pays for physician services—up to 80% of "reasonable charges" as determined by the program (after an annual deductible). Physicians who accept "assignment" are paid directly by the program and agree to accept the sum as final payment.[45] Once a person is a resident in a nursing home, and the Medicare benefits run out, the resident then must spend down to a certain level to become eligible for Medicaid to pay the rest of the bills.

Medicare, however, remains principally an acute care coverage system. It is there to make sure that acute conditions are addressed and treated. It is not a provider of long-term coverage. Indeed, the system is set up in such a way that, for all intents and purposes, long-term coverage is effectively blocked. Thus as part of assessing coverage, the health care provider needs to determine the overall state of the client's finances and to query him or her about long-term care insurance or other insurance supplements that may provide for either community-based or institutional long-term care. Moreover, by understanding the nature of the client's income state, it may be possible to determine his or her eligibility for Supplemental Security Income and Medicaid benefits. The Medicaid system with its specific support of indigent long-term care may at times be the only system that permits the person to receive the needed community-based or institutional long-term care he or she requires.

The final element to consider when assessing economic well-being in the client is retirement. For most older adults this represents a significant life event, and for some it marks an important rite of passage to a new status with new privileges. The loss of social contact at work may leave the older adult with a void difficult to fill, and without planning, he or she may suddenly have much time at home with little to do. While many older workers retire for reasons of health, the issues surrounding retirement are intimately related to occupation and financial considerations. A significant number of retirees may not have personally fulfilling jobs and so welcome the chance to leave a boring or even dangerous occupation, wishing to retire as early as financially possible. Better economic conditions, including the proliferation of pension plans and the increased benefits from Social Security, allow a more comfortable retirement with less reluctance on the part of most people.[53,54]

Planning for retirement, and ensuring appropriate arrangements are made, is a field in its own right.[55] For most persons, income falls after retirement, but at the same time, retirees expect that their standard of living will not change. Indeed, this is the desirable goal toward which retirement planning strives. It is estimated that about 64% of preretirement income would be needed from interest and dividend income, pensions, and Social Security in order to maintain the same living standard as before retirement.[52]

Older adults constitute a largely untapped resource. This is true from an economic perspective as well as from a personal and societal one. The care of some frail older adults might be partially provided by healthy older people with special training. Teachers' aides and foster grandparent are other roles for retirees. Retired adults might choose to continue working, performing tasks not yet paying full market wages.[56] Since many older adults can expect to live one to two decades following retirement, such options could provide more opportunities for the productive use of time.

Retirement in the future will reflect changing careers, mobility of the work force, flexible work hours, shortened work weeks, and favorable attitudes toward work and retirement (see Chapter 1). In some settings, retirement is gradually phased in, as the older adult has a shorter and shorter workweek. Some older workers may remain as temporary consultants. Mental and physical functioning may be maintained through the pursuit of volunteer activities and hobbies, which should be actively encouraged by health professionals.

Anticipatory guidance with regard to the use of time, maintaining self-esteem, attitudes toward household tasks, and the moderate use of alcohol and tobacco may be useful to the retiree. Dr. Gene Cohen, former Director of the National Institute on Aging, suggests that older adults develop a "social portfolio" containing four compartments: (1) group active (activities that involve others actively, such as tennis or travel); (2) group passive (such as discussion groups centered around movies or books); (3) individual active (walking and gardening are examples); and (4) individual passive (like reading, woodworking, or knitting). Then when occupational roles wane, the older adult is ready with a portfolio of other activities that keep the mind and body active.

The clinician may feel uncomfortable asking questions about financial status; clues that indicate economic difficulty are sometimes overlooked or attributed to other causes. Note can be taken of the condition of shoes, handbags, and clothing (including the undergarments). In addition, economic reasons for noncompliance with the treatment regimen should be considered. A home visit may provide a more complete picture of the economic status of the older adult than is possible elsewhere. A rough indication of the adequacy of financial resources is the ability to spend money on small luxuries. Out-of-pocket expenses for health care may cut significantly into the elderly person's ability to use money for other purposes.

Although the total assets of an older person, such as a paid-for house, may be substantial, frequently such assets are not available to pay day-to-day bills. If income is low, the older person may choose deprivation rather than sell a familiar house. A home may have fallen into disrepair since taxes and maintenance costs have increased. What the older person once thought were adequate savings for his or her later years may no longer even pay the bills.

Many elders who need financial help do not receive it simply because they are unaware of where or how to receive it. The bureaucracy, with its endless forms to complete and numerous telephone calls necessary to coordinate services, can be overwhelming, even for a younger person. Some older persons may be illiterate, uneducated, and have a poor command of English; these characteristics further hamper their efforts to obtain help. The person may not understand written material even if it is in his or her native language. The stigma of public assistance may keep some older people from even making an inquiry about obtaining it.

The clinician may also choose to use a more formal assessment instrument. One of the domains assessed as part of the Older Americans Resources and Services (OARS) Multidimensional Functional Assessment Questionnaire (Exhibit 6–3) estimates the economic resources of older people.[48] Items deal with employment, sources of income, annual income, home ownership, and the client's subjective estimates of the adequacy of financial resources. The OARS Economic Resources section is an extensive questionnaire.

The primary goal for this part of the assessment is that the clinician learn whether the older person will be hindered in following the treatment plan because of financial difficulty. Providers should offer assistance to older adults in obtaining information and benefits, or should be prepared to refer them to someone who can.

ASSESSMENT OF THE ENVIRONMENT

A health care provider needs to be aware of problems in the client's environment that may limit his or her ability to carry out a care plan. In many cases, the assessment of the home brings out problems that are not readily apparent during an office interview.[57] A thorough environmental assessment should include such issues as the condition of the living arrangements; the nature of the neighborhood, including the physical infrastructure; and the transportation system. Steel and his colleagues[57] note there is a prima facie belief that understanding environment is critical when working with older adults. At the same time, they note little attention has been paid to how best to implement such an evaluation. Moreover, while there are several instruments available for assessment of the home,[57] there are few instruments that cover such issues as the physical infrastructure of the house, its foundation, and the sidewalks around the home, as well as available transportation systems.

Steel[57] offers a checklist (Exhibit 6–4) for assessing the client's home environment as well as solutions for addressing likely hazards that put the person at risk for physical harm requiring medical intervention.

While this checklist identifies hazards in the home, it does not cover issues of the home's or the neighborhood's infrastructure, which may affect the patient's ability to carry out proposed care plans. The lack of wheelchair ramps may make it impossible for a person to easily egress from their home. Broken or the lack of walkways and sidewalks may make it difficult for the person to get to public transportation. The assessor needs to determine by inspection whether there is appropriate

Exhibit 6–3 Economic Resources Assessment Scale of the Older Americans Resources and Services Multidimensional Functional Assessment Questionnaire

1. Are you presently employed full-time, part-time, retired, retired on disability, not employed and seeking work, or not employed and not seeking work? Or are you a full-time student or a part-time student?
2. What kind of work have you done most of your life?
3. Does your spouse work or did he or she ever work?
4. Where does your income (money) come from (that is, yours and your spouses')?
   - Earnings from employment
   - Income from rental, interest from investments, etc.
   - Social Security (but not Supplemental Security Income)
   - Veterans Administration Benefit
   - Disability payments not covered by Social Security, Supplemental Security Income, or the Veterans Administration
   - Unemployment compensation
   - Retirement pension from job
   - Alimony or child support
   - Scholarships or stipends
   - Regular assistance from family members
   - Regular financial aid from private organizations and churches
   - Welfare payments
   - Other
5. How much income do you and your spouse have in a year?
6. How many persons live on this income (that is, it provides at least half their income)?
7. Do you own your own home?
8. Are your assets and financial resources sufficient to meet emergencies?
9. Are your expenses so heavy that you cannot meet the payments, or can you barely meet the payments, or are your payments no problem to you?
10. Is your financial situation such that you believe you need financial assistance or help beyond what you are already getting?
11. Do you pay for your own food or do you get any regular help at all with costs of food or meals?
12. Do you believe that you need food stamps?
13. Are you covered by any kinds of health or medical insurance?
14. Please tell me how well you think you and your family are now doing financially as compared with other persons your age—better, about the same, or worse?
15. How well does the amount of money you have take care of your needs—very well, fairly well, or poorly?
16. Do you usually have enough to buy little extras, that is, those small luxuries?
17. Do you believe that you will have enough for your needs in the future?

Source: Reprinted with permission from Fillenbaum, G., *Multidimensional Functional Assessment of Older Adults: The Duke Older Americans Resources and Services Procedures*, Lawrence Erlbaum Associates, Inc., Hillsdale, NJ, 1988. (pp. 130–135).

means for exiting the home and accessing needed transportation. The assessor also needs to develop an understanding of the available public and private transportation services, particularly if the client is no longer able to drive, or if he or she no longer has any one to assist with transportation. It is also critical to understand how a person accesses and pays for the use of that system. The assessor must document all of these in order to place them in the context of the client's ability to get to needed services or treatments.

SEXUAL HEALTH ASSESSMENT

The sexual health of older adults is an important component of the overall health assessment. Unfortunately this area may inadvertently be omitted because of stereotypic beliefs regarding aging and sexuality.

Exhibit 6–4 Environmental Checklist

1. Where does the patient spend most of his or her time during the day (in what part of the house)?
2. How accessible are other parts of the house from this central location, especially toileting facilities, telephones? Does the person have sufficient mobility to reach other parts of the house if necessary?
3. If the person is using a walker or wheelchair, are rooms accessible to this equipment? Can the person enter and exit the house and get safely away from the house if necessary using these implements?
4. What type of floor coverings are used in the house? Is the house carpeted? Does it have wood or tile floors? What affect does this have on mobility? Are there throw rugs?
5. Is the lighting sufficient so the objects are easily visible to someone with poor vision?
6. Are there sufficient electrical outlets? If not, and extension cords are used, how are these laid out? Do they constitute an obstacle?
7. Consider stairs both inside and outside the house. How steep are they? Can someone with mobility problems traverse them?
8. Are heating and cooling sufficient for the needs of the person? Consider extremes in temperature, either hot or cold.
9. What other hazards may there be because of the person's disabilities, either physical or mental?
10. Consider the external environment. Are sidewalks available? Is parking available? What is the state of repair of the sidewalks?
11. Can the home be made accessible, and what would it take to make the home accessible?

There is clear evidence that while certain physiologic functions related to sexuality change with aging, healthy sex lives among older adults are the norm. In the 1940s and 50s, with the groundbreaking work of Kinsey and colleagues,[58,59] we began to understand sexuality in later life. While those early studies documented sexual functioning and capacity in older adults, they also documented changes in sexual capacity with aging. A recent study on sexual activity and satisfaction among 1,216 older adults (mean age 77.3) found that almost 30% engaged in sexual activity in the past month with 67% noting satisfaction with their sexual activities. That study noted that men were more likely to be sexually active but less apt than women to be satisfied with their sexual activity.[60,61] It is also true, however, that sexual activity is affected by declining health and selected medications. Libido and sexual response are inhibited when individuals are ill or on medications that may blunt sexual arousal response. In conducting a sexual health history, it is important to review systematically the individual's regular patterns of sex, expectations related to sex, and any changes in capacity or enjoyment, as well as to elicit the client's goals for a healthy sex life. Once the clinician understands these goals, he or she can recommend appropriate treatment and/or actions such as counseling, adjunct therapy, or physical aides to increase sexual capacity.[62]

It is key that the clinician understand that sexuality in late life is a normal and positive experience of aging. Clinicians need to assess their own level of comfort in eliciting a sexual history from the older adult, in that any discomfort on their part is likely to inhibit the older adult's ability to discuss his or her sexual life frankly. Key components of a sexual history should include an understanding of what the older adult's normal sexual patterns and interests have been over the course of his or her life, and if any changes have transpired that now affect sexual capacity and performance. Biologic factors, illness, and medication (Table 6–1) should all be reviewed. Medications are often contributors to sexual dysfunction. (In fact, individuals over age 65 take 25% of all prescription drugs and account for over half of all adverse drug reactions.)[63] Certain biologic factors that affect sexual interests and behaviors relate to normal aging. For men, the duration and intensity of sexual response changes with aging. Older men may take longer to achieve an excitement phase and experience a shortened, less forceful orgasm phase (Exhibit 6–5). Their resolution phase is more rapid with an increased refractory period between erections. In older women, the time needed to experience a sexual cycle (excitement, orgasm, and resolution) is increased with decreased vaginal expansion and lubrication. In some cases, uterine atrophy can cause painful intercourse.[62] Sexual desire is thought to be controlled by a dopamine-sensitive excitatory center along with serotonin-sensitive inhibitory centers.[64] True sexual dysfunction is described as the absence of one or more phases of the sexual response cycle: desire, excitement, orgasm, and/or resolution. Clinically, dysfunction could be further subdivided into: (1) primary sexual dysfunction, which is defined as realistic sexual expectations that have never been met under any circumstances; (2) secondary dysfunction, all phases have functioned in the past, but are no longer doing so; or (3) situational dysfunction, defined as the response cycle functions under some circumstances, but not others (Table 6–2).[64]

The clinician should elicit any sexual concerns or chief complaints during the course of the overall health assessment. At this juncture, there is the opportunity to educate the client about myths related to sexuality in aging: specifically, the myth that sexual behavior is aberrant in older individuals, and that there is no longer an opportunity for a healthy sex life in aging. Most important, the clinician must determine whether the individual's sexual activities are meeting his or her expectations and whether that person perceives there to be any sexual difficulties. In some cases, it might be useful to interview the older adult's partner; his or her responses may be different. The clinician can

Table 6–1 Drugs That Can Diminish Sexual Function in Women

Type of Agent	Example
Hypnotic agents	Alcohol, barbiturates
Tranquilizers	Chlordiazepoxide, diazepam
Narcotics	Heroin, methadone
Antipsychotic agents	Phenothiazines, butyrophenones
Antidepressants	Tricyclic agents, monoamine oxidase inhibitors
Stimulants	Cocaine, amphetamines
Anorectic agents	Fenfluramine
Hallucinogens	THC, LSD, PCP, mescaline
Hormones	Progestins, oral contraceptives
Antihypertensive agents	Reserpine, propranolol, methyldopa
Anticholinergic agents	Propantheline bromide
Diuretics	Acetazolamide

Note: *THC, tetrahydrocannabinol; LSD, lysergic acid diethylamide; and PCP, phenylcyclohexylpiperidine

Source: Reprinted with permission from AE Reading and JR Bragonier, Human Sexuality and Sexual Assault, in NF Hacker and JG Moore, Eds., Essentials of Obstetrics and Gynecology, 3rd ed., pp. 534–536, W.B. Saunders Company.

Exhibit 6–5 Sexual Problems That Occur in Older Patients

Women

Arousal

- Foreshortening of the vagina
- Slower and decreased vaginal lubrication
- Delayed and reduced vaginal expansion

Orgasm

- Fewer contractions
- Occasional painful uterine spasms
- Greater need for direct clitoral stimulation

Postorgasm

- No dilation of external cervical orifice
- Vaginal irritation and clitoral pain as a result of the thinner and more atrophic vaginal epithelium, which is more susceptible to mechanical trouble

Men

Arousal

- Delayed and less firm erection
- Longer interval to ejaculation
- Impaired sense of timing of orgasm

Orgasm

- Shorter ejaculation event
- Fewer expulsion contractions
- Less forceful expulsion of semen
- Reduced volume of seminal fluid

Postorgasm

- Rapid loss of erection
- Longer refractory period

Source: Reprinted with permission from A.E. Reading and J.R. Bragonier, Human Sexuality and Sexual Assault, in N.F. Hacker and J.G. Moore, Eds., *Essentials of Obstetrics and Gynecology*, 3rd ed., pp. 534–536, W.B. Saunders Company.

---

then recommend counseling for couples who have different expectations. Once a problem is identified, it should be fully documented with regard to perception, duration, precipitating events, and change. Once the nature of the problem has been discerned, the provider can reassure and educate the client as well as institute counseling and referral. The provider may be able to treat certain conditions such as vaginismus, which is pain with penile penetration, or lack of desire, which may be due to psychological distress or biologic conditions.

In summary, the clinician needs to understand whether the older adult perceives there to be any sexual dysfunction, what his or her expectations are of normal sexuality in later life, and any existing diseases or medication that may affect sexual function. The clinician then needs to develop strategies for resolving sexual concerns that are noted during the sexual assessment. Sexual options for older adults are as varied as they are for younger adults. Finally, homosexuality; unsafe intercourse resulting in venereal disease, including HIV infection; sexual trauma from rape; and other types of sexual assault are all issues that should not be overlooked because of stereotypes held about older people.

SPIRITUAL ASSESSMENT

A systematic approach to spiritual assessment is a key feature to understanding the overall well-being of an older adult. Spiritual assessment encompasses a broad range of concepts, and it is important to obtain from the older adult what spirituality means to him or her. Maas and colleagues[65] have proposed a definition for spiritual distress as well as summarized ideological factors and defining characteristics that can help guide the clinician in conducting a spiritual assessment. Kelly[66] has defined spiritual distress as a feeling of despair or alienation related to religious, moral, or other beliefs/values. Possible reasons for spiritual distress noted in that work include the following:

- disruption in usual religious activity
- personal and family disasters

Table 6–2 Classification of Sexual Dysfunction*

Category	Characteristics	Etiology
Primary	Sexual expectations have never been met	Usually psychogenic
Secondary	All phases functioned in the past, but one or more no longer do so	May be organic or pharmacologic
Situational	Response cycle functions under some circumstances, but not others	May be psychogenic or relationship-related

*Any of the dysfunctions may involve desire, excitement, or orgasm.

Source: Reprinted with permission from A.E. Reading and J.R. Bragonier, Human Sexuality and Sexual Assault, in N.F. Hacker and J.G. Moore, Eds., *Essentials of Obstetrics and Gynecology*, 3rd ed., pp. 534–536, W.B. Saunders Company

- loss of significant others
- behaviors contrary to society/cultural norms

Defining characteristics of spiritual distress are noted to be[66]:

1. feeling separated or alienated from the deity
2. dissatisfaction with personal past or present
3. depression
4. crying
5. self-destructive behavior or threats
6. fear
7. feelings of abandonment
8. feelings of hopelessness

There are a number of spiritual assessment instruments available in the literature.[67] (An example is shown in Exhibit 6–6.) Assessment tools elicit assessment information related to the following key concepts:[65]

1. the older person's concept of God or deity
2. religious practices
3. beliefs about spirit and hell
4. values and meaning of life

Recent literature related to spirituality and aging notes the associations between intrinsic religiosity and spiritual well-being with hope and positive mood states,[68] and the positive correlation between religious well-being with social support and hope.[69] Gerwood, Le Blanc, and Piazza[70] noted that spirituality is related to positive high scores on the Purpose-in-Life Test, which may therefore be a clinically useful indicator for spiritual well-being.

SUICIDE ASSESSMENT

Suicide rates among older adults are the highest of any age group, and may be double the rate seen in the general population.[71] It has been noted that white men over the age of 85 are at the greatest risk and a key target for intervention.[72] All clinicians play a key role in recognizing depression and treatment in order to prevent suicide.[72-74] Social isolation, losses, and physical illness along with any past history of suicide attempts or psychiatric illness are risk factors for suicide in later life. It should also be noted that suicide in older people is more often lethal than in any other age group. In one study, a Tele-Help/Tele-Check ser-

Exhibit 6–6 Spiritual Scale

	Strongly Agree	Agree	Neutral	Disagree	Strongly Disagree
1. In the future, science will be able to explain everything.	1	2	3	4	5
2. I can find meaning in times of hardship.	5	4	3	2	1
3. A person can be fulfilled without pursuing an active spiritual life.	1	2	3	4	5
4. I am thankful for all that has happened to me.	5	4	3	2	1
5. Spiritual activities have not helped me become closer to other people.	1	2	3	4	5
6. Some experiences can be understood through one's spiritual beliefs.	5	4	3	2	1
7. A spiritual force influences the events in my life.	5	4	3	2	1
8. My life has a purpose.	5	4	3	2	1
9. Prayers do not really change what happens.	1	2	3	4	5
10. Participating in spiritual activities helps me forgive other people.	5	4	3	2	1
11. My spiritual beliefs continue to evolve.	5	4	3	2	1
12. I believe there is a power greater than myself.	5	4	3	2	1
13. I probably will not reexamine my spiritual beliefs.	1	2	3	4	5
14. My spiritual life fulfills me in ways that material possessions do not.	5	4	3	2	1
15. Spiritual activities have not helped me develop my identity.	1	2	3	4	5
16. Meditation does not help me feel more in touch with my inner spirit.	1	2	3	4	5
17. I have a personal relationship with a power greater than myself.	5	4	3	2	1
18. I have felt pressure to accept spiritual beliefs that I do not agree with.	1	2	3	4	5
19. Spiritual activities help me draw closer to a power greater than myself.	5	4	3	2	1
20. When I wrong someone, I make an effort to apologize.	5	4	3	2	1
21. When I am ashamed of something have done, I tell someone about it.	5	4	3	2	1
22. I solve my problems without using spiritual resources.	1	2	3	4	5
23. I examine my actions to see if they reflect my values.	5	4	3	2	1

continues

Exhibit 6–6 continued

24. During the last week I prayed (check one)
    □ 10 or more times
    □ 7–9 times
    □ 4–6 times
    □ 1–3 times
    □ 0 times

25. During the last week I meditated (check one)
    □ 10 or more times
    □ 7–9 times
    □ 4–6 times
    □ 1–3 times
    □ 0 times

26. Last month I participated in spiritual activities with at least one other person
    (check one)
    □ more than 15 times
    □ 11–15 times
    □ 6–10 times
    □ 1–5 times
    □ 0 times

Source: R.L. Hatch et al., The Spiritual Involvement and Beliefs Scale, Development and Testing of a New Instrument, Vol. 46, No. 6, pp. 476–486d, © 1988, Dowden Publishing Company, Inc. Reproduced with permission from *The Journal of Family Practice*.

vice was used to contact older adults at risk twice a week for assessment needs and emotional support.[75] Suicide rates for the group connected to this telemedicine group were significantly lower than for the group without the intervention, which supports telemedicine interventions for prevention of suicide in older adults. In another study, health status variables were identified for relationships to suicide in older adults.[76] Those individuals who committed suicide were more likely to have a history of cancer, use alcohol moderately or heavily, and be white and male. Finally, in an analysis of 100 cases of attempted suicide, it was documented that older people who attempt suicide have a high mortality rate from later completed suicides.[77] All of these data would indicate that suicide is a very real risk in older adults. White men over 85 years of age commit suicide at an annual rate of 67 per 100,000 with white women in the same category at 6 per 100,000. Suicide rates for white men and white women over age 75 have slightly but steadily increased since 1980 with older African Americans having a much lower suicide rate than older Whites.[78] Ebersole and Hess[79] note that a suicide assessment should include the following:

1. frequency of suicidal ideation
2. formulated plan for suicide
3. availability of means to carry out the plan
4. specificity regarding details (eg, time and place)
5. lethality of the method chosen

Additional factors they suggest include[79]:

1. internal resources (ie, personality factors and coping strategies)
2. external resources (ie, money, family, friends, and services)
3. communication skills (ie, ability to ask for help and express feelings)

A thorough suicide assessment can provide vital information to use in preventing suicide (Exhibit 6–7). Fear of nursing home placement and pain have been noted as leading reasons for suicide in the elderly.[80] In screening for suicidal thoughts, the clinician should be alert to individuals who express feelings of sadness, hopelessness, despair, or grief. If those feelings are reflected in the assessment, more specific questions should follow such as[73,81]:

1. Have you ever felt so blue, you thought you would hurt yourself?
2. Do you feel like hurting yourself now?
3. Do you have a plan to hurt yourself?

Exhibit 6–7 Recognition of Risk and Recovery Factors of Suicide

Risk factors

Depression

Paranoia or a paranoid attitude

Rejection of help; a suspicious and hostile attitude toward helpers and society

A major loss, such as the death of a spouse

A history of major losses

A recent suicide attempt

A previous history of suicide attempts

A major mental, physical, or neurological illness

Major crises or transitions, such as retirement or imminent entry into a nursing home

Major crises or changes in others, especially among family members

Typical age-related blows to self-esteem, such as loss of income or loss of meaningful activities

Loss of independence, when dependency is unacceptable

Expressions of feeling unnecessary, useless, and devalued

Increased irritability and poor judgment, especially after a loss or some other crisis

Alcoholism or increased drinking

Social isolation; living alone; having few friends; the social isolation of the couple is also associated with suicide

Expression of the belief that one is in the way, a burden, or harmful to others

Expression of the belief that one is in an insoluble and hopeless situation

Communication of suicidal intent: the direct or indirect expression of suicidal ideation or impulses, including symptomatic acts, such as giving away valued possessions, storing up medications, or buying a gun

Intractable, unremitting pain, mental or physical, that is not responding to treatment

Feelings of hopelessness and helplessness in the family and social network

Feelings of hopelessness in the therapists or other helpers or a desire to be rid of the older adult

Expression of a belief in ageism, especially that the aged should not be

Acceptance of suicide as a solution

Recovery factors

A capacity for:
    Understanding
    Relating
    Benefiting from experience
    Benefiting from knowledge
    Acceptance of help
    Loving
    Wisdom
    A sense of humor
    Social interest

A caring and available family

A caring and available social network

A caring, available, and knowledgeable professional and health network

Source: Reprinted with permission from J. Richman, A Rational Approach to Rational Suicide. In A. Leemars et al., Eds., Suicide and the Older Adult, © 1992, The Guilford Press/American Association of Suicidology.

4. What would happen to you, if you were dead?
5. How would other people react if you were dead?

CONCLUSION

In conclusion, a comprehensive social assessment is the context in which to understand disease and disability. The adage, "if you have seen one old person, you have seen one old person," could never be more accurate than when considered through the lens of the social assessment.

REFERENCES

1. Paveza GJ. Social services and the Alzheimer's disease patient: An overview. *Neurology.* 1993;43(8, suppl 4):11–15.

2. Fengler AP, Goodrich N. Wives of elderly disabled men: The hidden patients. *Gerontologist.* 1979;19:175–183.

3. Stone R, Cafferata GL, Sangl J. Caregivers of the frail elderly: A national profile. *Gerontologist.* 1987;27:616–626.

4. U.S. Senate Special Committee on Aging. *Developments in Aging.* Vol 1. Washington, DC: U.S. Government Printing Office, 1988.

5. Preston SH. Children and the elderly in the US. *Sci Am.* 1984;250:44–49.

6. Berkman L. The assessment of social networks and social support in the elderly. *J Am Geriatr Soc.* 1983;31:743–749.

7. Brown LJ, Potter JF, Foster BG. Caregiver burden should be evaluated during geriatric assessment. *J Am Geriatr Soc.* 1990;38:455–460.

8. Fisk AA, Pannill FC. Assessment of the elderly for long-term care. *J Am Geriatr Soc.* 1987;35:307–311.

9. Lindsey AM, Hughes EM. Social support and alternatives to institutionalization for the at-risk elderly. *J Am Geriatr Soc.* 1981;29:308–315.

10. Sloane PD. Nursing home candidates: Hospital inpatient trial to identify those appropriately assignable to less intensive care. *J Am Geriatr Soc.* 1980;28:511–514.

11. Wachtel TJ, Fulton JP, Goldfarb J. Early prediction of discharge disposition after hospitalization. *Gerontologist.* 1987;27:98–103.

12. Williams TF, Williams ME. Assessment of the elderly for long-term care. *J Am Geriatr Soc.* 1982;30:71–75.

13. Rzetelny H, Mellor J. *Support Groups for Caregivers of the Aged.* New York: Community Service Society; 1981.

14. Zarit SH, Pearlin LI, Schaie KW, eds. *Caregiving Systems: Informal and Formal Helpers.* Hillsdale, NJ: Lawrence Erlbaum Associates; 1993.

15. Gallo JJ, Franch MS, Reichel W. Dementing illness: The patient, caregiver, and community. *Am Fam Phys.* 1991;43:1669–1675.

16. Hooyman NR, Lustbader W. *Taking Care: Supporting Older People and Their Families.* New York: Free Press; 1986.

17. Reichel W. Care of the elderly in rural America. *Md Med J.* May 1980:75.

18. Lozier J, Althouse R. Retirement to the porch in rural Appalachia. *Int J Aging Hum Dev.* 1975;6:7–15.

19. Norbeck JS, Lindsey AM, Carrieri VL. The development of an instrument to measure social support. *Nurs Res.* 1981;30:264–269.

20. Norbeck JS, Lindsey AM, Carrieri VL. Further development of the Norbeck Social Support Questionnaire: Normative data and validity testing. *Nurs Res.* 1983;32:4–9.

21. Pillemer KA, Wolf RS, eds. *Elder Abuse: Conflict in the Family.* Dover, MA: Auburn House; 1986.

22. Lubben JE. Assessing social networks among elderly populations. *Fam Community Health.* 1988;11:45–52.

23. Kane RA. Assessment of social functioning: Recommendations for comprehensive geriatric assessment. In: Rubenstein LZ, Wieland D, Bernabei R, eds. *Geriatric Assessment Technology: The State of the Art.* New York: Springer Publishing Co; 1995: 91–110.

24. Seeman TE, Berkman LF. Structural characteristics of social networks and their relationship with social support in the elderly: Who provides support? *Soc Sci Med.* 1988;26:737–749.

25. George LK, Blazer DG, Hughes DC, Fowler N. Social support and the outcome of major depression. *Br J Psychiatry.* 1989;154:478–485.

26. George LK, Gwyther LP. Caregiver well-being: A multidimensional examination of family caregivers of demented adults. *Gerontologist.* 1986;26:253–259.

27. Paveza GJ, Cohen D, Eisdorfer C, et al. Severe family violence and Alzheimer's disease: Prevalence and risk factors. *Gerontologist.* 1992;32(4):493–497.

28. Poulshock SW, Deimling GT. Families caring for elders in residence: Issues in the measurement of burden. *J Gerontol.* 1984;39:230–239.

29. Zarit SH, Orr NK. *Working with Families of Dementia Victims: A Treatment Manual.* Washington, DC: U.S. Government Printing Office; 1984. Publication no. 84–20816.

30. Drinka TJK, Smith JC, Drinka PJ. Correlates of depression and burden for informal caregivers of patients in a geriatric referral clinic. *J Am Geriatr Soc.* 1987;35:522–525.

31. Gallo JJ. The effect of social support on depression in caregivers of the elderly. *J Fam Pract.* 1990;30:430–436.

32. Kiyak HA. *Coping with Alzheimer's Disease: Patient and Family Responses.* (Paper presentation). Chicago: Gerontological Society of Ameria; November 11, 1986.

33. Pearlin LI, Schooler C. The structure of coping. *J Health Soc Behav.* 1978;18:2–21.

34. Pearlin LI, Skaff MM. Stressors and adaptation in late life. In: Gatz M, ed. *Emerging Issues in Mental Health and Aging.* Washington, DC: American Psychological Association; 1995:97–123.

35. Stephens MAP, Crowther JH, Hobfoll SE, Tennenbaum DL, eds. *Stress and Coping in Later-Life Families.* New York: Hemisphere Publishing Corporation; 1990.

36. The National Center on Elder Abuse at The American Public Human Services Association in collaboration with Westat I. *The National Elder Abuse Incidence Study—Final Report.* Washington, DC: The Administration on Aging; 1998.

37. Steinmetz SK. *Duty Bound: Elder Abuse and Family Care.* Vol 166. Newbury Park, CA: Sage Publications; 1988.

38. Pillemer K, Finkelhor D. The prevalence of elder abuse: A random sample survey. *Gerontologist.* 1988;8:51–57.

39. Coyne AC, Reichman WE, Berbig LJ. The relationship between dementia and elder abuse. *Am J Psychiatry.* 1993;150(4):643–646.

40. Pillemer K, Suitor JJ. Violence and violent feelings: What causes them among family caregivers? *J Gerontology: Soc Sci.* 1992;47(4):S165–S172.

41. Strauss MA, Gelles RJ, Steinmetz SK. *Behind Closed Doors: Violence in the American Family.* New York: Anchor Books; 1980.

42. Fulmer T, Wetle T. Elder abuse screening and intervention. *Nurse Practitioner* 1986; 11(5):33–38.

43. Pritchard J. *Working with Elder Abuse: A Training Manual for Home Care, Residential and Day Care Staff.* London, England: Jessica Kingsley Publishers; 1996.

44. Quinn MJ, Tomita SK. *Elder Abuse and Neglect.* 2nd ed. New York: Springer Publishing Co; 1997.

45. Schulz JH. *The Economics of Aging.* Belmont, CA: Wadsworth Publishing Co; 1985.

46. Applegate WB. Use of assessment instruments in clinical settings. *J Am Geriatr Soc.* 1987;35:45–50.

47. Kane RA, Kane RL. *Assessing the Elderly: A Practical Guide to Measurement.* Lexington, MA: Lexington Books; 1981.

48. Fillenbaum GG. The OARS multidimensional functional assessment questionnaire. In: *Multidimensional Functional Assessment of Older Adults: The Duke Older Americans Resources and Services Procedures.* 2nd ed. Durham, NC: Duke University Center for the Study of Aging and Human Development; 1978:7–12.

49. Williams T. Comprehensive functional assessment: An overview. *J Am Geriatr Soc.* 1983;31:637–641.

50. Achenbaum WA. *Social Security: Visions and Revisions.* New York: Cambridge University Press; 1986.

51. Holzman D. Closing Medicare's coverage gaps. *Insight.* January 26, 1987;3:52–53.

52. England R. Greener era for gray America. *Insight.* March 2, 1987;3:8–11.

53. Atchley RC, Robinson JL. Attitudes toward retirement and distance from the event. *Res Aging.* 1982;4;299–313.

54. Foner A, Schwab K. Work and retirement in a changing society. In: Riley MW, Hess BB, Bond K, eds. *Aging in Society: Selected Reviews of Recent Research.* Hillsdale, NJ: Lawrence Erlbaum Associates; 1983.

55. Dennis H, ed. *Retirement Preparation: What Retirement Specialists Need To Know.* Lexington, MA: Lexington Books; 1984.

56. Morris R, Bass SA. The elderly as surplus people: Is there a role for higher education? *Gerontologist.* 1986;26:12–18.

57. Steel K, Musliner M, Berg K. Assessment of the home environment. In: Rubenstein LZ, Wieland D, Bernabei R, eds. *Geriatric Assessment Technology: The State of the Art.* New York: Springer Publishing Co; 1995:135–145.

58. Kinsey AC, Pomeroy WB, Martin CE. *Sexual Behavior in the Human Male.* Philadelphia: WB Saunders Co; 1948.

59. Staff of the Institute for Sex Research, Indiana University. *Sexual Behavior in the Human Female.* Philadelphia: WB Saunders Co; 1953.

60. Matthias RE, Lubben JE, Atchison KA, Schweitzer SO. Sexual activity and satisfaction among very old adults: Results from a community-dwelling Medicare population survey. *Gerontologist.* 1997;37:6–14.

61. Helgason AR, Adolfsson J, Dickman P, et al. Sexual desire, erection, orgasm and ejaculatory functions and their importance to elderly Swedish men: A population-based study. *Age Aging,* July 1996;25:285–291.

62. Levy JA. Sexuality and aging. In: Hazzard WR, Bierman EL, Blass JP, Ettinger WH, Halter JB, Reubin A, eds. *Principles of Geriatric Medicine.* 3rd ed. New York: McGraw-Hill; 1994:115–123.

63. Besdine RW, Beers MH, Bootman JL. *When Medicine Hurts Instead of Helps: Preventing Medication Problems in Older People.* (Congressional Briefing) Washington, DC: Alliance for Aging Research; 1998.

64. Reading AE, Bragonier JR. Human sexuality and sexual assault. In: Hacker MJ, NF, eds. *Essentials of Obstetrics and Gynecology.* 3rd ed. Philadelphia: WB Saunders Co; 1998: 532–542.

65. Maas M, Buckwalter KC, Hardy MA, eds. *Nursing Diagnoses and Interventions for the Elderly.* Redwood City, CA: Addison-Wesley Publishing Co; 1991.

66. Kelly MA. *Nursing Diagnosis Source Book: Guidelines for Clinical Application.* Norwalk, CT: Appleton-Century-Crofts; 1985.

67. Fehring RJ, Rantz M. Spiritual distress. In: BK, Maas M, Hardy MA, eds. *Nursing Diagnoses and Interventions for the Elderly.* Redwood City, CA: Addison-Wesley Publishing Co; 1991:598–609.

68. Fehring RJ, Miller J, Shaw C. Spiritual well-being, religiosity, hope, depression, and other mood states in elderly people coping with cancer. *Oncol Nurs Forum.* May 1997; 24:663–671.

69. Zorn CR, Johnson M. Religious well-being in noninstitutional elderly women. *Health Care Women Int.* May–June 1997;18:209–219.

70. Gerwood JB, Le Blanc LM, Piazza N. The Purpose-in-Life Test and religious denomination: Protestant and Catholic scores in an elderly population. *J Clin Psychol.* January 1998;54:49–53.

71. Devons CA. Suicide in the elderly: How to identify and treat patients at risk. *Geriatrics.* March 1996;51:67–72.

72. Conwell Y. Management of suicidal behavior in the elderly. *Psychiatr Clin North Am.* September 1997;20:667–683.

73. Johnston M, Walker M. Suicide in the elderly. Recognizing the signs. *Gen Hosp Psychiatry.* July 1996;18:257–260.

74. Moscicki, EK. Epidemiology of suicide. *Int Psychogeriatric.* Summer 1995;7;137–148.

75. De Leo D, Carollo G, Dello Buono M. Lower suicide rates associated with a Tele-Help/Tele-Check service for the elderly at home. *Am J Psychiatry.* April 1995;152:632–634.

76. Grabbe L, Demi A, Camann MA, Potter L. The health status of elderly persons in the last year of life: A comparison of deaths by suicide, injury, and natural causes. *Am J Public Health.* March 1997;87:434–437.

77. Hepple J, Quinton C. One hundred cases of attempted suicide in the elderly. *Br J Psychiatry.* July 1997;171:42–46.

78. US Bureau of the Census. *Statistical Abstracts of the United States: 1995.* 115th ed. Washington, DC: US Bureau of the Census; 1995.

79. Ebersole P, Hess P. *Towards Healthy Aging*. 5th ed. St Louis, MO: Mosby; 1998.

80. Loebel JP, Loebel JS, Dager SR, Centerwall BS, Reay DT. Anticipation of nursing home placement may be a precipitant of suicide among the elderly. *J Am Geriatr Soc*. April 1991;39:407–408.

81. Jarvis C. *Pocket Companion for Physical Examination and Health Assessment*. 2nd ed. Philadelphia: WB Saunders Co; 1996.

7

Using the Values History To Enhance Advance Directive Communication

David J. Doukas and Laurence B. McCullough

THE VALUES HISTORY: ASSESSING PATIENT VALUES AND DIRECTIVES REGARDING LONG-TERM AND END-OF-LIFE CARE

Geriatric assessment is a multidimensional process. For physicians, addressing life's ethical concerns may be just as important as helping patients with their medical ailments. Physicians have a prime responsibility to identify those values relevant in the execution of an advance directive. This responsibility has become of paramount importance since physicians have been less than forthright in discussing advance directives, or using them when executed.[1,2] Physicians have stated that they tend to not address advance directives because of their own discomfort, as well as troubling the minds of their patients and families.[1] Further, as the SUPPORT study revealed, even when such discussions do take place, there is no guarantee that these preferences will be implemented in the form of physician orders.[2]

Both the living will and the durable power of attorney for health care (DPA/HC) are intended to address preferences for future health care. The Patient Self-Determination Act of 1990 is federal legislation meant to enhance utilization of these instruments by requiring provision of information about them in health care institutions that receive

Medicare and Medicaid. However, studies revealed that signing rates did not increase as much as hoped.[3] While people liked the concept of advance directives, they did not rush to their doctors to discuss them. While these legal instruments are valuable if used appropriately, they are hampered in that they fail to acknowledge people's values in their formulation and execution. Preferences about future health care management are not decided in a moral or historical vacuum. Physicians understand that past events, and how people view their lives and health care will influence the decision-making process of advance directives. What has been proposed to make this process more systematic is an instrument that can amplify and acknowledge the values of patients in end-of-life health care planning—namely, the Values History.[4-7] The Values History enhances autonomy through open discussion of values and, in turn, those preferences that are to be carried out when decision making by the patient is no longer possible. The Values History is intended to facilitate the communication process by identifying value-based preferences before the patient can no longer speak for himself or herself. As such, the Values History is a valuable adjunct in fulfilling the Patient Self-Determination Act's aim of informing patients about their right to refuse medical therapy (including the use of advance directives).[8] By addressing values and preferences with the Values History in the outpatient setting, the probability of encountering uncertainty about the person's preferences for end-of-life care is greatly lessened. As a result, addressing values and preferences in determining advance directives makes explicit their intrinsic role in geriatric care. The person must be informed about advance directives to be able to consider and consent or refuse to execute them. The Values History eases this process by addressing those values that underlie the informed consent process for these directives.

THE LIVING WILL

The living will is a written statement or oral declaration (as provided in relevant statutory law) that documents a person's competent decision to withhold or withdraw mechanical and other artificial means of health care in circumstances of terminal illness (and in many states, irreversible comatose and vegetative states) when the person can no longer make decisions. The living will allows the person to decide in advance which drugs, procedures, and therapies available to treat a terminal disease process and its complications should not be administered. The individual may revoke the living will even when he or she is incompetent. The instrument cannot be overturned or interfered with by third parties so long as it has been executed according to the procedures defined in the state's statute.

Sometimes a living will is vague about which particular medical procedures are to be refused. This imprecision can lead to misinterpretation of what the person has refused.[9] Adherence to a living will can therefore vary with the physician's interpretation of the person's intent, as well as the physician's assessment of the probability of recovery.[9] Furthermore, in many states, the living will must be in the precise form mandated by the statute.[10]

As noted above, physicians also have been less than forthright about offering the living will because of their own personal reservations and concerns of upsetting the patient and family.[11] This undermining of the informed consent process disenfranchises the patient, who needs to understand what options for end-of-life care are available and that they can be refused. Further, even when living wills are offered by physicians, this is no guarantee that they also work with their patient to identify their values regarding terminal treatment and care, or to make decisions about terminal care that are based on those values. While the living will is a helpful first step in allowing older adults to declare themselves noncandidates for some means of life support, it does not address those fundamental values that help them articulate explicit end-of-life preferences. The physician's ability to understand the person's reasoning and motivation needs to be augmented in order to help extrapolate the living will's meaning at life's end and, thus, increase the clinical utility of the living will.

THE DURABLE POWER OF ATTORNEY

The DPA/HC is a legal transfer of power from one person to another person (termed an agent) in order to make health care decisions when that person is incapacitated. Its "durability" illustrates that the power begins and continues despite the person's incapacity. The durable power of attorney allows a person to assign a legally enforceable surrogate decision maker when the person has lost decision-making capacity. The individual does not have to be terminally ill for the DPA/HC to take effect, in contrast to living wills, only incapacitated (see Exhibit 7–1). Most states have DPA/HC laws focusing this authority for health-related decision making. The duty of the designated surrogate decision maker is to consider the available medical options and then select those options that most closely adhere to the previously

Exhibit 7–1 Conditions for Applicability of Advance Directives

---

Living Will
- The patient is, in reasonable medical judgment, terminally ill or, in some state statutes, persistently vegetative (as this phrase is defined in applicable statute or, as in the case of the Department of Veterans Affairs, in applicable policy).
- The patient, in reasonable medical judgment, has lost the capacity to make decisions about his or her own care.

Durable Power of Attorney for Health Care
- The patient, in reasonable medical judgment, has lost the capacity to make decisions about his or her own care.

Source: D. Doukas and L. McCullough, The Values History: The Evaluation of the Patient's Values and Advance Directives, Vol. 31, No. 1, pp. 145–153, © 1991, Dowden Publishing Company, Inc. Reproduced with permission from *The Journal of Family Practice.*

---

stated or written preferences of the individual. The use of a DPA/HC may allow for greater flexibility and accuracy in following the person's preferences than the living will, providing that he or she has expressed his or her health care preferences. Though the living will avoids the potential burden of placing decision making on another's shoulders, the DPA/HC may be a better approach as it can accommodate a wider spectrum of future medical conditions and possible medical responses.

The main objection to the DPA/HC is whether the agent can understand all of the person's health care preferences.[11] Can the agent possibly anticipate the individual's likely responses in all health care circumstances? Many persons may not have ever discussed their values regarding terminal care or their specific preferences based on those values with their surrogate decision makers.

THE VALUES HISTORY

The Values History (Appendix 7–A) has been offered as a means to identify end-of-life health care values and health care preferences on the basis of those values. The Values History is a useful clinical adjunct to other advance directives. The Values History consists of two sections: the first inviting the individual to identify his or her values and beliefs regarding terminal care; and the second asking him or her to make explicit decisions in advance about such care, given these values. The goals are to clarify end-of-life values and assist health care providers in understanding, respecting, and implementing the value-based decisions expressed in the Values History. The physician's goal is to better understand the person's reasons for his or her future health care decisions, not to gauge validity of the person's values, and, to implement these preferences in the future.

The Preamble

The Values History's preamble explains that the Values History is a supplement to the person's preexisting advance directive(s) by providing him or her with the opportunity to articulate explicit, value-based preferences. As with other advance directives, the values and directives of the Values History are reversible as long as the person is competent. Further, these directives are revokable under the terms of the living will or DPA/HC legislation existing in each jurisdiction. These values and preferences act as a guide to health care providers when an individual without decision-making capacity has been documented as terminally ill and the withholding or withdrawing of life-sustaining measures is being contemplated.

The Values Section

The person identifies his or her values that are relevant to the decisions that must be made. A fundamental decision in this process is between length of life and quality of life. The person is then asked to identify those values most important to him or her from a list of 13 common end-of-life values. He or she can also add to the list, as well as elaborate on the chosen values. The values discussion then can help the individual formulate his or her advance directives toward medical care in the next section.

The Preferences Section

The Preferences Section contains a list of health care interventions that are potentially used in end-of-life care. Acute care decisions are dealt with first, and are highly pertinent to code/no code decision making. Of note, directives two through eight broach the concept of "trials of intervention," either limited by time or benefit. This approach allows for a course of action to attempt a therapy for a designated period of time or to ascertain if medical benefit is present and continued once a therapy is initiated. This option allows the person to request to see if a therapy might be useful, yet allows for discontinuation at a later date. Discussing the use of cardiopulmonary resuscitation (CPR) is fundamental in considering end-of-life care since withholding of resuscitation will usually result in death. Discussion on CPR is important to reduce ambiguity because many physicians presume that persons want this medical therapy unless told otherwise. Code status is of particular importance when the person may be soon hospitalized, and such decisions are increasingly relevant. Many states now have at-home, do not resuscitate orders so that these wishes can be respected in home and hospice care. Respirator and endotracheal tube use is also important to consider, especially for persons with chronic pulmonary disease. Discussing endotracheal tube use can often clarify concerns or misconceptions about the first two directives.

The chronic care designations include the use of total parenteral nutrition, intravenous hydration and medication, all medications necessary for the treatment of illnesses by other routes (eg, by mouth or by intramuscular injection), enteral feeding tubes, and dialysis. Pain medications should be assured as viable therapy when any of the above are refused. Each directive requires discussion both in the context of long-term recuperative or vegetative care.

The next advance directives address autopsy, proxy negation, and organ donation. The option of autopsy allows the person to voice his or her preference regarding the investigation of the causes of death. The physician should explain that an autopsy could benefit the person's family by their learning about diseases with a genetic pattern of inheritance. The next directive is an opportunity to add other preferences not otherwise addressed (eg, specific types of allowable or refused surgery). The proxy negation directive allows the individual to name a person(s) who is (are) to be excluded from the person's health care decision making should he or she become incompetent. This directive is useful for the person with a family member who has a different philosophy about medical care or who may have a conflict of interest. The last directive concerns the Uniform Donor Card (specific to state), which should be considered to allow for the postmortem use of organs in transplantation, medical therapy, and medical research or education. As noted with the autopsy directive, it is urged that the family respect this personal decision.

Each directive is signed and dated as the individual consents to them over time. Preferences expressed after initial signing can be subsequently articulated, then signed and dated, in the Values History. The physician should make note of any later changes in the medical record for that date. Importantly, each of these directives requests that the person discuss reasons for his or her decision, based on the values from the Values Section, as well as other relevant concerns. It is important to understand that while the values in the first section may be the obvious rationale for a directive, other values may also emerge in this discussion.

This information allows for a more meaningful understanding of the individual's reasoning while also probing possible inconsistent values. This process may also expose psychological ideation that could constrain the person's ability to formulate an informed consent. After learning of such an impediment, the physician can help the person therapeutically to restore his or her decision-making capacity. Throughout this evolving advance directive process, the assumption is that the person is able to consent to these decisions unless he or she is reliably shown to be incompetent to do so. The burden of proof is on the physician to establish and document in the medical record that the individual is unable to make these decisions.

Clinical Use of the Values History

All adult competent persons should be considered candidates for the Values History since it can easily be made part of geriatric assessment. In the primary care office, preliminary questioning on end-of-life care should be directed toward the older adult on the living will, and a DPA/HC should be initiated by the physician. It cannot be emphasized strongly enough that this task is the duty of the physician. It is the equivalent of disclosure in informed consent. Because people cannot make decisions on things they know nothing about, the physician must quell any personal reservations if he or she intends to promote the person's autonomy. When the individual decides to execute a living will or DPA/HC, this decision should be documented with forms according to the laws effective in that jurisdiction, copies should be placed in the medical record, and an appropriate note should be written in the record, especially to document oral declarations.

The physician should then initiate a discussion on the individual's perspectives on quality of life versus length of life (ie, the Values Section of the Values History). After the Values Section has been completed, the physician should discuss the preferences listed in the Values History. A helpful starting point for these discussions is the person's own medical problems. For example, the physician should explain the use or refusal of a ventilator to someone with chronic lung disease, as well as the meaning of a trial of intervention. This method makes for a more relevant discussion, and the specific life-sustaining therapy that could be implemented in a person's near future would be discussed first. Also, the options of acute care therapy (eg, CPR, intubation, and ventilation) would also be discussed early. The physician can discuss the remainder of the Values History during follow-up visits as part of other health maintenance exams, thereby noting preferences and decisions as they are articulated.

The Values History is a dynamic guide for the DPA/HC agent if an individual becomes incapacitated and can serve to initiate important health care discussions. The assignment of an agent is very helpful for the person who has been undecided in his or her Values History. Preferably, the person would understand that it is desirable to make his or her own decisions rather than obliging a relative or friend to figure them out later. If the individual has not signed a Values History or living will and has not assigned an agent, the physician should inform him or her that using any of these advance directive methods would best ensure that his or her wishes will be carried out. In several states (ie, Delaware, Michigan, Missouri, and New York), cases that have gone to a court have required "clear and convincing" standards of evidence (ie, explicit written or oral declarations) prior to withholding or withdrawing life-prolonging care. The physician should alert the person that, in the absence of any health care directive, a health care institution could be forced to act on a presumption in favor of treatment, which could violate his or her autonomous wishes. In summary, when an individual has signed a living will and/or a DPA/HC, he or she should discuss his or her values and advance directives of the Values History with his or her physician over time. As decisions are reached, directives are signed and dated.

Barriers in Using the Values History

Potential barriers may arise in using the Values History. First, as noted above, the physician may perceive that revealing the possibility of approaching death to the person is harmful or that he or she wants to wait until the "right time."[1] This lack of informed consent inappropriately truncates the person's ability to make free decisions about his or her future health care. Such an undermining of future care based on paternalistic concerns serves neither the patient nor the physician. Both could lose a valuable opportunity to discuss values regarding end-of-life care before the patient becomes ill and decisions need to be made in the absence of helpful exchanges.

The patient could be a barrier to the Values History by being ambivalent or refusing to discuss the notion of advance directives. Individuals who are indecisive or resistant to advance directives (by not wanting to talk about them, or more commonly by not signing them when discussed) can impair efforts to elicit a Values History. In response to these circumstances, physicians should attempt continued, sensitive probing of the person's end-of-life values and preferences.

An individual's family can impede the Values History's implementation. A family member may disagree with a person's autonomous request to withhold or withdraw certain therapies and attempt to circumvent these preferences. When such a challenge to competent decisions occurs, it is helpful to acknowledge the family member's concerns and values, while informing him or her that advance directives are intended to safeguard the person's liberty-based rights to stop therapeutic intrusiveness. Such education and acknowledgment of autonomy in refusing specific interventions can be helpful.

The possibility of legal barriers to the Values History must also be considered. First of all, while almost every state now has a living will statute, some still do not. However, common law still supports use of living wills. Moreover, of those states that do have the living will statute, nearly all allow for directives to be appended to them.[10] Therefore, in a state without a living will statute with this stipulation, it is prudent to append the Values History to a DPA/HC. Specific applicable state laws should be consulted in this regard. Both instruments are still quite helpful since they help the medical team by clarifying the individual's values and preferences regarding end-of-life care. Organ donation statutes vary according to jurisdiction. Again, appropriate statutory wording should be substituted in the Values History according to the jurisdiction where it will be used. If deemed legally necessary, directives may be deleted from the Values History (upon consultation with counsel) by the health care provider prior to presentation to the patient if required by the jurisdiction. With the investment of some effort in tailoring the Values History in this way, the clinician will be able to use the Values History with his or her patients, confident it complies with the state laws.

CONCLUSION

The Values History is an adjunct to the living will and the DPA/HC. It intends to bring advance directives to a deeper level of meaning. The physician possesses a tool of considerable clinical utility to facilitate discussion and consent to a variety of value-based preferences. The most important step in the process is the initial broaching of the subject followed by continued, sensitive dialog in order to best help the patient articulate his or her own values and preference toward life-sustaining treatment.[12] As a result, the physician can safeguard the patient's autonomy by translating these preferences into physician orders.

REFERENCES

1. Doukas D, Gorenflo D, Coughlin S. The living will: A national survey. *Fam Med.* 1991;123:354–356.

2. The SUPPORT Investigators. A controlled trial to improve outcomes for seriously ill hospitalized patients: The study to understand prognoses and preferences for outcomes and risks of treatment. *JAMA.* 1995;274:1591–1598.

3. Teno JM, Lynn J, Wenger N, et al for the SUPPORT Investigators. Advance directives for seriously ill hospitalized patients: Effectiveness with the patient self-determination act and the SUPPORT intervention. *J Am Geriatr Soc.* 1997;45:500–507.

4. Doukas D, McCullough L. Assessing the Values History of the aged patient regarding critical and chronic care. In: Gallo J, Reichel W, eds. *The Handbook of Geriatric Assessment.* 1st ed. Rockville, MD: Aspen Publishers; 1988:111–124.

5. Doukas D, Lipson S, McCullough L. Value History. In: Reichel W, ed. *Clinical Aspects of Aging.* 3rd ed. Baltimore: Williams & Wilkins; 1989:615–616.

6. Doukas D, McCullough L. The Values History: The evaluation of the patient's values and advance directives. *J Fam Pract.* 1991;3:145–153.

7. Doukas D, Reichel W. *Planning for Uncertainty: A Guide to Living Wills and Other Advance Directives for Health Care.* Baltimore: Johns Hopkins University Press; 1993.

8. Omnibus Budget Reconciliation Act, Pub L. No. 101–508 §§4206, 4751 (1990).

9. Eisendrath S, Jonsen A. The living will: Help or hindrance? *JAMA.* 1983;249:2054–2058.

10. Society for the Right to Die. *The Physician and the Hopelessly Ill Patient: Legal, Medical, and Ethical Guidelines.* New York: The Society for the Right to Die; 1985.

11. Wanzer S, Adelstein J, Cranford R, et al. The physician's responsibility toward hopelessly ill patients. *N Engl J Med.* 1984;310:955–959.

12. Doukas D. If you ask them . . . They will sign. *Am Fam Phys.* In press.

Appendix 7–A
The Values History

Patient name: _____

This Values History serves as a set of my specific value-based directives for various medical interventions. It is to be used in health care circumstances when I may be unable to voice my preferences. These directives shall be made a part of the medical record and used as supplementary to my living will and/or durable power of attorney for health care.

I. VALUES SECTION

Values are things that are important to us in our lives and our relationships with others—especially loved ones. There are several values important in decisions about terminal treatment and care. This section of the Values History invites you to identify your most important values.

A. Basic Life Values

Perhaps the most basic values in this context concern length of life versus quality of life. Which of the following two statements is the most important to you?

____ 1. I want to live as long as possible, regardless of the quality of life that I experience.
____ 2. I want to preserve a good quality of life, even if this means that I may not live as long.

B. Quality of Life Values

There are many values that help us to define for ourselves the quality of life that we want to live. Review this list (and feel free to either elaborate on it or add to it), and circle those values that are most important to your definition of quality of life.

Source: D. Doukas and L. McCullough, The Values History: The Evaluation of the Patient's Values and Advance Directives, Vol. 31, No. 1, pp. 145–153, © 1991, Dowden Publishing Comany, Inc. Reproduced with permission from *The Journal of Family Practice*.

1. I want to maintain my capacity to think clearly.
2. I want to feel safe and secure.
3. I want to avoid unnecessary pain and suffering.
4. I want to be treated with respect.
5. I want to be treated with dignity when I can no longer speak for myself.
6. I do not want to be an unnecessary burden on my family.
7. I want to be able to make my own decisions.
8. I want to experience a comfortable dying process.
9. I want to be with my loved ones before I die.
10. I want to leave good memories of me to my loved ones.
11. I want to be treated in accord with my religious beliefs and traditions.
12. I want respect shown for my body after I die.
13. I want to help others by making a contribution to medical education and research.
14. Other values or clarification of values above:

_____

_____

_____

_____

_____

II. PREFERENCES SECTION

Some directives involve simple yes-or-no decisions. Others provide for the choice of a trial of intervention. Use the values identified above to explain why you made the choice you did. The information will be very useful to your family, health care surrogate (or proxy), and health care providers.

Initials/Date

_____ _____ 1. I want to undergo cardiopulmonary resuscitation.
        _____ Yes
        _____ No

Why?

_____

_____

_____

_____

____ ____ 2. I want to be placed on a ventilator.

     ____ Yes
     ____ Trial for the time period of _____
     ____ Trial to determine effectiveness using reasonable
         medical judgment.
     ____ No

Why?

_____

_____

_____

_____

____ ____ 3. I want to have an endotracheal tube used in order to
perform items 1 and 2.

     ____ Yes
     ____ Trial for the time period of _____
     ____ Trial to determine effectiveness using reasonable
         medical judgment.
     ____ No

Why?

_____

_____

_____

_____

____ ____ 4. I want to have total parenteral nutrition administered
for my nutrition.

____ Yes
____ Trial for the time period of _____
____ Trial to determine effectiveness using reasonable
medical judgment.
____ No

Why?

_____

_____

_____

_____

____ ____ 5. I want to have intravenous medication and hydration
administered; regardless of my decision, I understand
that intravenous hydration to alleviate discomfort or
pain medication will not be withheld from me if I so
request them.

____ Yes
____ Trial for the time period of _____
____ Trial to determine effectiveness using reasonable
medical judgment.
____ No

Why?

_____

_____

_____

_____

_____ _____ 6. I want to have all medications used for the treatment of my illness continued; regardless of my decision, I understand that pain medication will continue to be administered including narcotic medications.

_____ Yes
_____ Trial for the time period of _____
_____ Trial to determine effectiveness using reasonable medical judgment.
_____ No

Why?

_____

_____

_____

_____

_____ _____ 7. I want to have nasogastric, gastrostomy, or other enteral feeding tubes introduced and administered for my nutrition.

_____ Yes
_____ Trial for the time period of _____
_____ Trial to determine effectiveness using reasonable medical judgment.
_____ No

Why?

_____

_____

_____

_____

____ ____ 8. I want to be placed on a dialysis machine.

    ____ Yes
    ____ Trial for the time period of _____
    ____ Trial to determine effectiveness using reasonable
    medical judgment.
    ____ No

Why?

_____

_____

_____

_____

____ ____ 9. I want to have an autopsy done to determine the cause(s) of my death.

    ____ Yes
    ____ No

Why?

_____

_____

_____

_____

____ ____ 10. I want to be admitted to the intensive care unit if necessary.

    ____ Yes
    ____ No

Why?

_____

_____

_____

_____

____ ____ 11. If I become a patient in a long-term care facility or I receive care at home and experience a life-threatening change in health status, I want 911 called in case of a medical emergency.

____ Yes
____ No

Why?

_____

_____

_____

_____

_____

____ ____ 12. Other directives:

_____

_____

_____

_____

_____

I consent to these directives after receiving honest disclosure of their implications, risks, and benefits by my physician, free from constraints and being of sound mind.

_____
Signature   Date

_____
Witness

_____
Witness

____ ____ 13. Proxy negation:

I request that the following persons NOT be allowed to make decisions on my behalf in the event of my disability or incapacity:

_____

_____

_____

_____

_____
Signature   Date

_____
Witness

_____
Witness

____ ____ 14. Organ donation:
Specific state version inserted/attached here

8

Physical Assessment

Functional, social, value, and economic evaluations lie outside the traditional medical model's catenation of complaint, history, physical examination, investigations, diagnosis, treatment, and cure that permeates medicine and generally serves quite well. In dealing with older adults, however, things may not be so clearly and neatly packaged. Illness presentation in older adults corresponding to a single disease process (the medical presentation) is unusual.[1] Other types of presentations include: (1) the *synergistic morbidity* presentation (multiple conditions result in functional decline), (2) the *attribution* presentation (the patient attributes problems to a previously diagnosed condition while a new condition progresses), (3) the *causal chain* presentation (one illness causes another and precipitates decline), and (4) the *unmasking event* presentation (a stressful event exposes an underlying, previously hidden morbidity).[1] The concept of illness presentations facilitates thinking about multiple and interacting illnesses and the inclusion of social, psychological, and other factors.

Functional assessment, in particular, may be especially relevant to an older adult's circumstances and best suited to delineate the decisions facing him or her regarding appropriate placement or to define how physical problems interfere with the ability to live independently. The social assessment and evaluation of the caregiver play a pivotal role in making assessments about function as well. Emphasis on multiple aspects of assessment, however, is in no way meant to disparage a thorough and thoughtful physical examination. In most respects, the physical examination of an older adult is no different from the examination of a young adult.

The increasing rates of disease and infirmity with advancing age require a greater vigilance on the part of the examiner to discover abnormalities and to judge the relevance for a particular patient (separating pathologic processes from aging processes). The assessment process is complicated because the presenting symptom in the older person may be a red herring; that is, a nonspecific signal that something is amiss somewhere, but not necessarily in the system expected. Dysfunction in any organ system may only manifest as deteriorating mental status, for example, so that pneumonia (respiratory), appendicitis (gastrointestinal), or congestive heart failure (cardiac) cause confusion (central nervous system). The physical examination of the older person therefore needs to be as complete and systematic as possible, particularly at the time of admission to the hospital or nursing home or prior to surgery.[2,3]

Frequently the precise sequence and timing of the examination must be modified when dealing with an older person because of impaired hearing, sight, comprehension, or mobility. Rather than rush through the history and physical examination, it may be better to complete the entire process over two or more visits, along with an assessment of other domains. Unfortunately, physicians, if anything, may spend less time with older patients than with younger ones.[4]

What makes examination of older persons different, then, is not the content of the examination, but rather the need to develop an approach that does the older adult justice without undue discomfort or embarrassment. The approach must patiently take into account the older adult's impaired special senses or diminished mobility and must consider his or her slowed response time in answering questions. The physician must respectfully allow concerns that the person thinks are most important to be expressed. Caregivers and family may have concerns that need to be addressed within this context as well. Indeed, the chief complaint may be formulated by the family rather than by the person being examined.

COMMUNICATION AND RAPPORT

Because older persons frequently have impaired communication skills as a result of illness or lack of schooling, the examiner must pay special attention to communication issues in history taking and physical examination. When introducing him- or herself, the physician must take special note of communication problems. For many older adults, particularly the very old, English may be a second language; consequently, the examiner must keep in mind that the person may have difficulty in providing or understanding information during the interview. A hearing problem may be easily disguised and can result in misunderstanding if not recognized. Someone who is hearing impaired may respond to questions inappropriately, and an erroneous evaluation could result. If the individual uses a hearing aid, the volume of both the hearing aid and the examiner's voice must be adjusted. The physician should speak clearly and articulate rather than shout.

Eye contact, handshake, use of last name, and physical contact are the rudiments of good communication with all persons, but particularly for older adults. Eye contact is important to establish a relationship. Prolonged eye contact can seem like staring, however, and, in some cultures, eye contact is believed to be inappropriate. Addressing the individual by the last name is a sign of respect. Most of today's older adults grew up in a time when one would not think of addressing an older person or the physician by his or her first name. Using the last name is no barrier to friendliness; professional caregiving relationships are not less loving and warm as a result of using the last name. A touch on the hand or shoulder is appreciated by many older persons. Done in a sincere and caring manner, a touch may allay some of the anxiety associated with a trip to the physician's office or with a home visit by a nurse or social worker.

Speak to the older adult directly, not through others who may have accompanied him or her to the visit. For all but the most cognitively impaired, the clinician should talk to the caregiver only with the permission of the individual. The family members may appreciate some time alone with the practitioner to express their concerns without feeling embarrassed by the older person's presence. A natural time for this to occur is while the person undresses in preparation for the physical examination. The environment of the encounter must be comfortable with a minimum of noise, distractions, and interruptions. Provide the patient and family with a brief explanation and description of what is to be accomplished during the visit and subsequent visits (if the evaluation is to be spread out over several visits).

The writing of Viktor Frankl and others suggests that having meaning and purpose in life contributes to a healthy life.[5-7] At times when older persons experience loss of health, family and friends, vocation, or home, they are more apt to succumb to depression, alcoholism, hypochondriasis, or other disorders. The physician can contribute to hope by asking about what offers meaning in the patient's life. Meaning may derive from seeing a grandchild get married or to be assured that an adult child's marriage is stabilized. Feeling connected to family, neighborhood, or a faith community can support meaningfulness. In assessing older patients, the physician can discreetly and noncoercively enter these areas. By raising hope related to certain circumstances (ie, that with appropriate social supports the person may be able to remain at home rather than to be admitted to a nursing home), the physician may facilitate healing and increase motivation to improve. Practitioners rarely enter the areas of religious or spiritual beliefs, which are often thought to be taboo. However, in completing the history, practitioners might ask the older person the following questions (avoiding a coercive or intrusive tone)[8–10]: What role does religion play in your life? Are you a member of a faith community? Do you participate actively with this community? Spirituality is discussed in more detail in Chapter 6, Social Assessment. Asking questions pertaining to meaning, purpose, as well as spiritual and religious issues, can open up a dialog that will benefit the patient and enhance his or her relationship with the doctor.

EXAMINATION OF OLDER ADULTS WITH DEMENTIA

The physical examination of the person with Alzheimer's disease poses special challenges because the person may not be able to pinpoint what is wrong. Mental impairment severely limits the ability of many to express themselves. One danger is that mental deterioration will be automatically ascribed to the Alzheimer's disease and a reversible superimposed factor might consequently be overlooked. Therefore, the physical examination of the older person with mental impairment needs to be particularly thorough. Not only may a person with the Alzheimer's disease have communication difficulties, but he or she may not be cooperative. Because of memory difficulties, the individual may need to be gently but firmly reminded of what is expected. These persons may be extraordinarily restless. A firm and reassuring touch, such as in holding the hand or a shoulder; giving clear and simple, one-step requests; and maintaining eye contact, may forge the necessary links to communication and cooperation. Often the presence of a family member or friend can have a calming, orienting effect on the person being examined.

HISTORY TAKING

During the initial examination, an older person might present to the practitioner a barrage of complaints and difficulties. The family might inform the practitioner of problems of which their relative is unaware. The physical and laboratory evaluation may uncover yet other undisclosed problems. The practitioner could easily begin to feel frustrated and overwhelmed. Where to begin? What is important to address now, and what can wait? Just collecting adequate data with which to make a decision, let alone implementing a treatment plan, can be difficult within the time constraints of a primary care practice. At the initial interview it is probably best to attend to the specific problem, if there is one, be it medical or social, that prompted the evaluation,[11] with careful listing of other problems that may be addressed at subsequent visits.

Although some older persons are reluctant to give information to the interviewer, others are more than willing to share, at length, numerous irrelevant incidents that happened long ago. Without showing disinterest or disrespect, the interviewer must strive to help the person focus on the issues at hand. Functional assessment helps to direct the clinician's initial efforts to the solution of the problems that have a direct impact on the ability to perform the tasks of daily living.

The trouble is that there often are multiple chief complaints, or the chief complaint is unclear (eg, "Mom just doesn't seem herself"), or the chief complaint does not fit the usual mold (eg, "Mom just doesn't cook anymore"). The physician should use good problem-oriented medical records to help sort things out over time. Although not all the "problems" recorded will be addressed in a single visit, spelling them out, even if expressed as undifferentiated medical problems or functional difficulties, helps to organize the problems. For older people this is particularly important because the "parsimony of diagnosis" rule may not apply—several diseases (and their treatments) may coexist and interact. By keeping track of diagnosed and undifferentiated medical, social, and functional problems in this way, each visit will build on the information and rapport obtained in previous encounters. The physician should negotiate with the patient and family regarding which problems are the most salient to be addressed at each visit.

Although it is generally a good idea to use open-ended questions to obtain information (and older adults are no exception), it is sometimes necessary to supply the older person with specific words to choose from to help describe the problem. For example, "Describe your chest pain" is open-ended; "Was the pain sharp, stabbing, dull, or crushing?" may help the older individual describe the pain. Older adults have the reputation of answering yes to all the questions in the review of systems. Still, there are problems that may otherwise remain hidden unless specifically asked about by the examiner. Ham[12] has identified several: sexual dysfunction, depression, incontinence, musculoskeletal stiffness, alcoholism, hearing loss, and dementia. A suggested review of systems is presented in Exhibit 8–1. Some problems such as dyspnea may not be new, but rather altered in quality or frequency. The older person may always have had trouble on the stairs with shortness of breath, but now must rest three times instead of negotiating the stairs without resting.[13] Such a change in the degree of disability will be discovered by the careful interviewer.

Trying to confirm the diagnosis of every abnormality in every case may not be in the patient's best interest. The physician–patient relationship may be undermined if it depends solely on discovering reversible disease, rather than on optimal management of chronic disorders. Older adults often have multiple chronic illnesses that, although incurable, have aspects that can be modified to enhance function and limit discomfort.[14,15] Of course, a balance must be struck. The clinician must not be too quick to assume the symptoms are fully explained by the most serious, advanced, or chronic disease. Less seri-

Exhibit 8–1 Geriatric Review of Systems

General	Weight change	Genitourinary	Incontinence
	Fatigue		Dysuria
	Falls		Nocturia
	Anorexia		Hematuria
	Anemia		Sexual
	Poor nutrition		functioning
Special senses	Visual changes	Musculoskeletal	Morning
	Cataract		stiffness
	Hearing changes		Joint pain
	Imbalance		Joint swelling
	Vertigo		Limitation of
Mouth and teeth	Dentures		movement
	Denture discomfort	Neurology	Memory
	Dry mouth		problems
Respiratory	Cough		Headaches
	Hemoptysis		Syncope
	Dyspnea		Gait
Cardiovascular	Chest pain on exertion		Sensory function
	Orthopnea		Sleep disorders
	Ankle edema		Transient focal
	Claudication		symptoms
Gastrointestinal	Dysphagia		Voice changes
	Melena	Psychiatric	Depression
	Change in stool caliber		Alcoholism
	Laxative use		Anxiety
	Constipation		

Source: Reprinted from J. Gallo, Ed., Physical Assessment, *Handbook of Geriatric Assessment,* 2nd ed., pp. 151, © 1994, Aspen Publishers, Inc.

ous but treatable conditions may contribute to disability. Blind pessimism is unwarranted and can be counterproductive.

OVERVIEW OF THE PHYSICAL EXAMINATION

The physical assessment really begins when the physician first meets the patient and observes how he or she behaves and how well the patient is dressed and groomed. Does the person seem well nourished or thin and emaciated? Does he or she move about easily or unsteadily and unbalanced? How easily does the person arise from a chair to the examining table? During the taking of the history, the physician should observe the patient for involuntary movement, cranial nerve dysfunctions, and difficult respiration. The physician should also listen for the pace and clarity of speech.

The examination should require as few changes in position as possible. With the patient seated, the head, eyes, ears, nose, throat, neck, heart, lungs, joints, and neurologic examinations follow in turn. The patient is then positioned supine for examination of the abdomen, peripheral pulses, breasts, genitalia, and inguinal regions. The patient can then be turned to the lateral decubitus position for rectal examination. Finally, the patient is brought to a standing position so orthostatic blood pressure and pulse changes can be detected. Balance and gait can then also be tested.

COMPONENTS OF THE EXAMINATION

Pulse

The measurement of vital signs, temperature, and height and weight has been basic to physical assessment for centuries. The Chinese methods of diagnosis, thousands of years old, include questioning, feeling the pulse, and observing the voice and body. The radial artery is convenient for the determination of the heart rate. When the pulse is irregular, it is further characterized as regularly irregular or irregularly irregular. A *regularly irregular* pulse may indicate consistently dropped beats, as in the Wenckebach phenomenon, or added beats, such as with premature ventricular contractions. An *irregularly irregular* pattern often represents atrial fibrillation, but can also be caused by premature ventricular or atrial contractions. Palpation of the carotid pulse with simultaneous auscultation of the heart is helpful in timing murmurs or other sounds emanating from the heart.

Blood Pressure

Blood pressure should be taken both with the patient supine and standing, especially if he or she is taking medication for hypertension. Some fall in the systolic blood pressure is fairly common in older persons, particularly those with chronic disease or those on medication.[16] In one study of orthostatic blood pressure, after 1 minute of quiet standing, 24% of 494 persons over age 65 sustained a fall of 20 mmHg or more in systolic blood pressure. Five percent had decreases of 40 mmHg or more.[17] When older patients without risk factors for postural hypotension (such as chronic disease or medication use) were tested, only 8 of 125 persons (6.4%) had a 20 mm Hg or greater fall in systolic blood pressure on standing.[18]

The fall in blood pressure on standing can be exaggerated if the blood volume is low or if the reflex orthostatic mechanisms are impaired due to age or medication. Even mild sodium depletion (eg, serum sodium levels of 142 mEq/dL down to 137 mEq/dL) secondary to diuretics can result in marked postural hypotension in older adults although no such change occurs in younger subjects.[19]

The balloon of the blood pressure cuff should encircle about two thirds of the arm's circumference. If the person is obese, a wide cuff is used since a smaller cuff may overestimate the blood pressure. Conversely, a frail person with a thin arm may need a smaller than normal-sized cuff, perhaps a pediatric cuff, to avoid a spuriously low reading. Palpation of the cuff pressure at which the radial pulse disappears is a way to check the accuracy of the auscultated systolic blood pressure.

The Korotkoff sounds are listened for with the bell of the stethoscope pressed lightly over the brachial artery. The pressure at which the sounds are first heard is the systolic pressure. The sounds may become muffled before they disappear, and the pressure at the point where the muffling occurs should be recorded between the systolic and diastolic pressures (eg, 165/88/74 mmHg). Occasionally, an auscultatory gap is found, in which the sounds disappear only to reappear again at a lower pressure. If the auscultatory gap is not recognized, the diastolic pressure may be erroneously recorded as higher than its true value, or the systolic pressure may be erroneously recorded as lower than its true value.

Atherosclerosis may result in misleading blood pressure readings. The blood pressure reading may vary from one arm to the other because atherosclerosis involvement may be slightly asymmetrical. Stiff peripheral arteries may result in spuriously high readings. William Osler used a simple maneuver to detect its presence. Osler's maneuver is performed by inflating the blood pressure cuff above systolic pressure and then palpating the radial or brachial artery. If the pulseless artery is palpable, the true intra-arterial blood pressure reading may be lower than the blood pressure obtained by auscultation. Persons whose arteries remained palpable (Osler positive) when the cuff was inflated above systolic pressure had a blood pressure reading taken by auscultatory methods that was 20 percent higher than the intra-arterial measured pressure.[20] Some subjects had a diastolic cuff reading of 120 or 100 mmHg while a simultaneous intra-arterial pressure was 80 mmHg. Such persons with pseudohypertension might be erroneously diagnosed as hypertensive and treated. Perhaps older hypertensive persons are particularly susceptible to the adverse effects of antihypertensive drugs because this overestimation and overtreatment of blood pressure occurs.[20]

Antihypertensive drugs can sometimes be withdrawn from older adults without the return of hypertension. For example, of 169 patients withdrawn from therapy in one study, 51 patients had blood pressure increases immediately, and medication was reinstituted. Of the 118 remaining patients, 43 (25% of the original group) were still normotensive 1 year later, 16 required treatment for hypertension, 34 were treated with diuretics for congestive heart failure or angina pectoris, and 12 were lost to follow-up.[21] This evidence should not deter appropriate treatment of hypertension in older adults. Studies of older subjects have demonstrated reduction in cardiovascular mortality and stroke with treatment.[22-25]

Isolated systolic hypertension is defined as a blood pressure of greater than 160 mmHg systolic whereas the diastolic blood pressure remains less than 90 mmHg. Isolated systolic hypertension is quite common and is estimated to be present in 20% of persons over the age of 80 and in about 13% of those aged 70 to 79.[26] Isolated systolic hypertension will not be found in up to one third of cases when the blood pressure measurement is repeated.[27] Although believed by many in the past to represent a normal phenomenon in older adults, sustained isolated systolic hypertension is associated with increased risk of stroke and cardiovascular risk, even in the elderly.[28-32] Reduction of the cardiovascular risk may not be the only benefit of hypertension control. When the systolic blood pressure was controlled so that the measurement fell between a window of 135 to 150 mmHg, cognitive improvement was noted in persons with vascular dementia.[33]

Low blood pressure may be associated with some additional risk in older people,[31] namely, exposing the older person to falling hazard and injury. The condition may be only evident if the person is examined for orthostatic changes in blood pressure. Low blood pressure should prompt a search for a remedial condition such as overmedication, anemia, or Addison's disease.[34]

Respirations

After assessment of the pulse and blood pressure, the respirations are observed and counted to assess their rate and depth. Observe for use of accessory muscles of respiration and for retraction in the supraclavicular fossae. During the history taking does the person have to interrupt speaking to catch his or her breath? The usual rate in adults is about 12 to 18 breaths per minute.

Temperature

Older adults frequently do not have a normal febrile response to infections. That pneumonia may present without fever, for example, was observed by Osler, who remarked, "in old age, pneumonia may be latent, coming on without chill." Indeed, older persons are prone to *hypothermia* even from mildly cool ambient temperatures. Body temperatures of less than 95°F may not be readable on most clinical thermometers, and emergency departments are usually equipped with special thermometers that register the lower temperatures. Medications that interfere with the thermoregulatory mechanism, such as tranquilizers, antihypertensives, vasodilators, and antidepressants, as well as ingestion of alcohol, put the older person, who may already have numerous predisposing chronic conditions, at increased risk for hypothermia.

Height, Weight, and Nutrition

Older persons are at increased risk of malnutrition because of inappropriate food intake, social isolation, disability, and chronic medical conditions and medications.[35] Good nutritional status underlies adequate functioning and a sense of well-being. Height and weight are initial elements of the nutritional assessment. Four components of the nutritional assessment can be remembered as ABCD: A for anthropometric measurement such as height and weight, B for biochemical parameters such as serum albumin and the hemoglobin, C for clinical assessment (medical history, physical examination, and other domains discussed in this book), and D for dietary history, such as the content and adequacy of the diet and the use of nutritional supplements.

Although measurement of weight is standard for every patient encounter, measuring the height is not. Measurement of height is useful to evaluate the person's weight with standard weight-height tables. Height may be estimated using landmark measurements on arm and leg.[36] Serial height measurements may be useful. Recording serial height measurements in an aging woman who has a vertebral compression fracture due to osteoporosis may reveal loss of height and kyphosis from other asymptomatic fractures or bone loss. Therapy might then become more aggressive to prevent further bone loss (eg, hormonal therapy). Serial height measurements may also increase the person's awareness of osteoporosis and improve compliance with regimens of calcium, vitamin D, and, if prescribed, hormonal replacement.

The body mass index (BMI) can be calculated to improve interpretation of the height and weight. To calculate BMI, divide the weight of the person in kilograms by the square of the height in meters. Since 1 kg is equivalent to 2.2 lb, the person's weight in pounds must be divided by 2.2 to convert the weight to kilograms. Similarly, because 1 m equals 39.4 in, the person's height in inches must be divided by 39.4 to convert the height to meters. For example, a 72-year-old woman weighs 154 lb and is 5 ft 6 in (66 in). Her weight is 70 kg (154/2.2), and her height is 1.68 m (66/39.4). Her BMI is then calculated as $70/(1.68 \times 1.68) = 24.8$. Overweight was defined as a BMI equal to or greater than 27.8 for males and equal to or greater than 27.3 for females using data from the National Health and Examination Survey II (1976–1980).[37] Recent Clinical Guidelines of the National Heart, Lung, and Blood Institute in cooperation with the National Institute of Diabetes and Digestive and Kidney Diseases, working with many other professional organizations, defined overweight as a BMI between 25 to 29.9 and obesity as 30 and higher.[38]

Biochemical parameters that are useful for assessing nutritional status include the hemoglobin count, serum albumin, and serum cholesterol level. A reduced serum albumin (lower than 3 to 5 g/dL) may be a significant indicator of malnutrition. Clinical assessment of nutrition includes notation of changes in weight. Change in weight is an important parameter to follow in hospitalized or institutionalized patients who may be at increased risk of malnutrition.[39] Loss of subcutaneous fat, muscle wasting, and edema on physical examination may signal chronic malnourishment.[40]

The last component of the nutritional assessment is signified by a "D," the dietary history.[35,38] How does the person obtain and prepare meals? Does the daily diet contain appropriate proportions of food from the Food Guide Pyramid's five food groups: bread, cereal, rice, and pasta (6 to 11 servings); vegetables (3 to 5 servings); fruit (2 to 4 servings); milk, yogurt, and cheese (2 to 3 servings); and meat, poultry, fish, dried beans, eggs, and nuts (2 to 3 servings); fats, oils, and sweets (sparingly)? Does the person take any nutritional supplements, such as multivitamins? Does he or she take any medication that affects appetite or nutrients? Does he or she have a special diet, such as a diabetic diet, or does the person's diet contain an unusual amount of alcohol, sweets, or fried foods? Consider the ABCD components when assessing nutritional status.

Skin

Assessment of the skin should occur as other areas are examined, and the patient is disrobed. Changes in skin condition are generally believed to constitute the quintessential mark of aging itself. Older adults generally have less subcutaneous fat, and, consequently, the skin is thinner, especially on the dorsa of the hands and on the forearms. Elasticity is lost, and the skin turgor is routinely diminished even in patients who are adequately hydrated. Wrinkling and creasing occur, resulting in "crow's feet" at the corners of the eyes and lines on the forehead. Since older adults often have decreased sweat and sebaceous gland production, dry skin is a common finding. The tendency toward dryness can be exaggerated by disease (hypothyroidism) or medication (such as antidepressants with significant anticholinergic effects). Dry skin contributes to conditions such as nummular eczema and "winter itch."

The normal skin changes that occur in aging include the development of hyperpigmented macular lesions called senile freckles or lentigines, sometimes called age or liver spots. Cherry hemangiomas, small red or violet growths, are most often seen on the trunk or extremities and are very common. Skin tags are fleshy soft growths, typically with a pedicle, and are frequently ignored unless injured by clothing or jewelry.

Seborrheic keratoses are pigmented lesions with a waxy or greasy surface that have a stuck-on appearance and generally occur on the trunk and face. Seborrheic keratoses may become secondarily infected. Early lesions could resemble melanoma or other conditions.

Solar lentigo is a brown, flat lesion that is believed to be related to chronic exposure to sunlight. Solar lentigo is to be distinguished from *lentigo maligna*, which is an insidious flat lesion with irregular borders and a distinct variegated color that may include flecks of black. It is believed to represent melanoma in situ; raised areas may represent invasion into the dermis. Doubt about the nature of any lesion should be resolved by biopsy or excision.

Actinic keratoses occur on sun-exposed areas of the skin. The lesions are usually multiple and scaly, enlarging slowly over many years. Some can develop into squamous cell carcinoma, and a sudden spurt of growth in a senile keratosis should raise that possibility. A cutaneous horn is a very proliferative hyperkeratotic form of senile keratosis in which the hyperkeratosis resembles a horn. Such lesions can become quite large.

Basal cell carcinoma is the most common cancer of the skin. Fortunately, basal cell carcinomas only rarely metastasize. Over 90% occur on the head and neck and may take the form of an ulcer or a nodule. A characteristic feature of the ulcerative type is a firm, rolled border. One 65-year-old woman had such a lesion behind her ear for 6 months that she ascribed to irritation from her glasses. *Squamous cell carcinoma* has the potential for metastasis, and sometimes regional lymphadenopathy is found. Typically these lesions arise on sun-exposed areas, especially the face, and are hard and fixed. The lesion eventually becomes erythematous and scaling, initially resembling an actinic keratosis. Unchecked, however, squamous cell carcinoma and basal cell carcinoma, although eminently treatable, may be devastating and disfiguring.

Nummular eczema is generally seen in the winter, and is characterized by coin-shaped areas, resembling ringworm, on the arms and legs that may become secondarily infected. The lesions are intensely pruritic and chronic. The etiology of nummular eczema is unknown, but the low indoor humidity of winter dries the skin and intensifies the itch.

Seborrheic dermatitis also affects older adults. Seborrhea symmetrically involves the scalp, face, and body folds with scaly indistinct macules and papules. These lesions are often greasy and sometimes pruritic. Seborrheic dermatitis is particularly common in persons with Parkinson's disease. *Psoriasis* affects all age groups. The characteristic lesions in psoriasis are the scaly patches that typically involve the scalp, elbows, and knees. Psoriasis may also cause pitting of the nails and may be associated with arthritis.

Herpes zoster causes a painful eruption in the distribution of a peripheral nerve. After a primary infection that causes chickenpox, the virus remains dormant, possibly for decades, until it erupts as shingles. The pain may precede the rash, causing confusion with other conditions.

Herpes zoster involving the first branch of the trigeminal nerve can involve the eye, resulting in corneal scarring. A clue that this is occurring is the presence of vesicles at the tip of the nose. Unfortunately, pain can persist in the involved area even after the lesions have resolved.

Clues to physical abuse of an older adult may come from the examination of the skin. Bruises and welts on the chest, shoulders, back, arms, or legs, perhaps in various stages of healing, can be found in such cases. Unusual patterns, such as bruises that are clustered, might reflect the use of an instrument, a hand, or even biting. Lacerations and abrasions on the lips, eyes, or parts of the face may be associated with infection. Hemorrhages beneath the scalp may have resulted from hair pulling. Of course, frail older persons will be more prone to injuries from falls as well, making detection of real abuse more difficult. In addition, many older persons also bruise easily due to capillary fragility or poor nutrition. In any case, the possibility that such abuse is occurring should be considered when the pattern of injury does not fit the history obtained.[41-44]

Decubitus Ulcers

Impaired mobility puts the older adult at risk for the development of decubitus ulcers, or pressure sores. Other risk factors include malnutrition, dehydration, anemia, cardiovascular disease, edema, and urinary or fecal incontinence.[45] A pressure ulcer can develop over a short period of time (eg, as a result of several hours of surgery). Constant vigilance is required to prevent the development of pressure ulcers in institutionalized or hospitalized older adults.[46] Recurrent or extensive decubiti in older adults might signal abuse or neglect. Patients with decreased mobility, especially older patients admitted to the hospital or nursing home, should be evaluated for risk of decubiti using a standard assessment tool such as that shown in Exhibit 8–2.[47] Once present, treatment should be based on stage of ulceration, and measures to prevent further development of pressure sores should be instituted.[45]

Hair and Nails

Among the most notable indicators of age are changes in the color and distribution of hair. Hair color becomes gray or whitened. Progressive thinning of all body hair, including hair of the axillae and

Exhibit 8–2 Braden Scale for Predicting Risk of Pressure Ulcers

Patient's Name _____ Evaluator's Name _____

				Date of Assessment			

Category	1	2	3	4				
Sensory perception Ability to respond meaningfully to pressure-related discomfort	*1. Completely limited:* a. Unresponsive (does not moan, flinch, or grasp) to painful stimuli, due to diminished level of consciousness or sedation, OR b. Limited ability to feel pain over most of body surface.	*2. Very limited:* a. Responds only to painful stimuli. Cannot communicate discomfort except by moaning or restlessness, OR b. Has a sensory impairment that limits the ability to feel pain or discomfort over 1/2 of body.	*3. Slightly limited:* a. Responds to verbal commands but cannot always communicate discomfort or need to be turned, OR b. Has some sensory impairment that limits ability to feel pain or discomfort in 1 or 2 extremities.	*4. No impairment:* Responds to verbal commands. Has no sensory deficit that would limit ability to feel or voice pain or discomfort.			
Moisture Degree to which skin is exposed to moisture	*1. Constantly moist:* Skin is kept moist almost constantly by perspiration, urine, etc. Dampness is detected every time patient is moved or turned.	*2. Moist:* Skin is often but not always moist. Linen must be changed at least once a shift.	*3. Occasionally moist:* Skin is occasionally moist, requiring an extra linen change approximately once a day.	*4. Rarely moist:* Skin is usually dry; linen requires changing only at routine intervals.			
Activity Degree of physical activity	*1. Bedfast:* Confined to bed.	*2. Chairfast:* Ability to walk severely limited or nonexistent. Cannot bear own weight and/or must be assisted into chair or wheelchair.	*3. Walks occasionally:* Walks occasionally during day but for very short distances, with or without assistance. Spends majority of each shift in bed or chair.	*4. Walks frequently:* Walks outside the room at least twice a day and inside room at least once every 2 hours during waking hours.			
Mobility Ability to change and control body position	*1. Completely immobile:* Does not make even slight changes in body or extremity position without assistance.	*2. Very limited:* Makes occasional slight changes in body or extremity position but unable to make frequent or significant changes independently.	*3. Slightly limited:* Makes frequent though slight changes in body or extremity position independently.	*4. No limitations:* Makes major and frequent changes in position without assistance.			

continues

Exhibit 8–2 continued

	1.	2.	3.	4.
Nutrition Usual food intake pattern	*Very poor:* a. Never eats a complete meal. Rarely eats more than 1/3 of any food offered. Eats 2 servings or less of protein (meat or dairy products) per day. Takes fluids poorly. Does not take a liquid dietary supplement, OR b. Is NPO[1] and/or maintained on clear liquids or IV[2] for more than 5 days.	*Probably inadequate:* a. Rarely eats a complete meal and generally eats only 1/2 of any food offered. Protein intake includes only 3 servings of meat or dairy products per day. Occasionally will take a dietary supplement, OR b. Receives less than optimum amount of liquid or tube feeding.	*Adequate:* a. Eats over half of most meals. Eats a total of 4 servings of protein (meat, dairy products) each day. Occasionally will refuse a meal, but will usually take a supplement if offered, OR b. Is on a tube feeding or TPN[3] regimen, which probably meets most	*Excellent:* Eats most of every meal. Never refuses a meal. Usually eats a total of 4 or more servings of meat and dairy products. Occasionally eats between meals. Does not require supplementation.
Friction and shear	*Problem:* Requires moderate to maximum assistance in moving. Complete lifting without sliding against sheets is impossible. Frequently slides down in bed or chair, requiring frequent repositioning with maximum assistance. Spasticity, contractures, or agitation leads to almost constant friction.	*Potential problem:* Moves feebly or requires minimum assistance. During a move, skin probably slides to some extent against sheets, chair, restraints, or other devices. Maintains relatively good position in chair or bed most of the time but occasionally slides down.	*No apparent problem:* Moves in bed and in chair independently and has sufficient muscle strength to lift up completely during move. Maintains good position in bed or chair at all times.	
				Total score

[1]NPO: Nothing by mouth.   [2]IV: Intravenously.   [3]TPN: Total parenteral nutrition.

Source: Courtesy of Barbara Braden and Nancy Bergstrom. Copyright © 1988. Reprinted with permission.

pubis, occurs with age. The growth of facial hair in older women can sometimes be quite distressing, but measures to reduce the problem, such as depilatory agents, can be recommended. Lack of hair on the lower extremities may indicate diminished peripheral circulation but is often a normal finding in older adults. The nails are frequently afflicted by onychomycosis, a chronic fungal condition of the nail. The thickened, brittle, and crumbling nail is difficult to treat and is a common problem for neglected persons living alone.

Head

The patient is examined in the sitting position starting with the head and working down. The head and skull should be examined for evidence of trauma especially in cases of delirium or sudden changes in level of consciousness. Besides palpation for tenderness and deformity of the skull, the temporal artery is examined for tenderness. Changes in the skull that are characteristic of Paget's disease should be sought, such as frontal bossing or an increase in hat size. Temporal arteritis (or giant cell arteritis) is a condition in which the temporal arteries become tender and may lose their pulsations. This disorder may present as a headache that is unilateral and classically temporal. There may be dimness of vision. Temporal arteritis is an important condition to recognize because if untreated it can lead to blindness. Fever and elevated white blood cell count may occur. The sedimentation rate is markedly increased in advanced cases. Symmetrical pain and weakness of shoulders and hips can accompany temporal arteritis (polymyalgia rheumatica).

Eyes

After the cranium is assessed, the eyes are examined. Age-related changes in the eyes include darkening of the skin around the orbits, crow's feet, slower pupillary light reflex (which still, however, ought to be equal bilaterally), decreased tearing, and decreased adaptation to the dark. The older person, perhaps because of diminished pupil size and increased thickness and opacity of the lens, needs more illumination to compensate than someone younger.

The structures surrounding the eye itself are inspected first. Xanthomas are fat deposits sometimes seen in the skin near the eyes and may be associated with elevated levels of blood lipids. Loss of the lateral third of the eyebrows, although a classic sign of hypothyroidism, may be a normal finding in some older persons. On each eyelid, the examiner will find a central, relatively rigid tarsal plate that, in advancing age, may become lax, leading to ectropion (eversion of the lids), thereby exposing the eyes to drying and infection. The margin of the lid may roll backward toward the eye as well, so that eyelashes brush against the cornea, causing entropion.

The sclera is normally white but is uniformly yellow in patients with jaundice. In older persons, the periphery of the sclera may be yellow due to deposits of fat showing through thinned scleral membranes. Pingueculae are thin fatty structures that usually lie laterally on the eyeball. They may increase in size with advancing age, but are benign and generally cause no problem with vision. The conjunctiva, or lining of the eye, can become inflamed or infected. This is a common eye problem in older adults, particularly since they are prone to having dry eyes. Such drying may predispose them to infection of the conjunctiva by bacterial or viral agents. Conjunctivitis is associated with a red eye and purulent discharge, but discomfort is minimal. A painful red eye may signal iritis, glaucoma, or an abrasion.

Arcus senilis is a striking finding in some older persons. Initially, a thin line that is limited to the upper portion of the eye, it becomes thicker and denser and completely encircles the cornea. While arcus is found with other stigmata in persons with familial hypercholesterolemia, many persons with arcus will have normal cholesterol levels. Arcus senilis is a very common finding in persons aged 65 years and older.

The lens of the eye produces new fibers throughout life, but none are lost. These accumulate in the center of the lens, increasing its density and contributing to the development of senile cataracts that are generally bilateral. The lens loses its elasticity with advanced age so that the eye is more farsighted (presbyopia). Before ophthalmoscopy, the person's visual acuity is checked for reading and distance, with and without glasses. The pupils may react more sluggishly to light but should be equal in size. Many disorders may cause asymmetry of the pupils, including central nervous system lesions and diabetes; drugs can have this effect as well. After iridectomy, the pupil may be irregular. The extraocular muscles are checked for full range of motion: up and down, left and right.

Ophthalmoscopic examination of each eye should begin by focusing on the most anterior structures first and then working back to the retina. A cataract may be best visualized by focusing on the lens with an ophthalmoscope. A cataract appears as a black area against the orange reflection from the retina. The precise significance of the cataract depends on how much it interferes with the person's vision, function, and work.

Increased lens opacity with advancing age allows less light to pass to the retina than at younger ages. The 60-year-old retina receives only a fraction of the amount of light as the 20-year-old retina. Improved lighting may be all that is required to allow an older person to read small print, such as that in a telephone directory or the newspaper. Provision of excellent lighting in waiting and examination rooms is essential.

Examination of the retina with the ophthalmoscope requires some practice. The normal fundus reveals the optic disc, the macula, and arteries and veins. Pigment in the retina usually corresponds to skin pigmentation. The normal optic disc is frequently outlined by pigment. In older adults with hypertension or arteriosclerosis, and sometimes in normal older adults, so-called copper-wire changes caused by thickening of the arteriolar walls may be seen. As the vessel walls become more thickened, the vessels appear white or silver. Nicking, or narrowing, of venules by crossing arterioles becomes evident as the process continues. Exudates, hemorrhages, and cotton-wool spots may also be seen on the retina as a result of hypertension or diabetes.

Macular degeneration is a major cause of visual disability in older persons. The macula, the region of the retina with sharpest acuity, is affected. Visual acuity is decreased, but peripheral vision is preserved. Special studies by an ophthalmologist may be required to make the diagnosis of senile macular degeneration.

In glaucoma, the intraocular pressure is elevated, and there is contraction of the visual field. On ophthalmoscopic examination, the optic cup, which is a depression in the optic nerve as it emerges on the retina, is accentuated. The visual field of the person with Alzheimer's disease is contracted when compared with that of persons who were demented from other causes. This may significantly alter the demented person's perception of the environment.[48]

Ears

After the practitioner examines the eyes, the otoscope is used to examine the ears. Painless nodules on the pinnae of the ears could be basal cell carcinomas, rheumatoid nodules, or even gouty tophi. Common changes seen with age include increased ear lobe length, hair growth in the canal, and accumulation of cerumen. Loss of hearing that is due to problems with the external ear include impacted cerumen, external otitis, or foreign body. External otitis can be due to allergic reactions or irritation due to hearing aids. Malignant otitis externa is a *Pseudomonas* infection that involves the ear canal and presents as granulation tissue at the juncture of bone and cartilage.

The normal tympanic membrane is gray or pink with a light reflex produced by its cone shape. The malleus, which is the first of the three small bones in the inner ear, can be seen indenting the membrane, pointing posteriorly. The tympanic membrane may be thickened in the older person (tympanosclerosis), possibly as a result of scarring from prior infections. Effusions occur in relation to eustachian tube dysfunction, as in allergy or upper respiratory tract infection.

Hearing is assessed during the history-taking session but can be grossly gauged by such techniques as whispering words in the person's ear. Hearing loss may, for the sake of simplicity, be divided into conductive loss and sensorineural loss. *Conductive hearing loss* implies interference in the conduct of sound energy into the inner ear. It can be due to foreign bodies, cerumen, abnormalities of the tympanic membrane, otitis media or externa, or involvement of the ossicles with Paget's disease, rheumatoid arthritis, or otosclerosis (in which the stapes becomes fixed to the oval window of the cochlea).[49] Cerumen in the canal may be the primary or a contributing cause of hearing loss that is easily remedied.

Sensorineural hearing loss means disease anywhere from the organ of Corti to the brain. The cells within the organ of Corti are not replaced; thus, there is a gradual loss as the person ages. The result is high-tone hearing loss because it is hair cells in the basal turn of the organ of Corti, those sensitive to high tone, that are lost. Presbycusis is sensorineural hearing loss due to aging of the inner ear.[49] Often both conductive and sensorineural hearing loss are present simultaneously and the precise nature of the defect requires sophisticated audiometric testing. The ability to hear high frequency sounds is affected first so that certain consonants and sibilants become unintelligible (for example, *f, s, th, ch,* and *sh*). Understanding speech depends in large measure on the clear perception of these high-frequency consonants rather than low-frequency vowel sounds. Sensorineural hearing loss can be due to toxic damage to the hair cells of the organ of Corti from aspirin, aminoglycoside antibiotics, or diuretics; from trauma; and a wide variety of disorders from vascular insufficiency (the inner ear is dependent on a single end artery for its blood supply) to central nervous system disease.

The combination of hearing loss and cognitive impairment can lead to social isolation and paranoia and may make mental status testing a real challenge. Three simple clinical tests using a tuning fork may help sort out the type of hearing loss. These are the Rinne test, Weber's test, and Schwabach's test. To perform the *Rinne test*, the tuning fork is struck and applied to the mastoid prominence behind the ear. When the person indicates he or she no longer hears the sound, the vibrating fork is immediately put near the external canal. Normally, the sound is then heard and the test is said to be positive. Put another way, air conduction is better than bone conduction. A negative test, one in which the person does not hear the tuning fork in air, suggests there is a conduction loss in that ear.

Whether there is a conductive hearing loss in one ear can then be confirmed by *Weber's test.* A vibrating tuning fork is placed on the vertex of the head and the patient is asked if the sound is heard better in one ear than the other. Normally, the sound appears to come from above, that is, in the middle. If a conductive defect is present in one ear, the sound is heard best in that ear (bone conduction makes up for the defect). On the other hand, if deafness in an ear is due to neural problems, that ear will not sense any sound, and sound will only be heard in the contralateral or good ear.

Schwabach's test confirms a diagnosis of sensorineural deafness by comparing the person's hearing with the examiner's. The vibrating tuning fork is put on the person's mastoid process. When the sound is no longer heard by the patient, the fork is put on the examiner's mastoid. If the sound is heard by the examiner, then a sensorineural deficit in the person is confirmed.

Nose

The otoscope can be used to examine the nasal mucosa and the internal nasal architecture. Nasal patency should be tested by occluding one nostril. Nasal congestion due to vasomotor rhinitis, characterized by postnasal drip, little sneezing, and no eosinophils on nasal smear, can be particularly disturbing and interfere with sleep.

Rhinophyma of the nose starts as a diffuse redness, followed by papules, pustules, and, later, dilated venules. Excess ingestion of alcohol may be associated. The paranasal sinuses may be palpated for tenderness. Any chronic drainage from the nose that does not respond to therapy should be investigated since chronic drainage can be a symptom of cancer in the sinuses.

The sense of smell decreases with age, and the decrease in smell is often experienced as a loss of taste. The loss of the sense of smell can be significant for nutrition and safety. Many older persons cannot enjoy the pleasant smell of food cooking—smells that stimulate the appetite and make eating enjoyable. The inability to smell leaking natural gas creates a risk of serious accident. With age, the anterior taste buds, which are sensitive to sweet and salt, deteriorate before the posterior taste buds, which are sensitive to bitter and sour; thus, older adult patients frequently complain that food tastes bitter or sour. When cooking, older people may add undesirable amounts of salt to food to compensate for the loss of taste. Progressive loss of the senses of smell and taste means that, for older persons, the appearance and consistency of food plays a proportionately greater role in food's appeal.

Mouth

Cheilosis, or fissures at the angles of the mouth, may be a sign of poor nutrition and vitamin deficiency. Carcinomatous lesions may occur on the lips, which are highly exposed to sunlight. The oral mucosa may be dry because of diminished sputum production or due to drugs the individual is taking, particularly those with anticholinergic side effects. The oral mucosa should be carefully inspected for lesions by using the tongue blade to move the buccal mucosa away from the teeth. Leukoplakia is a white patch or plaque on any of the mucous membranes of the mouth that may appear to be painted on the surface. These patches may be present for years and represent a premalignant condition. Such lesions should be biopsied for definitive diagnosis. Other lesions with a similar appearance are *Candida* (thrush) and lichen planus. Traumatic injury, in particular from ill-fitting dentures, may damage the oral mucosa, producing erythematous tissue changes. In addition to inspection, a moistened glove may be used to palpate the buccal cavity, including the lips and floor of the mouth, for areas of induration. Palpation is particularly important to evaluate complaints related to the oral region, to assess suspicious areas, or to evaluate persons at risk of oral cancer (eg, those with a history of tobacco or alcohol use).

A lesion of the hard palate with no particular clinical significance except that it be recognized as benign is the torus pallatinus. It must be reiterated, however, that any masses not in the midline are suspect as neoplasms. A slowly growing asymptomatic lesion with a rough surface, irregular margin, and firm consistency should be biopsied, no matter how long it has been there.

The examination of the tongue should not be neglected. A sore, red inflamed tongue may be found in persons with vitamin B-12 or iron deficiency. Hairy or black tongue is a condition in which it looks as if the tongue is growing short hairs. It is symptomless and appears during treatment with antibiotics that inhibit normal bacteria and permit fungal overgrowth. The tongue may also be observed for fasciculations, which indicate lower motor neuron disease, and for abnormal movements such as tardive dyskinesia.

Teeth

Tooth loss and periodontal disease are extremely common in older persons. As many as half of all persons over age 65 are edentulous. Older persons are likely to see their physician more frequently than their dentist.[50,51] For this reason, it is particularly important to remove the dentures and inspect the mouth surfaces for areas of irritation and for suspicious lesions. The upper and lower lips are examined including hidden surfaces. Poorly fitting dentures can have far-reaching consequences, such as malnutrition, and result in numerous problems, such as traumatic ulcers, denture stomatitis, and possibly even cancer.

Any dental malocclusion, as well as abnormal speech sounds, such as slurred "s," clicks, or whistles, which signal improperly fitting dentures, should be recognized. The person may fail to realize that a misfitting of dentures has developed. Older adults should be encouraged to visit the dentist every year or two so that dentures can be adjusted to account for changing mandibular bone structure.

Older persons who retain teeth need to have their oral hygiene assessed. Dental caries may appear as soft white, yellow, or brown areas on the tooth. The person may complain of sensitivity to extremes of temperature. Periodontal disease, a major cause of tooth loss, involves inflammation and destruction of the supporting structures of the teeth.[51] Foul breath odor is common with dental infections, retention of food particles in the teeth or dentures, or chronic periodontal disease. It can also result from sinusitis or pulmonary infection.

Neck

The neck presents several important structures for examination: the lymph nodes, the trachea, the thyroid gland, and the carotid arteries. The posterior and anterior cervical lymph node chains as well as the supraclavicular area should be carefully palpated. Virchow's node, enlargement of the lymph node in the left supraclavicular fossa, is a classic sign of metastatic gastrointestinal carcinoma. The trachea should be checked for lateral deviation, and a search made for jugular venous distention, which could be a sign of heart failure. Prominent pulsations above the clavicle may represent kinking of a carotid artery or prominence of the innominate artery.

The carotids should be gently palpated. The pulses should be symmetrical. A bounding or collapsing pulse, in which the upstroke of the pulse wave is very sharp and the downstroke falls rapidly, may be present in a person with essential hypertension, thyrotoxicosis, aortic regurgitation, or an extreme emotional state. The carotids may be auscultated using the bell of the stethoscope, listening for bruits that signify turbulent blood flow (and not necessarily hemodynamically significant narrowing). The presence of bruits may be a clue to atherosclerosis and could be an important finding in an individual with a history of syncope, stroke, or transient ischemic attack. In asymptomatic persons, bruits are probably more indicative of coronary artery disease than of cerebrovascular disease, at least in older men.[52]

Attempt to palpate the thyroid gland for enlargement from both in front and in back of the person, even though the gland is generally not easily palpated. If the gland is enlarged, it must be determined whether the gland is diffusely enlarged (goiter) or exhibits discrete nodularity. Sometimes a bruit may be heard over vascular thyroid lesions, and occasionally a thrill is felt. Thyroid disease in older adults is notorious for subtle presentation. For example, hypothyroidism may manifest solely as depression or mental deterioration. The symptoms of hypothyroidism are easily misinterpreted by the older adult or the physician and include dry skin, constipation, sleepiness, lethargy, cold intolerance, and fatigue. Periodic evaluation of serum thyroid-stimulating hormone levels has been suggested in order to detect impending hypothyroidism.[53,54]

Hyperthyroidism or thyrotoxicosis may present without the signs and symptoms usually found in younger persons, such as exophthalmos, restlessness, hyperactivity, and tachycardia. Atrial fibrillation occurs in half of older hyperthyroid persons, but in only 10% of younger persons, while ocular changes are less common in older adults who are hyperthyroid. The term "apathetic thyrotoxicosis" has been used to refer to hyperthyroidism in older persons with nonspecific signs and symptoms. Results of thyroid function tests may be falsely reassuring unless the triiodothyronine (T-3) value measured by radioimmunoassay is specifically requested. Constipation, weight loss, and anorexia of hyperthyroidism may resemble a gastrointestinal carcinoma. The hyperthyroid state may precipitate heart failure as the presenting illness.

Heart and Lungs

The heart and lungs may be examined next while the client is still seated. Cardiovascular disease and morbidity is very common in older adults.[55] In older persons angina pectoris may very well present as dyspnea rather than as pain. Other common presentations are palpitations or syncope on exertion.[56] Patients presenting with transient ischemic attack, stroke, or an episode of confusion should have myocardial infarction considered in the differential diagnosis. Even when the pain is typical, an older person may ascribe it to other causes, so that jaw pain is attributed to arthritis and epigastric pain to hiatal hernia or ulcer.[55] Heart disease may be associated with nonspecific fatigue or weakness.

The palm of the examiner's hand is placed over the apex of the patient's heart to palpate the apex pulsation. Normally the apex pulsation covers an area the size of a half-dollar. If the apex pulsation is not easily palpated, the person may be asked to lean forward or to move into a left lateral decubitus position. Cardiac hypertrophy as a result of hypertension, for example, produces a small vigorous apical beat. Dilated ventricles, as from mitral regurgitation, cause the apex beat to be lateral to the midclavicular line. The heart size probably remains unchanged in healthy older persons.[57]

In auscultating the heart, the examiner should start at the apex using the diaphragm, inch across to the left lower sternal border, and then to the left second intercostal space, then cross to the right and down the right sternal border. The first and second heart sounds are listened to first. Simultaneous palpation of the carotid pulse may help identify which sound is the first heart sound. Since the first heart sound is produced by the closure of the mitral and tricuspid valves, it sounds louder than the second heart sound over the mitral and tricuspid areas (the apex of the heart and the right lower sternal border, respectively).

The sequence of auscultation is repeated to listen for murmurs and for silence in systole and diastole. High-pitched clicks and many murmurs will best be heard using the diaphragm of the stethoscope. Lower-pitched sounds such as gallops and diastolic rumbles arising from the mitral and tricuspid valves will best be heard with the bell of the stethoscope. Diastolic murmurs are always significant and may be caused by mitral stenosis. Aortic or pulmonic regurgitation may also be associated with diastolic murmurs. Mitral stenosis may be silent in older adults. Atrial fibrillation, particularly when accompanied by mitral stenosis or an enlarged left atrium, is a significant risk factor for stroke.

Systolic murmurs are very common in persons over the age of 65 years. Functional flow murmurs from a dilated aortic annulus are short, early systolic murmurs heard at the cardiac base. The second heart sound is normally split, and the carotid upstrokes are normal. The murmur of aortic stenosis is a systolic ejection (diamond-shaped murmur) at the base classically with diminished carotid upstrokes, sustained apical impulse, and a fourth heart sound. These findings may not be present in the older person. Mitral regurgitation in the elderly is commonly due to ischemic heart disease and results in a holosystolic murmur.[55] Since systolic murmurs are so common in older adults, distinguishing benign murmurs from significant murmurs in asymptomatic patients can be difficult.

Abnormalities of the heart rhythm may be poorly tolerated by older adults who generally have less reserve capacity than younger persons. Atrial fibrillation, for example, may not be tolerated because early diastolic filling in the older heart is considerably diminished. The contribution of the atrial "kick" to ventricular filling, lost in atrial fibrillation, becomes critical to appropriate cardiac output.

Arrhythmias are apparently quite prevalent in otherwise healthy older persons, with prognosis and significance probably related to the presence of overt or unrecognized coronary artery disease.[58-62] In one study, of 106 older adults studied with 24-hour electrocardiographic monitoring, one fourth had multifocal premature ventricular contractions and four had ventricular tachycardia. After 18 months of follow-up, recordings showed no difference among the 13 persons who died compared with the group as a whole.[62] In another study, supraventricular tachycardia was present in 28% of 50 persons over the age of 80 who were studied with 24-hour ambulatory electrocardiographic monitoring. Every person exhibited supraventricular ectopic beats, and 65% had more than 20 ectopic beats per hour. Premature ventricular contractions were also quite common, occurring in 32% of the persons at a rate of greater than 10 premature beats per hour. In 18% of the persons, the premature contractions were multifocal.[63]

Following the cardiac examination, the lungs are examined by auscultation and percussion. Assessment of respiration should have begun when the person came into the examining room. The rate and depth of breathing, as well as any use of accessory muscles of respiration, were observed. The aged lung has less elasticity due to loss of elastin and to collagen crosslinking. While listening over the chest and asking the person to take a few deep breaths, the physician must be alert for signs of hyperventilation, such as dizziness, especially in the older person, to avoid inducing syncope. Normally, only so-called vesicular breath sounds are heard over the chest. Bronchial or tubular breath sounds can be heard over the trachea. If one hears such sounds over the peripheral lung fields, consolidation is suggested.

Rales are sounds produced by the movement of fluid or exudate in the airways. Small amounts of fluid may be detected as posttussive rales. For posttussive rales to be heard, the person must expire fully and cough. When he or she inspires with the next breath, fine crackles can be heard. The cough collapses some wet alveoli, which are then heard opening in inspiration. Moist rales or rhonchi are gurgling sounds arising from larger bronchi. Moist breath sounds at the bases in older adults often do not represent congestive heart failure. Such marginal or atelectatic rales are heard most frequently in aged, debilitated, or bedridden patients or in habitual shallow breathers. These sounds should disappear after the person takes a few deep breaths. Other adventitious sounds heard in the lungs are friction rubs and wheezes.

The lung fields are percussed for areas of dullness or hyperresonance as further maneuvers to detect any abnormality. An underlying consolidation or effusion will yield dullness or flatness on percussion. In chronic obstructive pulmonary disease the lungs are often hyperresonant (that is, the pitch on auscultation is higher than that over the normal lung). A check is then made for tactile fremitus: after the ulnar surfaces of both the examiner's hands are applied to either side of the person's chest, the patient is asked to speak ("say 99"). Differences in vibration from one side to another may be significant. Consolidation as in pneumonia increases fremitus. Sometimes it is helpful to auscultate the lung fields and simultaneously tap the sternum. Increased transmission of the sound through areas of consolidation is sometimes identified more readily when using this technique rather than simple percussion. The clinician listens over the lung fields and asks the person to say "E." The "E" will frequently sound like "A" over a pleural effusion (egophony).

Musculoskeletal System

At the time the lungs are auscultated, any kyphosis or scoliosis is noted. Severe kyphosis can interfere with breathing and cardiovascular function. Tenderness over the spinous processes may portend a vertebral fracture. The joints are inspected next, particularly the joints of the hands. Osteoarthritis is common and especially affects the distal interphalangeal joints of the hands as well as the knees. Bony overgrowths at the distal interphalangeal joint are called Heberden's nodes. Limitation of external rotation of the hip can be an early sign of osteoarthritic involvement. Indeed, the range of motion of all the joints should be assessed.

Rheumatoid arthritis in the hands tends to affect the proximal interphalangeal joints. Joint swelling seen in rheumatoid joints is not bone, but rather synovia and soft tissue swelling that can be felt along the dorsal surface of the involved interphalangeal joint. Progression of the disease produces ulnar deviation in the hands at the metacarpophalangeal joints, as well as a tendency for joints to sublux. Morning pain and stiffness may last several hours for the person with rheumatoid arthritis, whereas the person with osteoarthritis is relieved from pain after a short period of limbering up the affected joints.

Clubbing of the fingers may indicate an underlying chronic disorder resulting in hypoxia. A normal nail, when viewed from the side, forms an angle with the skin of the nail bed. Clubbing results when the angle is greater than normal, and the finger has a "rounded" appearance. Clubbing is seen in chronic lung disorders, carcinoma of the lung, and other disorders associated with chronic hypoxia. The feet may be examined for changes in the joints and for clubbing as well. Frequently, the examination of the foot reveals evidence of diabetes, neglect, or peripheral vascular disease. The examination of the lower extremities may be deferred until the abdominal examination when the person will be supine.

Abdomen

The patient is placed supine so that the abdomen, breasts, peripheral pulses, genitalia, and the rectum may be examined. It is important to make the older person as comfortable as possible for this part of the examination. A pillow can be used or the head of the examining table elevated slightly to support the head and upper back; a perfectly flat position is uncomfortable for some older adults.

Examination of the abdomen begins with inspection, noting any distention or scars from previous surgery. The examiner should listen to the abdomen before proceeding with palpation to avoid inducing peristaltic activity. Partial bowel obstruction produces rushing sounds, and when obstruction is complete, the sounds may become tinkling or very high pitched. Ileus produced by obstruction or from other causes, such as pneumonia or appendicitis, may result in absence of bowel sounds. Abdominal wall rigidity is not as common a sign of peritoneal irritation among the older as among younger persons.

Constipation may produce a mass of feces that can easily be palpated and mistaken for a tumor. Conversely, a silent abdominal mass may be the only sign of a gastrointestinal carcinoma. Tortuosity or aneurysm of the abdominal aorta may be felt as a pulsatile mass in the abdomen. An abdominal aortic aneurysm may have lateral as well as anteroposterior pulsation, which distinguishes it from a mass in front of the aorta, which merely transmits the pulsations to the examining hand. In thin persons the aortic pulsation may be felt normally and may be quite alarming to the unsuspecting examiner. An abdominal ultrasound is a noninvasive way to evaluate the person for the possibility of an aneurysm. Leaking aneurysm or mesenteric ischemia should be considered in the differential of abdominal pain in older adults.

In addition to palpating and percussing the liver to estimate its size, the midlower abdomen is palpated to check for bladder distention. Such a finding may be important in the evaluation of incontinence or as a sign of urinary retention from prostatic hypertrophy. Urinary retention may be the cause of otherwise unexplainable confusion. With the patient still supine, the peripheral pulses in the feet are checked. The femoral arteries may be palpated in the groin and auscultated for bruits. Bruits heard in the femoral arteries are evidence of diffuse atherosclerotic disease. While examining the area of the groin, the physician can check for lymph node swelling. The feet and lower legs can be examined for skin changes and skin breakdown. Diabetics are at increased risk for foot ulcers and infection. Decubiti and heel sores are common, particularly in those persons who are bedfast. The legs are examined for evidence of arterial insufficiency: namely, laterally placed ulcers, loss of the skin appendages, and poor circulation in the toes. Venous insufficiency may be manifest by pigmented, medially placed ulcers.

Breasts

Palpation and examination of the breasts should not be neglected. Ideally this examination is done both while the patient is sitting and again while the patient is supine during the abdominal examination. A search is made for nipple retraction, skin changes, and masses, which, because of loss of connective tissue and adipose, are often more easily appreciated in the older woman. Retraction of the nipple secondary to age-related changes can be everted with gentle pressure around the nipple. Retraction due to an underlying growth, however, cannot be everted by such gentle pressure. The nipples are palpated so as to express any discharge present. All four quadrants of both breasts are examined including the axillary tail and a careful inspection made for any asymmetry. The skin under large, pendulous breasts is examined for maceration due to perspiration. The male breasts are not exempt from disease and should also be examined. Gynecomastia (breast enlargement) in an older male can result from a variety of causes, including bronchiogenic carcinoma, thyroid disease, testicular tumors, drugs (such as spironolactone), liver cirrhosis, and other types of cancer.

Genitourinary System

The genitalia in both men and women may be conveniently examined in conjunction with the rectal examination. This part of the examination may be deferred but never neglected.

The male genitalia should be examined for sores, discharge, and testicular masses. The glans of the penis in an uncircumcised man is checked by retracting the foreskin. The prostate is palpated during the rectal examination. The prostate is frequently enlarged in older men but should normally feel soft and nonnodular. The two lobes of the prostate can usually be distinguished by the median furrow between them. Since lobes of the prostate not palpable by the examining finger may enlarge and cause obstruction, a normal-sized gland on physical examination does not rule out urinary obstruction from prostatic enlargement. Do not neglect the evaluation of the prostate in the workup of back pain.

The female genitalia should at a minimum be inspected for lesions of the skin, although a bimanual and speculum pelvic examination, which is often neglected, is mandatory if urinary incontinence is a problem or if the woman is due for a Papanicolaou smear. Note is made of any cystocele, rectocele, or uterine prolapse that may occur as the pelvic musculature becomes lax with age. After the menopause, the estrogen-responsive tissues of the genitalia and the lower urinary tract atrophy. This leads to dryness of the vagina, shrinkage of the vagina and its surrounding structures, altered bacterial resistance, and weakened uterine ligaments. Urinary incontinence and infections may result. Postmenopausal changes in the vagina cause itching, burning, and dyspareunia (painful intercourse), which are symptoms most older women are reluctant to spontaneously volunteer. The context of the pelvic examination, however, is a natural one in which to broach such subjects in a straightforward and supportive manner. Vaginal atrophy may also be associated with bleeding, but it should be emphasized that all postmenopausal bleeding must be suspect for uterine carcinoma until proved otherwise. Additionally, palpable ovaries are never normal in an older woman.

Rectal examination may be performed after the patient is helped into the lateral decubitus position (alternatively, the patient may be asked to bend over the examination table). The examiner should tell the patient what to expect and when. The anus is inspected for tears, irritation, and external hemorrhoids, and the tone of the anal sphincter, which may diminish with age, is noted. A gloved finger is used to make a sweep of the entire rectum, being sure to take in its entire circumference. The patient is asked to strain, as at stool, to bring down any lesions just outside the reach of the examining finger. A stool sample to test for occult blood is obtained.

Older adults may not want to bring urinary incontinence to the attention of their doctor, preferring instead to make adjustments on their own, such as decreasing fluid intake and using absorbent napkins. In addition to a neurologic examination that includes testing for perineal sensation and sacral reflexes, and a pelvic examination in women and prostate examination in men, examine the abdomen for grossly distended bladder and look for leaking of urine in the supine and standing position.[64] Fecal incontinence is a serious problem among institutionalized older adults and is a significant risk factor for formation of decubiti.[65] Guidelines for the evaluation and treatment of urinary incontinence provide detailed information on the office assessment.[66]

Sexual functioning in late life was formerly a taboo subject; yet older adults in good health may continue sexual expression and intimacy. Potentially treatable problems such as impotence in men or diminished vaginal lubrication in women can significantly diminish quality of life and should be addressed. Problems with sexual functioning may be at the root of depression or poor adherence to therapeutic regimens. Education regarding sexually-transmitted diseases, including AIDS, continues to be important for older adults.

Nervous System

The neurologic examination is performed after bringing the person to a sitting position. The neurologic examination is composed of six components: intellectual function, the cranial nerves, motor examination, sensory examination, reflexes, and cerebellar examination. The mental status examination was discussed at length in Chapter 3. The importance of the mental status examination should be emphasized again. Unless in an advanced stage, patients with Alzheimer's disease have a normal neurologic examination to an examiner who neglects to specifically test cognitive functioning.

Age-related changes in the nervous system include decreased vibratory sensation (especially in the legs), less brisk deep tendon reflexes, and decreased ability for upward gaze.[67] The Achilles tendon reflex is frequently unobtainable. The so-called pathologic reflexes such as the grasp, palmomental, glabellar, and snout reflexes are characteristic of release of cortical inhibition, but are fairly common in normal older persons. Concomitant presence of these release signs may signal arteriosclerotic changes in the brain or dementia.[68] Demented persons with pathologic reflexes may have more functional impairment and poorer prognosis, but the release signs may also be present in persons without dementia.[69,70]

Sensation may be tested by evaluation of the person's ability to feel a soft cotton-tipped applicator, sharp pinprick, and vibrating tuning fork. Such examination is often quite subjective, and sometimes deficits are not reproducible. Impaired mental status or aphasia may make sensory examination more difficult, prone to error, or even impossible. More complex sensory integration is examined by asking the patient to identify common objects placed in his or her hands, such as a coin, comb, or paper clip (stereognosis). Position sense (proprioception) is examined by asking the patient to identify the direction in which the toes or fingers are displaced by the examiner. Elderly persons asked to stand with their feet together and eyes closed (Romberg test) may have some difficulty, perhaps due to impaired proprioception.

Motor tone is frequently increased in older persons. Passive movement of the person's limb by the examiner may commonly demonstrate gegenhalten, or involuntary rigidity, which should not be mistaken for lack of cooperation. Strength is decreased as is muscle mass, especially in the small muscles of the hands. Coarse senile tremors may involve the head as well as the hands, may improve after alcohol use, and may worsen with stress or fatigue.

Gait and Balance

Falling is an example of a geriatric problem with multiple contributing causes and serious consequences requiring careful delineation of the circumstances of the fall and thorough search for underlying physical illness. The risk of falling increases with advancing age, and simple diagnostic evaluation may identify persons at increased risk.[71-73] The patient can be observed as he or she is requested to sit and rise from a chair, walk and turn around, and bend down to pick up an object off the floor.[74] Does the individual rise from a chair in a single movement? Is he or she steady in walking and turning without grasping for support, while using smooth continuous movement? Does the person seem sure of him- or herself when bending? Observe the patient climbing and descending a flight of stairs, if possible.[75] Testing balance and gait in a standard way (Exhibit 8–3) would be indicated for persons with neurologic disorders as well as to assess the effect of medications that might interfere with balance.

Exhibit 8–3 Tinetti Balance and Gait Evaluation

BALANCE
Instructions: Seat the subject in a hard armless chair. Test the following maneuvers. Select one number that best describes the subject's performance in each text, and add up the scores at the end.

1. Sitting balance
   Leans or slides in chair   = 0
   Steady, safe   = 1 ____

2. Arising
   Unstable without help   = 0
   Able but uses arms to help   = 1
   Able without use of arms   = 2 ____

3. Attempt to arise
   Unable without help   = 0
   Able but requires more than one attempt   = 1
   Able to arise with one attempt   = 2 ____

4. Immediate standing balance (first 5 seconds)
   Unsteady (staggers, moves feet, marked trunk sway)   = 0
   Steady but uses walker or cane or grabs other objects for support = 1
   Steady without walker, cane, or other support   = 2 ____

5. Standing balance
   Unsteady   = 0
   Steady but wide stance (medial heels more than 4 inches
    apart) or uses cane, walker, or other support   = 1
   Narrow stance without support   = 2 ____

6. Nudging (With subject's feet as close together as possible, push
    lightly on the sternum with palm of hand three times.)
   Begins to fall   = 0
   Staggers and grabs, but catches self   = 1
   Steady   = 2 ____

7. Eyes closed (at same position as in No. 6)
   Unsteady   = 0
   Steady   = 1 ____

8. Turning 360 degrees
   Discontinuous steps   = 0
   Continuous steps   = 1 ____
   Unsteady (grabs and staggers)   = 0
   Steady   = 1 ____

continues

Exhibit 8–3 continued

9. Sitting down
   Unsafe (misjudges distance, falls into chair)   = 0
   Uses arms or lacks smooth motion   = 1
   Safe, smooth motion   = 2 _____

GAIT
Instructions: The subject stands with the examiner, and then walks down hallway
or across room, first at the usual pace and then back at a rapid but safe pace, using
a cane or walker if accustomed to one.

10. Initiation of gait (immediately after being told to go)
    Any hesitancy or several attempts to start   = 0
    No hesitancy   = 1 _____

11. Step length and height
    Right swing foot:
       Fails to pass left stance foot with step   = 0
       Passes left stance foot   = 1 _____
       Fails to clear floor completely with step   = 0
       Completely clears floor   = 1 _____
    Left swing foot:
       Fails to pass right stance foot with step   = 0
       Passes right stance foot   = 1 _____
       Fails to clear floor completely with step   = 0
       Completely clears floor   = 1 _____

12. Step symmetry
    Right and left step length unequal   = 0
    Right and left step equal   = 1 _____

13. Step continuity
    Stopping or discontinuity between steps   = 0
    Steps appear continuous   = 1 _____

14. Path (Observe excursion of either left or right foot over
    about 10 feet of the course.)
    Marked deviation   = 0
    Milk to moderate deviation or uses walking aid   = 1
    Walks straight without aid   = 2 _____

15. Trunk
    Marked sway or uses walking aid   = 0
    No sway but flexion of knees or back or spreads arms out = 1
      while walking
    No sway, flexion, use of arms, or use of walking aid   = 2 _____

continues

Exhibit 8–3 continued

16. Walking stance
   Heels apart   = 0
   Heels almost touch while walking   = 1 _____

Balance score: _____ /16   Gait score: _____ /12
               Total score: _____ /28

Source: Adapted with permission from M Tinetti, Performance-Oriented Assessment of Mobility Problems in Elderly Patients, *Journal of the American Geriatric Society*, Vol. 34, pp. 119–126, © 1986, Lippincott Williams & Wilkins.

CONCLUSION

The physical examination of the older person is not markedly different than the physical examination of any adult. The focus on contributing factors to functional loss, the frequent barriers to communication present in older adults (such as impaired special senses), and the difficulty of many older adults in obtaining adequate access to medical care (because of their values or inadequate transportation) distinguish the examination of the older adult from examination of younger persons. In addition, the increased morbidity incurred as a person ages cannot be neglected. The physical examination is complementary to functional, social, economic, and values assessment. For the older adult, evaluation of these other domains is often the key to the solution of the multifaceted problems of living presented by older adults to the primary care practitioner and others who care for the elderly.

REFERENCES

1. Fried L, Storer DJ, King DE, Lodder F. Diagnosis of illness presentation in the elderly. *J Am Geriatr Soc.* 1991;39:117–123.
2. Galazka S. Preoperative evaluation of the elderly surgical patient. *J Fam Pract.* 1988;27:622–632.
3. Goldman L. Cardiac risks and complications of noncardiac surgery. *Ann Intern Med.* 1983;98:504–513.
4. Keeler E, Solomon D, Beck J. Effect of patient age on duration of medical encounters with physicians. *Med Care.* 1982;20:1101–1108.
5. Frankl VE. *Man's Search for Meaning.* Boston: Beacon Press; 1959.
6. Frankl VE. *The Doctor and the Soul.* New York: AA Knopf; 1995.
7. Yalom ID. *Existential Psychotherapy.* New York: Basic Books; 1980.

8. Sulmasy DP. *The Healer's Calling*. Mahwah, NJ: Paulist Press; 1997.

9. Matthews DA, McCullough ME, Larson DB. Religious commitment and health status. *Arch Fam Med*. 1998;7:118–124.

10. King DE, Bushwick B. Beliefs and attitudes of hospital inpatients about faith healing and prayer. *J Fam Pract*. 1994;39:349–352.

11. Cadieux R, Kales J, Zimmerman L. Comprehensive assessment of the elderly patient. *Am Fam Phys*. 1985;31:105–111.

12. Ham RJ. *Geriatrics I: American Academy of Family Physicians Home Study Self-Assessment,* Kansas City, MO: American Academy of Family Physicians; 1986. Monograph 89.

13. Besdine RW. The educational utility of comprehensive functional assessment in the elderly. *J Am Geriatr Soc*. 1983;31:651–656.

14. Williams TF. Assessment of the geriatric patient in relation to needs for services and facilities. In: Reichel W, ed. *Clinical Aspects of Aging*. 2nd ed. Baltimore: Williams & Wilkins; 1983:543–548.

15. Williams T. Comprehensive functional assessment: An overview. *J Am Geriatr Soc*. 1983;31:637–641.

16. Mader S. Aging and postural hypotension: An update. *J Am Geriatr Soc*. 1989; 37:129–137.

17. Caird F, Andrews G, Kennedy R. Effect of posture on blood pressure in the elderly. *Br Heart J*. 1973:527–530.

18. Mader S, Josephson K, Rubenstein L. Low prevalence of postural hypotension among community-dwelling elderly. *JAMA*. 1987;258:1511–1514.

19. Shannon R, Wei J, Rosa R. The effect of age and sodium depletion on cardiovascular response to orthostasis. *Hypertension*. 1986;5:438–443.

20. Messerli F, Ventura H, Amodeo C. Osler's maneuver and pseudohypertension. *N Engl J Med*. 1985;312:1548–1551.

21. Hansen A, Jensen H, Laugesen L. Withdrawal of antihypertensive drugs in the elderly. *Acta Med Scand*. 1983;676:178–185.

22. Amery A, Birkenhager WH, Brixko P, et al. Mortality and morbidity results from the European Working Party on high blood pressure in the elderly trial. *Lancet*. 1985; 1:1349–1354.

23. National Heart Foundation of Australia. Treatment of mild hypertension in the elderly: Report by the Management Committee. *Med J Aust*. 1981;2:398–402.

24. Dahlof B, Lindholm L, Hansson L. Morbidity and morality in the Swedish trial in old persons with hypertension (STOP-hypertension). *Lancet*. 1991;338:1281–1285.

25. MRC Working Party. Medical Research Council trial of treatment of hypertension in older adults. *Br Med J*. 1992;304:405–412.

26. Hulley S, Feigal D, Irelan C. Systolic Hypertension in the Elderly Program (SHEP): The first three months. *J Am Geriatr Soc*. 1986;34:101–105.

27. Gifford R. Isolated systolic hypertension in the elderly. *JAMA*. 1982;247:781–785.

28. Hypertension Detection and Follow-Up Program Cooperative Group. Five-year findings of the Hypertension Detection and Follow-Up Program: II. Morality by race, sex, and age. *JAMA*. 1979;242:2572–2577.

29. Hypertension Detection and Follow-Up Program Cooperative Group. Five-year findings of the Hypertension Detection and Follow-Up Program: I. Reduction in morality of persons with high blood pressure, including mild hypertension. *JAMA*. 1979;242: 2562–2571.

30. Kannel W. Implications of Framingham Study data for treatment of hypertension: Impact of other risk factors. In: Laragh JH, Buhler FR, Seldin DW, eds. *Frontiers in Hypertension Research*. New York: Springer-Verlag; 1981:17–21.

31. Applegate WB, Rutan GH. Advances in the management of hypertension in older persons. *J Am Geriatr Soc*. 1992;40:1164–1174.

32. SHEP Cooperative Research Group. Prevention of stroke by antihypertensive drug treatment for older persons with isolated systolic hypertension. *JAMA*. 1991;265: 3255–3264.

33. Meyer JS, Judd BW, Tawakina T, et al. Improved cognition after control of risk factors for multi-infarct dementia. *JAMA*. 1986;256:2203–2209.

34. Morley J, Solomon D. Major issues in geriatrics over the last five years. *J Am Geriatr Soc*. 1994;42:218–225.

35. The Nutrition Screening Initiative. *Report of Nutrition Screening: Toward a Common View*. Washington, DC: Nutritional Screening Initiative; 1991.

36. Haboubi N, Hudson P, Pathy M. Measurement of height in the elderly. *J Am Geriatr Soc*. 1990;38:1008–1010.

37. Dwyer JT. *Screening Older Americans' Nutritional Health: Current Practices and Future Possibilities*. Washington, DC: Nutritional Screening Initiative; 1991.

38. National Heart Lung and Blood Institute and the National Institute of Diabetes and Digestion and Kidney Diseases. *Clinical Guidelines on the Identification, Evaluation, and Treatment of Overweight and Obesity in Adults*. Bethesda, MD: National Institutes of Health; 1998.

39. Dwyer J, Gallo J, Reichel W. Assessing nutritional status in elderly patients. *Am Fam Phys*. 1993;47:613–620.

40. Detsky A, Smalley P, Chang J. Is this patient malnourished? *JAMA*. 1994;271:54–58.

41. O'Malley TA, Everitt DE, O'Malley HC, et al. Identifying and preventing family-mediated abuse and neglect of elderly persons. *Ann Intern Med*. 1983;98:998–1005.

42. Council on Scientific Affairs of the American Medical Association. Elder abuse and neglect. *JAMA*. 1987;257:966–971.

43. Taler G, Ansello E. Elder abuse. *Am Fam Phys*. 1985;32:107–114.

44. Rathbone-McCuan E, Goodstein RK. Elder abuse: Clinical considerations. *Psychiatr Ann*. 1985;15:331–339.

45. Allman R. Pressure ulcers among the elderly. *N Engl J Med*. 1989;320:850–853.

46. Brandeis G, Morris J, Nash D, Lipsitz L. The epidemiology and natural history of pressure ulcers in elderly nursing home residents. *JAMA*. 1990;264:2905–2909.

47. Clinical Practice Guidelines. *Pressure Ulcers in Adults*. Rockville, MD: US Dept of Health and Human Services, Public Health Service, Agency for Health Care Policy and Research; 1992.

48. Steffes R, Thralow J. Visual field limitation in the patient with dementia of the Alzheimer's type. *J Am Geriatr Soc*. 1987;35:198–204.

49. Mader S. Hearing impairment in elderly persons. *J Am Geriatr Soc*. 1984;32:548–553.

50. Gordon S, Jahnigen D. Oral assessment of the edentulous elderly patient. *J Am Geriatr Soc*. 1983;31:797–801.

51. Gordon S, Jahnigen D. Oral assessment of the edentulous elderly patient. *J Am Geriatr Soc*. 1986;34:276–281.

52. Sauve JS, Laupacis A, Ostbye T, Feagan B, Sackett DL. Does this patient have a clinically important carotid bruit? *JAMA*. 1993;270:2843–2845.

53. Livingston EH, Hershman JM, Sawin CT, et al. Prevalence of thyroid disease and abnormal thyroid tests in older hospitalized and ambulatory persons. *J Am Geriatr Soc.* 1987;35:109–114.

54. Cooper DS. Subclinical hypothyroidism. *JAMA.* 1987;258:246–247.

55. Wei J, Gersh B. Heart disease in the elderly. *Curr Problems Cardiol.* 1987;12:1–65.

56. Agency for Health Care Policy and Research. *Heart Failure: Evaluation and Care of Patients with Left Ventricular Failure.* Rockville, MD: US Dept of Health and Human Services, Public Health Service, Agency for Health Care Policy and Research; 1994.

57. Potter J, Elahi D, Tobin J, et al. The effect of age on the cardiothoracic ratio of man. *J Am Geriatr Soc.* 1982;30:404–409.

58. Martin A, Benbow L, Butrous G, et al. Five year follow-up of 101 elderly subjects by means of long-term ambulatory cardiac monitoring. *Eur Heart J.* 1984;5:592–596.

59. Heger J. Cardiac arrhythmias in the elderly. *Cardiovasc Clin.* 1981;12:145–159.

60. Fleg J, Kennedy H. Cardiac arrhythmias in a healthy elderly population: Detection by 24-hour ambulatory electrocardiography. *Chest.* 1982;81:302–307.

61. Dreifus L. Cardiac arrhythmias in the elderly: Clinical aspects. *Cardiol Clin.* 1986;4:273–283.

62. Camm A, Evans K, Ward D, et al. The rhythm of the heart in active elderly subjects. *Am Heart J.* 1980;99:598–603.

63. Kantelip J, Sage E, Duchene-Marullaz P. Findings on ambulatory electrocardiographic monitoring in subjects older than 80 years. *Am J Cardiol.* 1986;57:398–401.

64. Vernon M. Urinary incontinence in the elderly. *Primary Care.* 1989;16:515–528.

65. Madoff R, Williams J, Caushaj P. Fecal incontinence. *N Engl J Med.* 1992;326:1002–1007.

66. Urinary Incontinence Guideline Panel. *Urinary Incontinence in Adults.* Rockville, MD: US Dept of Health and Human Services, Public Health Service; 1992.

67. Katzman R, Terry R. *The Neurology of Aging.* Philadelphia: FA Davis Co; 1983.

68. Thomas R. Blinking and the releasing reflexes: Are they clinically useful? *J Am Geriatr Soc.* 1994;42:609–613.

69. Molloy D, Clarnette R, McIlroy W, et al. Clinical significance of primitive reflexes in Alzheimer's disease. *J Am Geriatr Soc.* 1991;39:1160–1163.

70. Hodges J. Neurological aspects of dementia and normal aging. In: Huppert F, Brayne C, O'Connor D, eds. *Dementia and Normal Aging.* Cambridge, England: Cambridge University Press; 1994:118–129.

71. Nevitt M, Cummings S, Kidd S, Black D. Risk factors for recurrent nonsyncopal falls: A prospective study. *JAMA.* 1989;261:2663–2668.

72. Tinetti M, Speechley M, Ginter S. Risk factors for falls among elderly persons living in the community. *N Engl J Med.* 1987;319:1701–1705.

73. Studenski S, Duncan P, Chandler J, et al. Predicting falls: The role of mobility and nonphysical factors. *J Am Geriatr Soc.* 1994;42:297–302.

74. Tinetti M, Speechley M. Prevention of falls among the elderly. *N Engl J Med.* 1989;320:1055–1059.

75. Tinetti M. Performance-oriented assessment of mobility problems in elderly patients. *J Am Geriatr Soc.* 1986;34:119–126.

9

Pain Assessment

James P. Richardson

cute and chronic noncancer-related pains are among the most common complaints of older adults. Acute pain may be caused by exacerbation of a chronic problem (eg, a vertebral fracture in a person with osteoporosis) or a new injury from a recent fall. Chronic pain may result from osteoarthritis, rheumatoid arthritis, chronic back pain, myalgias, other rheumatologic conditions, or from cancer. This chapter will review acute and chronic pain assessment in older adults. For a comprehensive review of pain therapy, the reader is referred to the clinical practice guidelines published by the American Geriatrics Society on the management of chronic pain in older persons and to other sources.[1-3]

While definitions of chronic pain vary, a common and useful operating definition is persistent pain that does not respond to usual treatments. Chronic pain in older adults is common. For example, a recent telephone survey found that one fifth of older adults surveyed took analgesic medications regularly. Patients who are taking analgesics regularly tend to see multiple physicians, usually primary care doctors.[4] Chronic pain also is common in nursing home residents.[5]

Multiple patient and physician barriers might interfere with the assessment and successful treatment of chronic pain in older adults (Exhibit 9–1). Some older individuals will deny having pain, but will

251

Exhibit 9-1 Patient/Physician Beliefs and Barriers to Effective Pain Assessment/ Treatment in Older Adults

---

Patient
- Pain is a normal part of aging
- Stoicism
- Complaining of pain represents a moral failing
- Fear of the cause of the pain (eg, cancer)

Physician
- Inadequate time for assessment
- Lack of interest in assessment and treatment
- Lack of expertise

---

admit to experiencing discomfort, aching, or pressure. In addition, older adults may not receive adequate treatment because they and their doctors fear addiction.

HISTORICAL ASSESSMENT OF PAIN

While it has long been postulated that older adults do not experience pain with the same intensity as younger adults due to age-related changes in the nervous system, it is doubtful that these changes are clinically significant. In particular, it is important to stress that there is no evidence that pain perception is decreased in older adults compared with younger adults.[3,6] Increasingly, it has been recognized that only the individual truly knows the severity of the pain he or she is experiencing. "Accurate pain assessment begins when the physician believes patients and takes their complaints of pain seriously."[5(p682)] Therefore, physicians should focus on quantifying the individual's subjective experience of pain.

Unidimensional Pain Scales

There are numerous means of recording pain. Unidimensional scales record the intensity of the pain, but do not address other pain characteristics, such as affective components. An example is a verbal descriptor scale, in which persons are asked to choose from five words that reflect increasing severity of pain: mild, discomforting, distressing, horrible, and excruciating.[7] The disadvantages of a verbal descriptor scale are the limited words to choose from and that individuals tend to choose moderate words rather than those expressing the extremes.[7]

In common use today in most care settings is the numeric rating scale (NRS). When an NRS is used, persons are asked to rate the pain from 0 to 10, with 0 representing absolutely no pain and 10 the worst possible pain the person can imagine. A visual analog scale (VAS) is similar to an NRS in that persons rate pain from 0 to 10,[7] but do so by marking a 10-cm line that is labeled on one end as "no pain" and on the other as "worst imaginable pain." VASs appear to be valid and reliable indicators of chronic pain in older pain patients attending a chronic pain clinic, but have not been extensively tested in the general population of older persons suffering pain.[8] NRSs and VASs are widely used in acute care settings such as hospitals because of their simplicity and because they are easily understood by patients. In addition, these scales can reflect small changes in pain. However, NRSs and VASs do not reflect changes in psychologic distress or physical function caused by pain.

Multidimensional Pain Scales

Multidimensional pain scales are useful because they assess more than just the intensity of pain, but also affective or other components of pain. The best known and most studied of these is the McGill Pain Questionnaire (MPQ).[3,9] The MPQ assesses pain along three dimensions: sensory, affective, and evaluative. The three components of pain are derived from the gate-control theory of pain.[10] Each of the three components is subdivided into 20 subclasses. A person is asked to classify his or her pain by picking words in each subclass that are closest to the person's experience of pain. Each category is scored, and a total score is calculated.

While the MPQ has been used in a variety of clinical settings, its complexity makes it most suitable for use in chronic pain clinics or as a research tool. As is true for many pain-assessment instruments or quality-of-life instruments, some controversy attends the use of the MPQ as well.[10]

Other Historical Data

The quality of the pain can guide the practitioner as to the type of pain; the type of pain may then be helpful in deciding treatment options.[1] *Nociceptive pain* is either visceral or somatic and is caused by stimulation of pain receptors, usually through tissue injury or mechanical deformation. Examples include pain from the arthritic conditions and mechanical back pain. Most often the degree of pain is proportional to the degree of tissue injury. All tissue types may cause nociceptive pain except the central nervous system. Nociceptive pain usually responds to traditional treatments for pain.

Neuropathic pain involves damage to either the central or peripheral nervous system. Neuropathic pain is often described as "burning," "aching," or "deep" in quality. Examples include poststroke pain, phantom limb pain, or painful extremities from diabetic neuropathy. The pain may continue without ongoing tissue damage. This type of pain may not respond to the usual analgesic therapies, but may respond to treatment with tricyclic antidepressants, anticonvulsants, or antiarrhythmic drugs.[1] So-called *central pain* is a special case of neuropathic pain that is caused by damage to pain transmission pathways, such as the spinothalamic tract or the thalamus itself. *Allodynia* (ie, a painful response to a nonpainful stimulus) or *hyperesthesia* (ie, increased sensitivity to a stimulus) may present due to neuropathic pain.[7]

Mixed pain, such as recurrent headaches or vasculitic pain, appears to be caused by unknown mechanisms. Treatment is often difficult and usually requires a combination of therapies. *Psychogenic pain*, the final category of pain, is said to be present when psychological influences (eg, somatization or conversion disorder) are a major factor in the etiology or persistence of the pain symptoms. In these cases, the usual pain treatments are not advised and psychiatric intervention is necessary.[1]

Once the intensity and the quality of the pain have been evaluated and quantified, the other usual descriptors of pain should be elicited: location and radiation, duration, frequency or pattern, and precipitating and ameliorating factors. The location of the pain can be described or marked on a body diagram by the person. Persons who cover a large part of a body diagram, especially when previous evaluation has shown involvement limited to one or two nerve roots, are more focused on their pain and may be more disturbed.[11] An attempt should be made to determine whether the pain is localized or referred from another site and whether it is superficial or visceral. Examples of referred pain include shoulder pain resulting from diaphragmatic irritation and back pain from kidney or prostate disease. Pain that is superficial is easily localized, while visceral pain is diffuse.

A pain diary helps clarify relationships between ameliorating and precipitating factors, pain duration, and frequency. Completion of a pain diary also helps to assess the relationship between pain and activity.[1] For example, persons who identify particular activities as pain producing rather than certain movements may be having their pain behaviors reinforced by activity avoidance.[11] On the other hand, when pain-relieving factors are limited to medications, activity avoidance, or massage by family members, these persons may be having their pain behavior reinforced.[11] In the pain diary, pain intensity can be recorded according to an NRS (from 0 to 10) during various activities. Other helpful information may be recorded, such as the effect of medicines or other therapies, or emotional state and interactions with family members.[7]

Additional history taking should focus on the sequence of events that led to the chronic pain, as well as the treatments, especially over-the-counter and prescription medicines, along with the person's assessment of the results of treatments. This type of information becomes especially important when evaluating persons with psychogenic pain. Persons with psychogenic pain will benefit from a full psychologic evaluation that includes an assessment of the impact of the pain on the person's life, his or her premorbid personality, and a consideration of the financial aspects.[11] Assessment of activities of daily living and instrumental activities of daily living is very helpful in delineating the impact of the person's pain on function (see Chapter 4).

PHYSICAL ASSESSMENT OF PAIN

The evaluation of the older person with pain, as with all medical evaluations, should include a comprehensive physical examination. The physical assessment may not always be completed on the first visit, since persons with pain often present as urgent visits and because more time usually is necessary to evaluate older adults. While the goal is a "complete" examination, the neurological and musculoskeletal systems will require more attention and time when considering the person with pain. Since physical examination of the older adult is explored in detail in Chapter 8, in this chapter only topics that are pertinent in assessing pain syndromes will be highlighted.

General observations are important and may begin with the person's entrance to the waiting area. Does the patient walk in unassisted, or is he or she using a wheelchair or other assistive device? Is the patient's gait normal or antalgic? Is the patient anxious or in obvious pain? Is the patient accompanied by a family member? What is the interaction between the patient and caregiver? Further general observations can occur in the exam room during history taking.[12] The patient's dress and body language are observed. Poor grooming and personal hygiene suggest depression and/or dementia. The patient's posture and side-to-side symmetry can be assessed.[12] Kyphosis or scoliosis could indicate osteoporosis with compression fractures. Odors suggestive of poor hygiene, recreational substance use, or metabolic abnormalities should be noted. The patient should be observed while she or he is undressing to see whether an extremity is favored due to pain.[7] While a person in acute pain may manifest elevated pulse rate and blood pressure, these may not be present in someone with chronic pain due to physiologic adaptation.[12]

Skin

In addition to the usual observations, surgical scars should be noted that may indicate procedures that patients do not recall during history taking. Other scars may indicate trauma or infections. Lesions that may indicate a systemic condition (eg, neurofibromatosis) should be noted.[12] Excoriations may be a sign of dysethesias or pruritis. Color changes over the extremities may mean arterial or venous insufficiency (see below). Signs of trauma could be evidence of elder abuse. Pressure sores may mean abnormal posture or poor mobility. Evidence of trophic skin and nail changes should be sought.

Head, Eyes, Ears, Nose, Throat, and Neck

Evidence of head trauma, systemic disease that affects the sclera or iris, and the results of ophthalmoscopy should all be noted. Examination of the ears may reveal cerumen, impaction, or otitis. The condition of the teeth may reveal caries or other painful dental conditions. Foul breath may result from periodontal disease or sinusitis. The carotid arteries should be palpated and auscultated. Enlarged or tender lymph nodes (cervical, submandibular, supraclavicular) should be noted. The thyroid should be examined as well.

Chest, Abdomen, Genitalia, Pelvis, and Extremities

Breasts and axillae should be examined for tenderness, masses, or discharge. The sternum and the sternocostal, costoclavicular, and costochondral joints should be palpated for swelling or tenderness. The heart, lungs, and abdomen are examined in the usual fashion. If urinary pathology is suspected, be sure to percuss the flanks. The bladder should be palpated for the possibility of urinary retention. Lower abdominal or back pain complaints may require examination of the genitalia. Women should have a careful pelvic examination, including bimanual examination for masses or tenderness. Men should have inspection and palpation of the scrotum and prostate. Both men and women should have rectal examinations for masses, tenderness, and, if applicable, to check stool for occult blood. Tenderness of the ischia and coccyx may be noted during rectal exam. The bones of the pelvis should be palpated for tenderness. Pulses should be palpated. Notation should be made of skin changes suggestive of ischemia (eg, pallor, coolness, or ulcers) or venous insufficiency (eg, edema, hyperpigmentation, or ulcers) or thrombophlebitis (eg, swelling or pain).

Musculoskeletal System

Along with the neurological exam, the musculoskeletal exam deserves the most emphasis in persons with chronic pain. In addition to the points raised in Chapter 8, a thorough musculoskeletal exam in older persons with pain should include palpation of muscles, looking for spasm and referred pain.[12] Trigger points may be identified. Active range of motion of symptomatic joints should be checked. If limited, then the person is gently assisted to determine passive range of motion. Joint disease limits both active and passive motion, while greater passive than active range of motion suggests disease of the muscle or tendon. If contraction of the muscles of the affected joint against sufficient resistance to prevent movement is painful, this may also indicate muscular or supporting structure pathology. Joints should be examined for swelling, erythema, sponginess (suggestive of synovitis), and bony enlargement.[13] The areas surrounding joints should be examined for soft tissue pathology that may produce pain, such as ganglion cysts, bursitis, or tenosynovitis.[13] The spine deserves special emphasis. The person is asked to stand for this exam, and the spine is viewed from behind for symmetry and symmetric muscle bulk of the paraspinal and shoulder muscles. The iliac crests should be level. Forward flexion and extension, as well as lateral flexion and rotation test range of motion. Pain on percussion of the spinous processes may indicate vertebral fractures, ligamentous pathology, or may represent referred tenderness.[12]

A few special maneuvers deserve mention.[11] Pain in the cervical spine with Valsalva's maneuver suggests increased intrathecal pressure due to a space-occupying lesion in the spinal canal. If pain occurs on the concave side with lateral flexion of the thoracic spine, intercostal nerve root compression is likely; if the pain is on the convex side, pleural pathology with fixation to the chest wall is more likely. Straight leg raising tests for sciatic nerve irritation. Observation of the person's gait should be included (see Chapter 8).

Neurological System

A careful neurological examination is necessary in many individuals with chronic pain, especially if neuropathic pain is suspected. The usual neurological examination is reviewed in Chapter 8. Parts of the neurological examination that are particularly important in the older adult with pain will be emphasized. Pain in an area of hypoesthesia, allodynia, and hyperpathia (ie, increased response to a repetitive, non-painful stimulus) are indicative of neural pathology. Peripheral lesions may be distinguished from central lesions if typical radicular findings of motor weakness, reflex changes, and hypoesthesia are present. The reader is referred to standard medical or neurological texts for detailed information on nerve root lesions and the expected motor, reflexes, and dermatome patterns.

Evidence of autonomic dysfunction may be alteration in skin temperature or color, or decreased or increased sweating. Abnormal hair or nail growth may occur. If these signs are present in a painful extremity, complex regional pain syndrome (formerly reflex sympathetic dystrophy) may be present.[12] Mental status testing is important since persons with dementia may complain of pain or other somatic symptoms (see Chapter 3). It is difficult to complete a precise examination of persons with pain and advanced dementia because so much of the exam requires the person's cooperation. Examiners may need to rely on nonverbal expressions of pain, such as grimacing, agitation, or withdrawal, discussed in more detail below.

PAIN ASSESSMENT IN COGNITIVELY IMPAIRED OLDER ADULTS

As noted earlier, pain is common in nursing home residents, the majority of whom are cognitively impaired.[14] Although nursing home residents are difficult to evaluate for pain, there is no evidence that cognitive impairment "masks" the pain. However, impaired cognition may be associated with reduced pain complaints, even after adjustment for comorbidities and altered function.[14] Reports of current pain in demented persons are usually valid and reliable.[5,14] Recall of past episodes of pain may be less reliable. Chronic pain complaints may be attributed to depression because depression is so common in nursing home residents. However, psychogenic pain is rare in long-term care residents.

When older persons have cognitive impairment or language barriers, the report of the caregiver or family should be sought.[5] Examples of information that caregivers may provide include changes in function, such as altered gait or falls, agitation, and moaning or crying. Functional decline may be the most noticeable change in a nursing home resident with pain.

CONCLUSION

Increased recognition of the problem of pain in older adults brings with it the need for new assessment techniques and knowledge. While much more research needs to be done for a more complete understanding of pain and its treatment, the geriatric practitioner can improve skills in this area by keeping in mind the principles of assessment discussed in this chapter. For more in-depth discussion, readers are referred to other sources.[1,3,7,10] Improving pain assessment and treatment in the hospital, nursing home, hospice, and in ambulatory care settings is a worthwhile effort with the potential for a considerable effect on the quality of life of older persons.

REFERENCES

1. American Geriatrics Society Panel on Chronic Pain in Older Persons. The management of chronic pain in older persons. *J Am Geriatr Soc.* 1998;46:635–651.

2. Ferrell BR, Ferrell BA, eds. *Pain in the Elderly.* Seattle, WA: IASP Press; 1996.

3. Wall PD, Melzack R, eds. *Textbook of Pain.* 3rd ed. New York: Churchill Livingstone; 1994.

4. Cooner E, Amorosi S. *The Study of Pain and Older Americans.* New York: Louis Harris and Associates; 1997.

5. Ferrell BA. Pain evaluation and management in the nursing home. *Ann Intern Med.* 1995;123:681–687.

6. Harkins SW. Geriatric pain: Pain perceptions in the old. *Clin Geriatr Med.* 1996;12: 435–459.

7. Kittelberger KP, LeBel AA, Borsook D. Assessment of pain. In: Borsook D, LeBel AA, McPeek B, eds. *The Massachusetts General Handbook of Pain Management.* Boston: Little, Brown, and Company; 1996:26–44.

8. Harkins SW, Price DD, Bush FM, Small RE. Geriatric pain. In: Wall PD, Melzack R, eds. *Textbook of Pain*. 3rd ed. New York: Churchill Livingstone; 1994.

9. Melzack R. The McGill Pain Questionnaire: Major properties and scoring methods. *Pain*. 1975;1:277–299.

10. Valley MA. Pain measurement. In: Raj PP, ed. *Pain Medicine—A Comprehensive Review*. St Louis, MO: Mosby; 1996:36–46.

11. Doleys DM, Murray JB, Klapow JC, Coleton MI. Psychologic assessment. In: Ashburn MA, Rice LJ, eds. *The Management of Pain*. New York: Churchill Livingstone; 1998:27–49.

12. Weinstein SM. Physical examination. In: Ashburn MA, Rice LJ, eds. *The Management of Pain*. New York: Churchill Livingstone; 1998:17–25.

13. Cash JM. History and physical examination. In: Klippel JH, ed. *Primer on the Rheumatic Diseases*. 11th ed. Atlanta, GA: Arthritis Foundation; 1997:89–94.

14. Parmelee PA. Pain in cognitively impaired older persons. *Clin Geriatr Med*. 1996; 12:473–487.

10

Health Promotion and Disease Prevention

A s Eubie Blake, the jazz composer and pianist, observed on his 100th birthday, "These docs, they always ask you how you live so long. I tell 'em, if I'd known I was gonna live this long, I'd have taken better care of myself."[1] Health maintenance and disease prevention begin with appropriate decisions concerning diet and lifestyle made in the early and middle years of life, yet there are ample opportunities for preventive interventions for older persons. For persons of advanced age approaching the limit of natural life expectancy, the goal of prevention becomes preservation of functional capacity and not simply prolonging life.[2] Approaches to prevention of cancer, cardiovascular disease, cerebrovascular disease, and infections (those preventable through immunization) are complemented by focusing on the problems specific to old age.[3] Geriatric problems such as falling, functional impairment, and polypharmacy may not easily fit into a disease model of illness. The aspects of mental status, functional status, social situation, Values History, and medical considerations act as a focus of preventive activities and as a guide for highlighting preventive activities that are appropriate for the individual patient. An individualized plan for health promotion and disability prevention should be informed by multidimensional assessment because older persons vary greatly in their medical and functional status.

261

Older people are a distinctly heterogeneous group. Older persons in good health, frail elders with functional disability living at home, and older persons residing in institutions each have a unique level of appropriate health promotion and disease prevention activities.[4] This heterogeneity in function must be considered in recommending a strategy for prevention of disability and preservation of health. In the past, many studies did not include older adults or failed to separate them (young old, middle old, and old old) from adults in general. Some interventions may actually be more efficacious with advancing age (Table 10–1).[5] Although many disorders of old age are chronic and not curable, early detection and treatment of problems that interfere with functioning should be the focus of assessment.[6]

Prevention is sometimes categorized as primary, secondary, or tertiary. Primary prevention involves forestalling the development of disease (eg, flu vaccine to prevent development of influenza). Secondary prevention involves early detection and treatment of disease during an asymptomatic phase (eg, detection of hypertension). In other words, the person already has the disease, and it is too late for primary prevention, but the condition has not yet declared itself with symptoms. Tertiary prevention is directed toward avoidance of negative consequences among person with the disease (eg, preventing complications of diabetes through meticulous control of blood sugar). Tertiary prevention is tantamount to providing good medical care that avoids complications. The evidence needed to recommend a procedure intended to prevent a disorder must be strong because otherwise persons may be exposed to a potentially harmful intervention with little potential for benefit.

Preventive measures may also be categorized as universal, selective, or indicated.[7] Universal measures are desirable for the entire group of elderly persons (eg, intake of an adequate diet). Selective measures are warranted when the individual belongs to a group with a higher than average risk of disease (eg, intensive examinations of persons with a family history of colorectal cancer). Indicated measures apply to persons who have a higher than average risk of disease based on history or examination (eg, control of hypertension). Persons in high risk groups may benefit most from preventive interventions. The alternative designations of universal, selective, and indicated are similar to the form of recommendations of the US and Canadian guidelines for clinical preventive services, to be discussed later. Targets for preventive interventions should be common, associated with significant morbidity, easily detected, and treatable.

Table 10–1 Preventive Services That Have Improved or Diminished Effectiveness in the Old Old (age 80 years and older)

Preventive Service	Improved Effectiveness	Diminished Effectiveness
Historical		
Accidents		
Falls prevention; particularly with a history of previous falls	X	
Motor vehicle		X
Mobility/ADL/IADL assessment	X	
Nutrition (undernutrition) screening or counseling	X	
Podiatry care	X	
Polypharmacy identification	X	
Dementia screening	X	
Urinary incontinence identification	X	
Physical examination		
Blood pressure		X
Cancer screening		
Breast		X
Cervical		X
Hearing screening	X	
Visual acuity screening	X	
Laboratory		
Cholesterol		X
Interventions		
Advance directives counseling	X	
Vaccinations		
Influenza immunization	X	

ADL denotes activities of daily living; *IADL* denotes instrumental activities of daily living.

Source: P Zazove, et al., A Criterion-Based Review of Preventive Health Care in the Elderly, Vol. 34, No. 3, pp. 320–347, © 1992, Dowden Publishing Company, Inc. Reproduced with permission from *The Journal of Family Practice.*

INCORPORATING PREVENTION INTO PRACTICE

The physician and others in primary health care are in an ideal position for promoting preventive care for older persons because older adults make several visits per year to the physician. Unfortunately, physician, patient, and health system barriers conspire to make implementing prevention-based practice difficult. Physician characteristics may affect recommendations. For example, in two studies, women were more likely to take advantage of preventive interventions if their physicians were also women.[8,9] Physicians may not feel that there is adequate time to address preventive issues; this tendency is exacerbated by the lack of evidence-based information including sufficient numbers of older persons in primary health care settings upon which to make firm recommendations.[10] The lack of evidence-based studies pertains not only to prevention guidelines in older adults, but to clinical guidelines dealing with medical conditions of older adults in general.[11] Patient factors associated with failure to adhere to prevention practices include lack of knowledge, attitudes toward cancer and other conditions, and fear that a serious condition will be uncovered. For example, Mexican American women aged 65 years and older who were more knowledgeable about screening guidelines and detection methods for breast and cervical cancer were more likely to report having undergone cancer screening.[12] Health system factors such as accessibility of primary care and acceptability of interventions may act as barriers to participation in prevention. Continuity of primary care, threatened by changes in the health care system, reduces the barriers to obtaining screening. For example, minority women who reported a regular source of care from the same clinician were more likely to have had a recent Pap smear, breast examination, or mammogram than were women who reported that they did not have a usual source of care.[13] Despite barriers, there is a need for careful consideration of how to integrate prevention into practice.

Kennie[2,14,15] and others[16,17] have suggested that primary care practitioners practice "opportunistic case finding"; that is use the problem-oriented patient visit to carry out a search for unreported illnesses. In pediatric practice "case finding" is routine—when a child is seen for an acute illness, a few moments are spent evaluating development, giving anticipatory guidance, and checking for compliance with vaccination schedules. Current reimbursement structures do not encourage this practice in adult medicine; however, the process may be facilitated through consideration of components of the multidimensional assessment in a "prevention-oriented medical record."[18] Opportunistic case finding integrates the traditional medical care delivery system with a process of continual review and search for unreported problems of health or function.[2,14,15,17]

Since lifestyle choices underlie so many preventive interventions (eg, stopping smoking or reducing the amount of fat in the diet), a number of models have been applied to guide and facilitate behavioral change (see *Health Behavior and Health Education: Theory, Research, and Practice*[19] for a review). Two models will briefly be reviewed here: (1) the health beliefs model and (2) the transtheoretical model (the stages of change model). Pertinent concepts of the health belief model include perceived susceptibility, severity, benefits, and barriers to behavioral change.[20] Under the health beliefs model, whether a patient undertakes behavioral change or decides to undergo a preventive intervention procedure depends on how much the patient believes they are susceptible to the disease, his or her opinion on the seriousness of the condition to be prevented, whether the patient thinks the advised action is likely to be effective, and whether he or she thinks the barriers to carrying out the intervention are too great. In other words, the physician may need to explore whether the patient has beliefs that hinder adherence to recommendations. For example, some older persons may consider themselves "too old" for prevention to be effective, or may be sure that receiving an influenza vaccination will give them the flu. Cultural beliefs about the nature and meaning of illness or symptoms may also be influential. Addressing these beliefs directly may improve willingness to participate in preventive activities.

A second model related to behavioral change considers that change occurs in steps, and the key to changing behavior is to match the stage of change with the nature of the intervention.[21] In the precontemplation stage, people have no intention of changing their behavior. Contemplation stage refers to a step in which persons know that there may be benefits to changing behavior, but are ambivalent. When people intend to make a change, they are said to be in the preparatory stage. Action is the stage when people have modified their behavior, and maintenance refers to preventing relapse. Interventions may be most effective when the intervention matches the stage. For example, providing information may be most influential among persons in the contemplation phase, but not in the maintenance phase. Social support, such as engaging the family in supporting behavioral change, may be most important for persons in the contemplation stage or among persons who are trying to prevent relapse of the undesired behavior. No single theory can account for human behavior, but application of simple techniques derived from a theoretical framework may make the clinician more effective in helping patients participate in health promotion and disease prevention activities.

EVIDENCE-BASED GUIDELINES

Although there are a number of sources of clinical preventive guidelines pertaining to older persons,[3,5,22–27] attention here is focused on the second edition of the *Guide to Clinical Preventive Services,* the Report of the US Preventive Services Task Force[28] and the Canadian Task Force on Preventive Health Care's *The Canadian Guide to Clinical Preventive Health Care.*[27] The second edition of the US guide is evidence-based as compared to the first edition in 1989, which was based on expert opinion.[29] The Canadian Task Force on Preventive Health Care (formerly the Canadian Task Force on the Periodic Health Examination) has done landmark work on the periodic health examination and continues to update recommendations intermittently.[27] Unlike the US version, the Canadian guide contains a chapter devoted specifically to older persons. The Cochrane Collaboration, which had its start in Great Britain, examines worldwide evidence for efficacy of treatment and preventive recommendations and makes the reviews available in the Cochrane Library on CD-ROM and on the Internet.[30] Recently, a section of the Cochrane Collaboration devoted to the health care of older people has been organized (the web site for the Cochrane Collaboration can be found at www.cochrane.co.uk).

Updated evidence-based reviews and recommendations from the second report of the US Preventive Services Task Force and the Canadian Task Force on Preventive Health Care are available on the World Wide Web. The US Task Force recommendations and clinical practice guidelines can be found on the Agency for Health Care Policy and Research's web site (www.ahcpr.gov) and the Canadian report can be found on the Canadian Task Force's web site (www.ctfphc.org). Through the Internet, the most recent reviews and recommendations are available to older persons and their families as well as to health care professionals.

In this chapter, the recommendations for persons aged 65 years and older of the US Preventive Services Task Force *Guide to Clinical Preventive Services* are highlighted and provided in Exhibit 10–1,[28] while the recommendations of the Canadian Task Force on Preventive Health Care are provided in Exhibit 10–2.[27] Reviewers who formulated the US recommendations included representatives from professional organizations (eg, the American Academy of Family Physicians and the American College of Physicians), federal agencies (eg, the Agency for Health Care Policy and Research and the Centers for Disease Control and Prevention), and the National Institutes of Health. Canadian reviewers were similarly diverse. For this reason, the work of the US and Canadian Task Forces merits special attention.

Exhibit 10–1 Recommendations for Persons 65 years and Older from the US *Guide to Clinical Preventive Services*

Interventions Considered and Recommended for the Periodic Health Examination

Leading Causes of Death
Heart diseases
Malignant neoplasms (lung, colorectal, breast)
Chronic obstructive pulmonary disease
Pneumonia and influenza

INTERVENTIONS FOR THE GENERAL POPULATION

Screening
Blood pressure
Height and weight
Fecal occult blood test[1] and/or sigmoidoscopy
Mammogram clinical breast exam[2] (women ≤ 69 yr)
Papanicolaou (Pap) test (women)[3]
Vision screening
Assess for hearing impairment
Assess for problem drinking

Counseling

Substance use
Tobacco cessation
Avoid alcohol/drug use while driving, swimming, boating, etc*

Diet and exercise
Limit fat & cholesterol; maintain caloric balance; emphasize grains, fruits, vegetables
Adequate calcium intake (women)
Regular physical activity*

Injury prevention
Lap/shoulder belts
Motorcycle and bicycle helmets*
Fall prevention*
Safe storage/removal of firearms*
Smoke detector*
Set hot water heater to <120 to 130°F*
CPR training for household members

Dental health
Regular visits to dental care provider*
Floss and brush with fluoride toothpaste daily*

Sexual behavior
STD prevention; avoid high-risk sexual behavior,* use condoms*

Immunizations
Pneumococcal vaccine
Influenza[1]
Tetanus-diphtheria (Td) boosters

Chemoprophylaxis
Discuss hormone prophylaxis (women)

INTERVENTIONS FOR HIGH-RISK POPULATIONS

Population	*Potential Interventions*
Institutionalized persons	PPD[†] (HR1); hepatitis A vaccine (HR2); amantadine/rimantadine (HR4)
Persons with chronic medical conditions, TB contacts, low income, immigrants, alcoholics	PPD (HR1)
Persons ≥ 75 yr; or ≥ 70 yr with risk factors for falls	Fall prevention intervention (HR5)
Persons with cardiovascular disease risk factors	Consider cholesterol screening (HR6)

continues

Exhibit 10–1 continued

Population	Potential Interventions
Family history of skin cancer; nevi; fair skin, eyes, hair	Avoid excess/ midday sun, use protective clothing* (HR7)
Native Americans/Alaskan Natives	PPD (HR1); hepatitis A vaccine (HR2)
Travelers to developing countries	Hepatitis A vaccine (HR2); hepatitis B vaccine (HR8)
Blood product recipients	HIV screen (HR3); hepatitis B vaccine (HR8)
Persons practicing high-risk sexual behavior	Hepatitis A vaccine (HR2), HIV screen (HR3), hepatitis B vaccine (HR8), RPR/VDRL (HR9)
Persons injecting or using street drugs	PPD (HR1), hepatitis A vaccine (HR2), HIV screen (HR3), hepatitis B vaccine (HR8), RPR/VDRL (HR9), advice to reduce infection risk (HR10)
Health care/laboratory workers	PPD (HR1), hepatitis A vaccine (HR2), amantadine/rimantadine (HR4), hepatitis B vaccine (HR8)
Persons susceptible to varicella	Varicella vaccine (HR11)

[1]Annually

[2]Mammogram every 1 yr to 2 yr, or mammogram every 1 yr to 2 yr with annual clinical breast exam.

[3]All women who are or have been sexually active and who have a cervix at least every 3 yr. Consider discontinuation of testing after age 65 yr if previous regular screening with consistently normal results.

*The ability of clinician counseling to influence this behavior is unproven.

†Purified protein derivative.

HR1 = HIV positive, close contacts of persons with known or suspected TB, health care workers, person with medical risk factors associated with TB, immigrants from countries with high TB prevalence, medically underserved low-income populations (including homeless), alcoholics, injection drug users, and residents of long-term care facilities.

HR2 = Persons living in, traveling to, or working in areas where the disease is endemic and where periodic outbreaks occur (eg, countries with high or intermediate endmicity; certain Alaskan native, Pacific Island, Native American, and religious communities); men who have sex with men; injection or street drug users. Consider for institutionalized person and workers in these institutions, and day care, hospital, and laboratory workers. Clinicians should also consider local epidemiology.

HR3 = Men who had sex with men after 1975; past or present injection use; persons who exchange sex for money or drugs, and their sex partners; injection drug-

continues

Exhibit 10–1 continued

using, bisexual, or HIV-positive sex partner currently or in the past; blood transfusion during 1978 to 1985; persons seeking treatment for STDs. Clinicians should also consider local epidemiology.

HR4 = Consider for persons who have not received influenza vaccine or are vaccinated late; when the vaccine may be ineffective due to major antigenic changes in the virus; for unvaccinated persons who provide home care for high-risk persons; to supplement protection provided by vaccine in persons who are expected to have a poor antibody response; and for high-risk persons in whom the vaccine is contraindicated.

HR5 = Persons aged 75 yr and older; or aged 70 to 74 with one or more additional risk factors including use of certain psychoactive and cardiac medications (eg, benzodiazepines and antihypertensives); use of 4 or more prescription medications, impaired cognition, strength, balance, or gait. Intensive individualized home-based multifactorial fall prevention intervention is recommended in settings where adequate resources are available to deliver such services.

HR6 = Although evidence is insufficient to recommend routine screening in elderly persons, consider cholesterol screening on a case-by-case basis for persons aged 65 to 75 yr with additional risk factors (eg, smoking, diabetes, or hypertension).

HR7 = Persons with a family or personal history of skin cancer; a large number of moles; atypical moles; poor tanning ability; or light skin, hair, and eye color.

HR8 = Blood product recipients (including hemodialysis patients), persons with frequent occupational exposure to blood or blood products, men who have sex with men, injection drug users and their sex partners, persons with multiple recent sex partners, persons with other STDs (including HIV), and travelers to countries with endemic hepatititis B.

HR9 = Persons who exchange sex for money or drugs and their sex partners, persons with other STDs (including HIV), and sexual contacts of persons with active syphilis. Clinicians should consider local epidemiology.

HR10 = Persons who continue to inject drugs.

HR11 = Healthy adults without a history of chickenpox or previous immunization. Consider serologic testing for presumed susceptible adults.

Source: Reprinted with permission from the U.S. Preventive Services Task Force, *Guide to Clinical Preventive Services: An Assessment of the Effectiveness of 169 Interventions,* 2nd ed., © 1996, Lippincott, Williams & Wilkins.

ETHICS OF PREVENTIVE INTERVENTIONS

In medicine, the notion of primary prevention of disease is attractive because it makes sense that patients will be better off if they don't become ill in the first place. At the same time, the recommendation of potentially hazardous, uncomfortable, or inconvenient maneuvers to persons who have no symptoms raises a number of ethical issues. First, avoiding coercion requires informed consent. Patient education materials that are tailored to the ethnicity and age of patients may

Exhibit 10–2 Recommendations for Older Men and Women from the Canadian Task Force on Preventive Health Care

RECOMMENDATIONS FOR OLDER MEN

Condition	Maneuver	Comments
"A" Recommendations		
Falls/injury	Multidisciplinary postfall assessment	
Hypertension	Pharmacologic treatment	
Influenza	Outreach strategies to reach high-risk groups	Specific groups (eg, diabetics)
"B" Recommendations		
Coronary heart disease	General dietary advice on fat and cholesterol	Men 30 to 69 yr
Diminished visual acuity	Snellen sight card	
Hearing impairment	Inquiry, whispered voice test, or audioscope	
Household and recreational injury	Legislation, safety aids, stairs, and bathtubs	
Hypertension	Blood pressure measurement	
Influenza	Annual immunization	
"C" Recommendations		
Age-related macular degeneration	Fundoscopy	
Bladder cancer	Urine dipstick or cytology	High-risk men >60 yr
Cognitive impairment	Mental status screening	
Elder abuse	Elder abuse questionnaire	
Glaucoma	Fundoscopy, tonometry or automated perimetry	
Household and recreational injury	Monitor medical impairment	
Household and recreational injury	Public education, nonflammable fabrics, self-extinguishing cigarettes	
Hypertension	Pharmacologic treatment	
Pneumococcal pneumonia	Immunization, one dose	Immunocompetent elderly living

continues

Exhibit 10–2 continued

Condition	Maneuver	Comments
Prostate cancer	Digital rectal examination	Men >50 yr
Testicular cancer	Physical exam or self-examination	

"D" Recommendations

Prostate cancer	Prostate specific antigen	Men >50 yr
Prostate cancer	Transrectal ultrasound	Men >50 yr
Testicular cancer	Tumor markers	
Urinary infection	Urine dipstick or culture	

"E" Recommendations

Urinary tract infection (asymptomatic)	Urine dipstick or culture	

RECOMMENDATIONS FOR OLDER WOMEN

"A" Recommendations

Breast cancer	Mammography and clinical exam	Women aged 50 to 69 yr
Falls/injury	Multidisciplinary postfall assessment	
Hypertension	Pharmacologic treatment	
Influenza	Outreach strategies to reach high-risk groups	Specific groups (eg, diabetics)

"B" Recommendations

Cervical cancer	Papanicolaou [smear]	
Diminished visual acuity	Snellen sight card	
Hearing impairment	Inquiry, whispered voice test, or audioscope	
Household and recreational injury	Legislation, safety aids, stairs, and bathtubs	
Hypertension	Blood pressure measurement	
Influenza	Annual immunization	
Osteoporotic fractures (and side affects)	Counseling, hormone replacement therapy	Perimenopausal

"C" Recommendations

Age-related macular degeneration	Fundoscopy	
Breast cancer	Teach breast self-examination (BSE)	
Cognitive impairment	Mental status screening	

continues

Exhibit 10–2 continued

Condition	Maneuver	Comments
"C" Recommendations		
Elder abuse	Elder abuse questionnaire	
Glaucoma	Fundoscopy, tonometry, or automated perimetry	
Household and recreational injury	Monitor medical impairment	
Household and recreational injury	Public education, nonflammable fabrics, and self-extinguishing cigarettes	
Hypertension	Pharmacologic treatment	
Osteoporosis; fractures	Counseling, weight bearing exercise	
Osteoporotic; fractures	History and physical examination	
Ovarian cancer	Pelvic exam, transvaginal ultrasound, CA 125, or combination	
Pneumococcal pneumonia	Immunization, one dose	Immunocompetent elderly living independently
Thyroid disorders	Thyroid stimulating hormone test	Perimenopausal women
Urinary infection	Urine dipstick or culture	
"D" Recommendations		
Cervical cancer	Human papillomavirus screening	
Osteoporotic fractures	Bone mineral density screening	
Ovarian cancer	Pelvic exam, transvaginal ultrasound, CA 125, or combination	
"E" Recommendations		
Urinary tract infection (asymptomatic)	Urine dipstick or culture	

Source: Adapted with permission from Canadian Task Force on Preventive Health Care *Guide to Clinical Preventive Health Care,* © 1997, Health Canada. Reproduced with the permission of the Minister of Public Works and Government Services Canada, 1999.

help impart information about potential benefits and risks of particular strategies. For example, of 100 persons screened, how many persons who are screened will have falsely positive or falsely negative results? Second, raising the specter of hidden disease or that one is at high risk for a disorder may engender anxiety or guilt out of proportion to the actual risk of disease for a specific individual. Health care information systems have the potential for breaches of confidentiality regarding risk factors, lifestyles, and family history that may result in denial of employment or insurance coverage. Third, in cases in which a preventive intervention is recommended, serious financial burden may be imposed on older persons if insurance or managed care denies payment. In addition, will persons who persist in potentially unhealthy behaviors be denied insurance coverage? Finally, how much evidence is required to make an assessment that the benefits outweigh the risk of the preventive intervention for a particular patient? Ethical implications of prevention research and practice are largely unexplored, and there are undoubtedly other ethical concerns not mentioned here.

The US and Canadian guides arm the clinician with an understanding of what is known to be effective, what is known not to be effective, and what uncertainty persists because of a lack of evidence that particular preventive interventions are effective. Physicians and other health care providers can be empowered by the guides to share the most current recommendations with patients and their families, including uncertainty about the value of specific interventions. Recommendations from disease-specific organizations or from published reviews can inform health care providers about the value of preventive interventions, but the careful methodology and wide representation make the recommendations of the task forces particularly compelling.

Where there is considerable certainty about the appropriateness of a preventive intervention, computer-assisted decision making and reminder systems can be organized to provide ticklers to perform specific interventions. Over the age of 65 years, for example, the patient should receive pneumococcal vaccine immunization. How often do older patients go in and out of physicians' offices or the hospital while the opportunity to receive pneumococcal vaccine immunization has been missed? In some cases, managed care health plans are developing systems to call patients in for specific procedures, such as immunizations or screening mammography, even without the physician's direct knowledge. However, the primary health care office of the future will have new means for illustrating where the patient stands in relation to preventive screening and health maintenance interventions and for the evaluation of risk to target preventive interventions to the individuals who are most likely to benefit. The National Cancer Institute, for example, has developed a "risk disk" to calculate risk of breast cancer based on patient characteristics.

RATING THE RECOMMENDATIONS

To develop recommendations based on current knowledge, the first job of the US task force was to rate the quality of evidence related to preventive interventions. To grade evidence, the task force employed a five-point scale adapted from the earlier Canadian Task Force on the Periodic Health Examination: (I) At least one randomized clinical trial (deemed to be the best kind of evidence of effectiveness), (II-1) evidence obtained from well-designed controlled trials but without randomizing participants, (II-2) evidence obtained from well-designed cohort or case-controlled analytic studies, probably from more than one center or research group, (II-3) evidence obtained in uncontrolled experiments or studies of natural history of persons with and without the intervention, and (III) opinions or reports from experts.[28]

After careful review of the literature, the US task force categorized recommendations into five levels: A, B, C, D, and E. An "A" recommendation was used if there was good evidence for the application of the preventive intervention in a periodic health examination. A "B" recommendation was given if there was fair evidence for the recommendation. If the evidence was poor from studies, but the recommendations could be made on other grounds, the task force reported a "C" recommendation. If there was fair evidence that the preventive intervention should be excluded from the periodic examination, a "D" recommendation was made. Finally, if there was good evidence to exclude the preventive intervention, an "E" recommendation was applied.

It is telling that, for many of the preventive services reviewed in the *Guide to Clinical Preventive Services,* there is insufficient evidence to determine whether routine interventions will improve clinical outcomes (the "C" recommendation). Several circumstances can result in the "C" recommendation: (1) very high-quality studies have resulted in conflicting results, (2) the studies performed were not adequate to determine effectiveness (eg, insufficient statistical power, samples studied were not representative, lack of clinically significant endpoints, or other study deficiencies), and (3) evidence of significant benefits from the intervention was offset by evidence of important harm that occurs at the same time. A "C" recommendation should not be interpreted as evidence that an intervention is not effective or beneficial, but simply reflects a lack of evidence on the question. In other words, just because a recommendation was rated as "C" does not mean that the maneuver or test is not worth doing, especially when other risk factors are present.

SPECIFIC RECOMMENDATIONS

In the summary that follows, preventive strategies will be discussed from the point of view of the US *Guide to Clinical Preventive Services* and *The Canadian Guide to Clinical Preventive Health Care*. The reader is advised, however, to consult the US task force's *Guide to Clinical Preventive Services* and the Canadian task force's *The Canadian Guide to Clinical Preventive Health Care* for the detailed rationale for the recommendations. In addition, the recommendations are periodically updated, and readers can now access the newest versions of the documents on the World Wide Web. Finally, tension and controversy persist regarding preventive measures in older persons, based on severe limitations in the evidence base pertaining to older adults. For this summary, "A" and "B" level recommendations are emphasized; however, there are many situations where physicians should participate in shared decision making with patients, especially when the evidence does not exist or there is conflicting evidence.

PROCEDURES AND MEASUREMENTS

Blood Pressure

Periodic screening for hypertension is recommended for all persons older than 21 years of age. . . . Hypertension should not be diagnosed on the basis of a single measurement; elevated readings should be confirmed on more than one reading at each of three separate visits.[28(p46)] ("A" recommendation)

Many studies now provide evidence that older persons with high blood pressure, including persons with elevated systolic blood pressure only, are at increased risk for adverse events, and that treatment is effective in lowering the risk of stroke, cardiac events, and death.

Height and Weight

Periodic height and weight measurements are recommended for all patients.[28(p234)] ("B" recommendation)

The calculation of the body mass index from the height and weight can assist in assessment of nutritional status, both in relation to obesity and undernutrition (discussed further in Chapter 8, Physical Assessment).

Vision Screening

Routine vision screening is recommended among the elderly, with Snellen acuity testing.[28(p379)] ("B" recommendation)

The optimal frequency for screening is not known and is left to clinical discretion. Selected questions about vision may also be helpful in detecting vision problems in older persons, but they do not appear as sensitive or specific as direct assessment of acuity.

Correction for refractive errors or surgery for cataract are highly effective in restoring vision. Although the US task force concluded there was insufficient evidence to recommend for or against routine screening ophthalmoscopy ("C" recommendation), persons with diabetes should be scheduled for ophthalmologic examination regularly. Both the US and Canadian task forces did not give a high priority to routine screening by primary care physicians to detect elevated intraocular pressure, but instead recommended that high-risk patients be referred for assessment (eg, African Americans over age 40 years, Whites over age 65 years, or patients with diabetes or a family history of glaucoma).[27,28]

Hearing Screening

Screening older adults for hearing by periodically questioning them about their hearing, counseling them about the availability of hearing aid devices, and making referrals for abnormalities when appropriate, is recommended. The optimal frequency of such screening has not been determined and is left to clinical discretion. An otoscopic examination and audiometric testing should be performed on all persons with evidence of impaired hearing by patient inquiry.[28(p401)] ("B" recommendation)

In a survey of older women from rural Idaho, the single question, "Would you say that you have any difficulty hearing?" had good sensitivity and specificity for hearing impairment as assessed by audiometry.[31] Examination strategies including whispering out of field of vision or using a tuning fork to assess hearing are also adequate to identify older persons who should receive further evaluation.[27]

Dental Care

> Counseling patients to visit a dental care provider on a regular basis is recommended based on evidence for risk reduction from such visits when combined with regular personal oral hygiene.[28(p717)] ("B" recommendation) . . . There is little evidence regarding the optimal frequency of visits; this recommendation should be made by the patient's dental care provider.

Good oral health is essential to quality of life, and patients should be encouraged to carry out oral hygiene practices such as brushing the teeth with a fluoride-containing toothpaste and cleaning between the teeth with dental floss to prevent dental caries and periodontal disease. Physicians can ask about gingival bleeding as an indicator of periodontal disease,[27] and can be alert for the oral lesions that might presage cancer (especially in patients who use tobacco or alcohol[27,28]).

Fecal Occult Blood Testing and Sigmoidoscopy

> Screening for colorectal cancer is recommended for all persons aged 50 or over.[28(p98)] ("B" recommendation)

To accomplish screening for colorectal cancer, several methods are available. The US task force recommended annual testing for fecal occult blood, but could not provide a firm recommendation for the frequency of sigmoidoscopy (a frequency of every 3 to 5 years was suggested,[28] consistent with recommendations of other groups). The US task force concluded that there was insufficient evidence to determine which of these two screening methods is preferable or whether the combination of both procedures produces greater benefits than either test alone. Randomized trials involving over 250,000 asymptomatic persons aged 50 years and older indicate that annual and biennial screening for fecal occult blood reduces mortality from colorectal cancer.[32] Because of the need to work up many false positive tests, the Canadian Task Force urged caution in application of screening for colorectal cancer, and rated the use of screening as a level "C" recommendation.[27] Patients at increased risk of colorectal cancer (family history of colorectal cancer and/or personal history of adenomas) warrant more frequent examinations.

Mammography and Clinical Breast Examination

> Screening for breast cancer every 1–2 years, with mammography alone or mammography and clinical breast examination (CBE) is recommended for women aged 50–69 years.[28] ("A" recommendation) . . . There is limited and conflicting evidence regarding clinical benefit of mammography or CBE for women aged 70–74 and no evidence regarding benefit for women over age 75; however, recommendations for screening women aged 70 and over who have a reasonable life expectancy may be made on other grounds.[28(p83)] ("C" recommendation)

The Canadian Task Force also rated the evidence related to women aged 50 to 69 years as an "A" recommendation.[27] In recent decades, nine prospective randomized trials have shown a clear benefit for women aged 50 to 69 years, but for women aged 40 to 49, the data are less clear.[33] The development of genetic markers for breast cancer raises additional questions about the role of such testing to stratify risk. Both the US and Canadian task forces stated that there was insufficient evidence to recommend teaching breast self-examination to women ("C" recommendation).

Papanicolau (Pap) Smear

> Regular Pap tests are recommended for all women who are or have been sexually active and who have a cervix.[28] ("A" recommendation) . . . There is insufficient evidence to recommend for or against an upper age limit for Pap testing, but recommendations can be made on other grounds to discontinue regular testing after age 65 in women who have had regular previous screening in which the smears have been consistently normal.[28(p112)] ("C" recommendation)

Beyond its function as a screening test for the detection of asymptomatic cancer of the uterine cervix, the Pap smear serves as the focal point for all the periodic health examinations women receive. The procedure affords an opportunity to examine the vagina and vulva for lesions and to broach issues related to sexuality. Younger women take health maintenance visits for granted, but an older woman may not consider that such examinations apply, since reproductive concerns seem far in the past. Older women are likely to be cared for by an internist or family physician, not a gynecologist, and may not specifically request a gynecologic examination.

Many women in the current older cohort have not had Pap smears at regular intervals.[34,35] Mandelblatt and colleagues offered a Pap smear to 1,542 women aged 65 years and older and found that 53% assented.[34] For 25% of this group, this was the first Pap smear, and only 26% gave a history of routine Pap smears. In addition to detecting cervical carcinoma, other gynecologic problems were uncovered, including breast cancer. Among 320 older women offered a Pap smear in primary health care, 24% reported never having had one, and only 24% gave a history of adequate screening.[36] No woman who was asked by their primary care provider refused to have a Pap smear, and 75% assented when asked by someone other than the primary care provider. In a large sample of women aged 55 years and older, 58% had never had a mammogram, and 87% had a Pap smear within 3 years of the interview.[37] Of the women who had not had a mammogram, over one third gave as the reason that their physicians had not recommended one. As the current cohort of women ages, more older women will have undergone screening with the Pap smear. Since many of the current cohort of older women have never had cervical screening, the Pap smear remains important.

Cognitive Impairment

Neither the US nor Canadian task force found sufficient evidence to recommend that asymptomatic persons be screened for dementia.[27,28] In addition, the Agency for Health Care Policy and Research's guidelines for the *Early Identification of Alzheimer's Disease and Related Dementias* recommended evaluation only when functional impairment or other clinical triggers were present[38] (discussed further in Chapter 3). Any benefit of finding early cases must be balanced against the anxiety and depression engendered in the patient and family and the uncertainty of diagnosis.[39,40] In contrast, screening for cognitive impairment would seem prudent at the time of admission to the hospital or nursing home, in the face of functional decline, when behavioral changes occur, or to monitor the effects of medication. Given the high rate of dementia among the oldest old and the potential for adverse effects on independence, persons over the age of 75 years could be tested at least once using a standard mental status examination.[5]

Clinicians should be aware that mild cognitive impairment accompanied by depressive symptoms may presage the onset of dementia.[41-44]

Whether screening for cognitive impairment should occur in primary health care is an empirical question for further research because finding incipient cases of dementia will be critical if new pharmacologic strategies for prevention and treatment are to be effectively employed. Recognition of cognitive impairment provides an opportunity to prevent complications arising from coexisting medical or psychiatric conditions, including extra care when medications that may affect mental status are prescribed.[45] Early diagnosis does afford the opportunity for discussion with the patient regarding advance directives and driving[5,46] although such discussions might best be considered universal interventions for older persons.

Laboratory Testing

Fasting Blood Glucose

Trials to assess whether screening and control of risk factors such as obesity in asymptomatic persons are underway (primary prevention), but secondary prevention of complications resulting from early diagnosis would be a rationale for screening. Neither the US nor Canadian task force recommended screening of asymptomatic persons (pregnancy excluded.)[27,28] Revised diagnostic criteria for diabetes mellitus include fasting plasma glucose greater than 126 mg/dl, with no distinction as to age.[47]

Serum Cholesterol

Periodic screening for high blood cholesterol, using specimens obtained from fasting or nonfasting individuals, is recommended for all men ages 35–65 and women ages 45–65 ("B" recommendation). There is insufficient evidence to recommend for or against routine screening in asymptomatic persons after age 65, but screening may be considered on a case-by-case basis ("C" recommendation). Older persons with major coronary heart disease (CHD) risk factors (smoking, hypertension, diabetes) who are otherwise healthy may be more likely to benefit from screening, based on their high risk of CHD and the proven benefits of lowering cholesterol in older persons with asymptomatic CHD. Cholesterol levels are not a reliable predictor of risk after age 75, however.[28(p29)]

Since older persons are at increased risk for cardiovascular events, even if the strength of the relationship of cholesterol as a risk factor is diminished for older adults compared with younger adults, evaluation and treatment of risk factors could have a large population effect on reducing the burden of cardiovascular illness. Intensity of treatment to reduce risk must be balanced, as in all interventions, with the potential for adverse effects on quality of life. Among older persons with a poor prognosis or poor quality of life, cholesterol screening is probably not warranted.[5]

Prostate-Specific Antigen

Routine screening for prostate cancer with prostate-specific antigen (PSA) (or digital rectal examination [DRE] and transrectal ultrasound for that matter) were not recommended for asymptomatic men by either the US or the Canadian task force[27,28] ("D" recommendation). If screening is to be carried out, the best evaluated procedure, according to the US *Guide to Clinical Preventive Services,* was DRE and PSA for men with a life expectancy of at least 10 years.[28]

Thyroid-Stimulating Hormone Level

Because of the subtle ways that hypothyroidism can present in older adults, either with few symptoms or with symptoms ascribed to aging,[48,49] screening elderly persons with thyroid-stimulating hormone (TSH) may be warranted every 2 to 3 years, at least in older women.[50–52] However, the US and the Canadian task forces concluded that there was not enough evidence to include routine TSH measurement ("C" recommendation). Instead, clinicians were encouraged to maintain a high index of suspicion when easy fatigability, weight gain, cold intolerance, trouble concentrating, and depression were present.[27,28]

BEHAVIORS AND LIFESTYLE

Tobacco Use

A complete history of tobacco use, and an assessment of nicotine dependence among tobacco users, should be obtained from all adolescent and adult patients. Tobacco cessation counseling is recommended on a regular basis for all patients who use tobacco products.[28(p602)] ("A" recommendation)

It goes without saying in a chapter on health promotion and disease prevention that patients should be encouraged to stop smoking since the evidence is overwhelming that tobacco use in any form is harmful. In a study of 2,674 persons aged 65 to 74 years, older smokers had a

52% increased mortality secondary to cardiovascular disease when compared to nonsmokers and former smokers. Persons who stopped smoking eventually reduced their mortality rate to the rate of non-smokers (in 1 to 5 years).[53] Counseling to stop smoking with adjunctive therapy employing nicotine gum or patches appears to be effective[27,28] (an "A" recommendation in reports from both the US and the Canadian task forces, although the relevant studies have included relatively few older persons). Caution must be exercised when using nicotine replacement therapy as an adjunct to counseling in older patients in whom cardiovascular disease is more common (but remember that continued smoking is not without risk either). When counseling patients about smoking cessation, consider the patient's readiness to change his or her behavior (eg, patients in the contemplation stage could be encouraged to take small steps such as delaying the first cigarette in the morning and so might be more prepared to quit[21]).

Problem Alcohol Use

Screening to detect problem drinking and hazardous drinking is recommended for all adult and adolescent patients.[28(p575)] ("B" recommendation) All patients should be counseled regarding the dangers of operating a motor vehicle while under the influence of alcohol or other drugs, as well as the risk of riding in a vehicle operated by someone who is under the influence of these substances.[28(p651)] ("A" recommendation)

Questions about amount and frequency of alcohol use may underestimate the extent of problem drinking, and it may be more productive to use one of the standardized assessment questionnaires described in Chapter 3, Mental Status Assessment. Counseling in primary care settings to decrease alcohol use appears to be effective.[54-56]

Diet and Nutritional Counseling

Adults should limit dietary intake of fat (especially saturated fat, "A" recommendation) and cholesterol ("B" recommendation), maintain caloric balance in their diet, and emphasize fruits, vegetables, and grain products containing fiber. ("B" recommendation) . . . Adults should reduce total fat intake to less than 30% total calories and dietary cholesterol to less than 300 mg/day. Saturated fat consumption should be reduced to less than 10% of total calories.[28(p633)]

In order to conform to these dietary recommendations, patients should emphasize fish, poultry (prepared without skin), lean meats, and low-fat dairy products in their diets. Daily consumption of at least five servings of fruit and vegetables and at least six servings of breads, cereals, or legumes will help patients achieve dietary goals related to fat. There was insufficient evidence to think that nutritional counseling by physicians is effective in changing the dietary habits of patients. In contrast, registered dietitians or other qualified nutritionists who obtain a complete dietary history, address barriers to improving dietary habits, and offer specific guidance on meal planning that may be more effective.

Regular Physical Activity

Counseling to promote regular physical activity is recommended for all adults. This recommendation is based on the proven efficacy of regular physical activity in reducing the risk for coronary artery disease, hypertension, obesity, and diabetes.[28(p619)] ("A" recommendation)

As a general strategy for all behavioral change, the clinician should ascertain the patient's baseline activity level, attitudes toward increasing physical activity, and perceived barriers to increasing activity, as well as provide information and encouragement to improve. Exercise has a number of beneficial effects that may include maintenance of function,[57] increased strength and fitness,[58] and sharpened memory and cognitive function.[59]

Use of Seat Belts and Helmets

Clinicians should regularly urge their patients to use lap/shoulder belts for themselves and their passengers.[28(p651)] (an "A" recommendation with regard to seat belt use and a "B" recommendation for counseling)

Patients who ride bicycles or motorcycles should be encouraged to use appropriate head protection[28] (an "A" recommendation). Helmet use has been legislated in some localities.

Sexual Behavior

All adolescent and adult patients should be advised about risk factors for sexually transmitted diseases and counseled appropriately about effective measures to reduce risk of infection.[28] ("B" recommendation)

Older adults may need information about sexual changes with aging as well as about sexually transmitted diseases, including the virus that causes the acquired immune deficiency syndrome. Screening for several conditions (such as breast examination for women) provides an opportunity to discuss topics related to sexual activity. High-risk patients who are sexually active may be candidates to test for chlamydia, gonorrhea, and other sexually transmitted diseases. Evaluation related to sexual issues is discussed in Chapter 6, Social Assessment.

Depression and Suicide

Neither the US task force nor the Canadian task force recommended screening for depression, but stated that clinicians should be alert for signs and symptoms that might stem from depression.[27,28] Psychiatric disorders including depression do not seem to fit the notion of detection during an asymptomatic phase of disorder because the presence of symptoms is the only way to make a diagnosis.[60] At the same time, symptoms that do not reach threshold for diagnosis appear to be a risk for development of depression[61-65] and functional impairment.[66] Visits in primary care settings provide opportunities for secondary prevention of depression, eg, monitoring patients with a history of depression to prevent recurrence.[45,67,68]

Older adults with chronic pain,[69,70] newly diagnosed medical illness,[71] stroke,[72-74] functional dependence,[75] cancer,[76] insomnia,[77] and who have experienced significant life events such as bereavement[78] or institutionalization[79,80] should be carefully assessed for development of depression. Caregivers,[81,82] persons who live alone,[83,84] and persons with less than a high school education[85] may also be considered to be a group at higher than average risk for depression.

Physicians should not be afraid to ask about suicidal ideation among older persons with symptoms that may be attributable to depression, especially among older adults who express helplessness or hopelessness about their circumstances (further discussion can be found in Chapter 3, Mental Status Assessment and in Chapter 6,

Social Assessment). Interventions targeted at general practitioners appear to be able to decrease suicide rates, at least in limited populations.[86,87] Both the US and Canadian task forces gave training of primary care physicians in recognition of suicide risk factors a "B" recommendation. Treatment of depression and other mental disorders, psychiatric consultation, increasing social support and identifying coping strategies, and educating the family about the illness are interventions that appear to be effective for persons who are having suicidal ideation.[27]

HOME AND HEALTH

Environmental factors probably play a role in falls and other injuries among older persons at home. For example, stairs, loose rugs, inadequate lighting, and lack of handrails on stairs and bathtub may contribute to falls in older persons with functional impairment. In the following paragraphs, considerations related to home safety are highlighted.

Falls and Other Injuries

Counseling elderly patients on measures to reduce the risk of falling, including exercise (particularly training to improve balance), safety-related skills and behaviors, and environmental hazard reduction, along with monitoring and adjusting medications, is recommended based on fair evidence that these measures reduce the likelihood of falling. ("B" recommendation) Intensive individualized home-based multifactorial intervention to reduce the risk of falls is recommended for high-risk elderly patients in settings where adequate resources are available to deliver such services.[28(p677)] ("B" recommendation)

High risk for falls is signaled by age 75 years and older, or at younger ages when additional risk factors are present, including use of psychoactive or cardiovascular medications (eg, benzodiazepines and antihypertensives), use of more than four medications, cognitive impairment, decreased strength in the hip, and poor balance when walking.[28] Several studies examining the outcomes of persons evaluated by a multidisciplinary falls clinic appeared to show benefit (primary prevention).[88–90] Prevention of falls in institutionalized older persons who had already fallen (secondary prevention) was not shown to be effective, but might be recommended on other grounds ("C" recommendation).

Older adults are at risk for injuries from burns, poisoning (from medications), suffocation (choking on food), and motor vehicle accidents, in addition to injuries as a result of falling. There is limited evidence of the effectiveness of counseling with regard to these additional kinds of injuries, but it seems prudent to consider whether risk factors, such as cognitive or functional impairment, are present that put the older person at increased risk. Assessment with respect to automobile driving is given special attention in Chapter 5, The Older Driver.

Firearms in the Home

Parents and homeowners should also be counseled to restrict unauthorized access to potentially lethal prescription drugs and to firearms within the home.[28(p552)] Clinicians should inform those identified as being at high risk for violence about the risks of violent injury associated with easy access to firearms and with intoxication with alcohol or other drugs.[28(p552)] ("C" recommendation)

Older men and others at increased risk for suicide should be asked about the availability of firearms in the home, and families may be asked to remove firearms to a safe place.

Smoke and Carbon Monoxide Detectors

Homeowners should be advised to install smoke detectors in appropriate locations and to test the devices periodically to ensure proper operation.[28(p676)] ("B" recommendation)

In addition to installation and maintenance of functioning smoke detectors, homeowners with fireplaces or wood-burning stoves should consider installing detectors that monitor the level of carbon monoxide. Older persons who cannot climb a ladder to reach the smoke detector and replace the batteries may need help doing so.

Hot Water Heater Settings

Hot water heaters should be set at 120–130°F.[28(p676)] ("B" recommendation)

Domestic Abuse and Violence

. . . including a few direct questions about abuse (physical violence or forced sexual activity) as part of the routine history in adult patients may be recommended on other grounds.[28(p562)] ("C" recommendation)

The American Medical Association defined elder abuse as: "Abuse includes intentional infliction of physical or mental injury; sexual abuse; or withholding of necessary food, clothing, and medical care to meet the physical and mental needs of an elderly person by one having the care, custody, or responsibility of an elderly person."[91] Currently, there is insufficient evidence to make a firm recommendation about screening for elder abuse,[27,28] but health care providers should be aware of the risk factors for abusive situations. Major factors predisposing to elder abuse include impairment and dependence of the older adult on the caregiver, caregiver stress, family dynamics, and history of violence and psychopathology in the caregiver such as substance abuse.[92–98] Cognitively impaired older patients may put extreme demands on the caregiver, exhibiting aggressive or violent behavior, thereby increasing the burden of care and the strain on the caregiver.[94,99,100] Mistreatment may start after some event that leaves the elder more dependent on the caregiver, so that health care professionals who deal with older patients should remain alert for functional changes in the elderly patient that can leave the caregiver unable to continue caregiving (see Chapter 6, Social Assessment).

SUPPLEMENTS AND CHEMOPROPHYLAXIS

Calcium

Women should be encouraged to consume recommended quantities of calcium . . . for post-menopausal women, 1000 to 1500 mg/day.[28(p634)] ("B" recommendation)

Hormone Replacement Therapy (Estrogen)

Clinicians should counsel all women around the time of menopause about the possible benefits and risks of post-menopausal hormone therapy and the available treatment options.[28(p839)] ("B" recommendation) Counseling should include asking about presence and severity of menopausal symptoms (hot flushes, urogenital symptoms), as well as assessing risk factors for heart disease, osteoporosis, and breast cancer. Women should be advised of the probable benefits of hormone therapy on menopausal symptoms, myocardial infarction, and fracture; the increased risks of endometrial cancer with unopposed estrogen; and a possible increased risk of breast cancer. Each woman should consider the relative importance of these benefits and risks, the possible side effects of treatment, and her willingness to take medication for an indefinite period.

Both the US and Canadian task forces recommended that all women should be counseled about the risks and benefits of hormone replacement therapy (at the "B" level of confidence).[27,28] However, neither task force felt that there was currently a role for techniques to measure bone density in screening asymptomatic persons for osteoporosis (specifically given a "D" recommendation by the Canadian Task Force).[27]

Aspirin

Neither task force felt that there was sufficient evidence, based on their review of the literature, to support or refute the use of aspirin to prevent the onset of cardiovascular disease.[27,28]

Other Substances

A number of other substances are being investigated for their potential roles in preventing a number of conditions, but for which there is not yet enough evidence to recommend widespread use. For patient groups at increased risk of disease (eg, first-degree relatives of persons with breast cancer), the use of agents with careful follow-up may be undertaken on an individual basis. Examples of substances purported to prevent various conditions include tamoxifen (breast cancer[101]), nonsteroidal anti-inflammatory drugs (Alzheimer's disease[102,103]), histamine-blockers (Alzheimer's disease[102]), and a variety of other substances (vitamin E, raloxifene, and antioxidants in red wine).

IMMUNIZATIONS AND INFECTIOUS DISEASE

Pneumococcal Vaccine

Pneumococcal vaccine is recommended for all immunocompetent individuals who are aged 65 years and older or otherwise at increased risk for pneumococcal disease.[28(p803)] ("B" recommendation)

Influenza Vaccine

Influenza vaccine should be administered annually to all persons aged 65 years and older, and to persons 6 months of age and older who are residents of chronic care facilities or suffer from chronic cardiopulmonary disorders, metabolic diseases (including diabetes mellitus), hemoglobinopathies, immunosuppression, or renal dysfunction. . . . In persons at high risk for Influenza A (eg, during institutional outbreaks), amantadine or rimantadine prophylaxis (200mg/day orally) may be started at the time of vaccination and continued for 2 weeks.[28(p802)] ("B" recommendations)

Caregivers of older persons should probably be immunized as well. Not all eligible older persons who should receive the vaccine are immunized—physicians forget to offer it or older patients refuse it. Some older persons refuse the vaccine because they fear an adverse reaction or they heard about neighbors or friends who "took sick" after receiving the vaccine. Asking specifically about such notions may dispel myths about the vaccine and enhance acceptance.

Tetanus-Diphtheria (Td) Boosters

The Td vaccine series should be completed for patients who have not received the primary series, and all adults should receive periodic Td boosters.[28(p804)] ("A" recommendation) . . . The optimal interval for booster doses is not established. The standard regimen is to provide a Td booster at least once every 10 years, but in the U.S., intervals of 15–30 years between boosters are likely to be adequate in persons who received a complete five-dose series in childhood. . . . For international travelers, an interval of 10 years between boosters is recommended.

Screening for Tuberculosis Infection

Screening for tuberculosis infection by tuberculin skin testing is recommended for all persons at increased risk of developing tuberculosis (TB).[28] ("A" recommendation) Asymptomatic persons at increased risk include persons infected with HIV, close contacts of persons with known or suspected TB (including health care workers), persons with medical risk factors associated with TB, immigrants from countries with high TB prevalence (eg, most countries in Africa, Asia, and Latin America), medically underserved low-income populations (including high-risk racial or ethnic minority populations), alcoholics, injection drug users, and residents of long-term care facilities (eg, correctional institutions, mental institutions, nursing homes).[28(p282)]

The Purified Protein Derivative test (0.1 mL containing 5 tuberculin units injected intracutaneously into the forearm) is the standard way to screen for exposure to the tubercle bacillus. The examination of the injection site should occur 48 to 72 hours later. For residents of long-term care facilities and other high-risk individuals, a 10-mm diameter reaction is considered a positive skin test. A 5-mm reaction may be significant among persons at very high-risk, such as persons who have been exposed to someone harboring an active infection. Assessment of conversion status in older nursing home residents may best be achieved with a two-step procedure, in which a negative skin reaction leads to a second skin test about 1 to 3 weeks later. Patients who react on the second skin test suggest previous exposure or infection (booster phenomenon). Negative reaction on the second skin test followed by a subsequent positive test delineates recent conversion.

OTHER CONSIDERATIONS FOR PREVENTION IN GERIATRICS NOT COVERED IN THE GUIDELINES

Functional Impairment

Functional status includes the ability to perform activities of daily living (ADL) and instrumental ADL (IADL), as well as the suitability of the older adult to drive, as discussed at length in other chapters of this book. In considering health promotion and disease prevention activities for older persons, the assessment of function deserves prominence from a number of perspectives. First, functional status is a consideration in recommending some preventive activities. For example, screening for colorectal cancer in an institutionalized and bed-bound patient with dementia may not serve the best interests of the patient. Functional impairment may be a signal that testing for another condition that remains undiagnosed is warranted (eg, cognitive impairment or depression, as discussed above). Second, it is conceivable that some preventive interventions may have an effect on functioning at least temporarily. Bowel preparation required for sigmoidoscopy may significantly impair the ability of an older person to perform caregiving tasks. Third, improved functioning may be an important ancillary outcome of effective preventive interventions directed at specific conditions. Primary prevention of a condition such as stroke should result in limitation of disability (at least that portion of functional impairment attributed to stroke). In addition, early detection of disorders may permit more complete and effective treatment before complications occur. Finally, functional impairment can be the chief target of preventive interventions. Physical frailty may be preventable if risk factors can be delineated and addressed.[104,105] The concept of "preclinical disability" suggests that an identifiable stage or stages may occur before overt functional impairment develops (namely, when older persons are able to perform an activity but have changed the way they do so[106]). Hebert and colleagues[107] employed a mailed questionnaire to stratify a sample of 842 community-dwelling adults aged 75 years and older into high- and low-risk groups; they found that the method was useful in predicting functional decline over the course of a 1-year follow-up. Preventive interventions may then be directed at the persons most at risk of functional decline in order to prevent disability.

Polypharmacy

Polypharmacy, use of multiple medications by older people, is an important problem not addressed by the US or Canadian guidelines. While abuse of illicit substances is uncommon among older persons, misuse of prescription medications such as hypnotics may be a significant problem.[108] The use of psychoactive drugs increases with advancing age,[109-117] despite increased hazard of cognitive impairment,[118] physical dependency,[119] unrecognized use of alcohol,[120] and injury.[121] Use of several drugs multiplies the risk for adverse reactions, and additional drugs may be prescribed in an effort to control symptoms that arise.[122] The review of *all* medications the patient is taking, including over-the-counter medications, should be part of virtually every contact with the patient.

Advance Directives

Despite progressive legal developments that permit and encourage advance directives, older adults typically do not make use of advance directives, assuming that family will be consulted and can make appropriate decisions in the event of critical illness and the loss of decision-making capacity. Even studies specifically designed to increase the use of advance directives have generally met with limited success, with some exceptions.[123,124] Although the primary care setting would be an excellent one for ongoing discussions regarding patient wishes in the event of terminal or irreversible illness, few older persons broach the subject with their doctors. The American College of Physicians recommended that these decisions should become part of the medical record.[125] Chapter 7 provides recommendations for incorporating advance directives into practice.

Advance directives are expected to extend patient autonomy, relieve patient anxiety about unwanted treatment, reduce family argument regarding treatment decisions, and increase physician confidence in treatment decisions.[126] Disadvantages of living wills include ambiguity, application only to terminal illness, and emphasis only on less aggressive treatment.[127] Instructional directives can be specific, but therefore are limiting and fixed when implemented. Instructions are also subject to interpretation at a later date when circumstances unforeseen by the patient have arisen.[128] Other problems with advance directives are that no one wants to think seriously about death, that advance directives may not be portable in a mobile society, that ideas of quality of life change with age, and that there is an inability to define all situations. Therapeutic advances and the patient's prognosis can change between execution of the directive and its implementation,[129] the patient may change his or her mind,[130] or the directive may not even be followed.[131–133] Designation of a proxy is not without difficulty since the proxy may not be available when decisions are made, or the proxy may not have discussed the patient's preferences.

Caregiver Stress and Knowledge

Children who find themselves caring for older parents may themselves be older. One fourth of all caregivers are 65 to 74 years of age, and 10% are over age 75.[134] The task that family caregivers undertake can be quite rigorous—both physically and emotionally. The extent of support provided by caregivers ranges from emotional support (such as telephone calls), to help with the IADL (eg, transportation, shopping, housekeeping, and meal preparation), to help with the ADL (eg, bathing, feeding, dressing, and toileting). Neither the US or Canadian guides addressed caregivers of older persons; however, persons who care for older persons were encouraged to learn cardiopulmonary resuscitation.[28]

Making the special effort to include an assessment of how the caregiver is coping validates the person's caregiving effort and sends the clear message that the physician is concerned with the caregiver, not just the older patient who is the center of attention.[81] Assessment of the physical health of the caregiver has practical value as well. The caregiver with cardiovascular problems or arthritis cannot be expected to do heavy lifting in the course of caring for an impaired older person. Caregivers reported three times as many stress-related symptoms and used more psychoactive drugs than similar control subjects.[135] The prevalence of depression in caregivers may be very high, and the perceived burden of care may be greater when depression is present.[82,136]

Increased knowledge and consideration of coping strategies may help caregivers continue to be effective in keeping older adults at home and in maintaining their own health. Information and support may be found in books (eg, *The 36-Hour Day*[137]), support groups (eg, Alzheimer's disease support groups or classes[138]), and education programs (eg, programs offered by some community colleges[139]). The primary care setting can develop partnerships with caregivers and social support agencies to sustain the caregiving role.[140]

ADDITIONAL NOTES

Neither the US or Canadian task forces found sufficient evidence for or against routine screening for abdominal aortic aneurysm (AAA) in older adults. Men over age 60 years might be at increased risk and could be targeted for physical examination to detect AAA.[27,28] Auscultation of the carotid arteries to detect silent cerebrovascular disease in asymptomatic persons has not been recommended.[27,28,141] While auscultation of the carotids provides an opportunity to educate the patient about the symptoms and risk factors for stroke, widespread screening would lead to unnecessary testing and potentially hazardous procedures. Symptoms suggestive of transient ischemic attack signal a high-risk group that should be evaluated.[142] Screening for asymptomatic bacteriuria in older persons was not recommended by either task force[27,28] ("D" rating for ambulatory older persons and "E" rating for institutionalized older persons). Ovarian cancer screening in elderly women was not recommended[27,28] ("D" recommendation). Although clinicians should keep vigilant for early symptoms of cancer that warrant work-up, the screening of asymptomatic persons for occult cancers was given a "C" recommendation (for skin and testicular cancers) or a "D" recommendation (for thyroid, lung, bladder, and pancreatic cancers) by the US task force.[28]

CONCLUSION

Because persons in good health at age 65 years can expect to remain functionally independent for 10 years or more,[143] health maintenance and promotion activities remain meaningful in late life. In considering health promotion and disease prevention for the older adult, the perspective must be shifted to include the domains of multidimensional assessment. A reasonable approach to screening for unrecognized problems in older persons would incorporate some screening activities within the context of routine, episodic patient encounters. The goal of screening becomes one of detecting conditions that could potentially disrupt the ability to maintain independence. Many potentially beneficial preventive interventions have been rated as a "C" because of a lack of evidence. Insufficient evidence related to older adults persists because few older adults are included in many studies. Preventive domains specific to older adults not addressed at all by the current guidelines belie the need for a life span approach, that is, the need to think about prevention in relation to the circumstances of the older adult in contrast to middle-age or youth. The older segment of the population may be considered to consist of several heterogeneous groups (eg, young old, middle old, and old old, to say nothing of the increasing numbers of older minority persons) for whom prevention strategies might emphasize different interventions and goals. Clearly, there is a pressing need for more research and consideration of preventive strategies appropriate to older persons.

REFERENCES

1. Sampson A, Sampson S. *The Oxford Book of Ages.* New York: Oxford University Press; 1985.

2. Kennie DC. *Preventive Care for Elderly People.* New York: Cambridge University Press; 1993.

3. Goldberg TH, Chavin SI. Preventive medicine and screening in older adults. *J Am Geriatr Soc.* 1997;45:344–354.

4. Stults BM. Preventive health care for the elderly. *West J Med.* 1984;141:832–845.

5. Zazove P, Mehr DR, Ruffin MT, Klinkman MS, Peggs JF, Davies TC. A criterion-based review of preventive health care in the elderly: Part 2. A geriatric health maintenance program. *J Fam Pract.* 1992;34:320–347.

6. Rubenstein LZ, Josephson KR, Nichol-Seamons M, et al. Comprehensive health screening of well elderly adults: An analysis of a community program. *J Gerontol.* 1986;41:342–352.

7. Gordon R. An operational classification of disease prevention. *Public Health Rep.* 1983;98:107–109.

8. German PS, Burton LC, Shapiro S, et al. Extended coverage for preventive services for the elderly: Response and results in a demonstration project. *Am J Public Health.* 1995;85:379–386.

9. Lurie N, Margolis KL, McGovern PG, Mink PJ, Slater JS. Why do patients of female physicians have higher rates of breast and cervical cancer screening? *J Gen Intern Med.* 1997;12:34–43.

10. Gallo JJ, Rabins PV, Iliffe S. The 'research magnificent' in late life: Psychiatric epidemiology and the primary health care of older adults. *Int J Psychiatry Med.* 1997;27:185–204.

11. Schwab EP, Forciea MA, Carson L, Aisner AM, Lavizzo-Mourey RJ. Clinical practice guidelines in geriatrics. In: Gallo JJ, Busby-Whitehead J, Rabins PV, Silliman R, Murphy J, eds. *Reichel's Care of the Elderly: Clinical Aspects of Aging.* 5th ed. Baltimore: Lippincott Williams & Wilkins; 1999:50–58.

12. Suarez L, Roche RA, Nichols D, Simpson DM. Knowledge, behavior, and fears concerning breast and cervical cancer among older low-income Mexican-American women. *Am J Prev Med.* 1997;13:137–142.

13. O'Malley AS, Mandelblatt J, Gold K, Cagney KA, Kerner J. Continuity of care and the use of breast and cervical cancer screening services in a multiethnic community. *Arch Intern Med.* 1997;157:1462–1470.

14. Kennie DC. Good health care for the elderly. *JAMA.* 1983;249:770–773.

15. Kennie DC. Health maintenance of the elderly. *J Am Geriatr Soc.* 1984;32:316–323.

16. US Public Health Service. Implementing preventive care. *Am Fam Physician.* 1994;50:103–108.

17. Spitzer WO, Mann KV. The public's health is too important to be left to public health workers: A commentary on *Guide to Clinical Preventive Services. Ann Intern Med.* 1989;111:939–942.

18. Sloane P. A prevention oriented medical record. *J Fam Pract.* 1979;9:89–96.

19. Glanz K, Lewis FM, Rimer BK, eds. *Health Behavior and Health Education: Theory, Research, and Practice.* 2nd ed. San Francisco: Jossey-Bass Publishers; 1997.

20. Strecher VJ, Rosenstock IM. The health belief model. In: Glanz K, Lewis FM, Rimer BK, eds. *Health Behavior and Health Education: Theory, Research, and Practice.* 2nd ed. San Francisco: Jossey-Bass Publishers; 1997:41–59.

21. Prochaska JO, Redding CA, Evers KE. The transtheoretical model and stages of change. In: Glanz K, Lewis FM, Rimer BK, eds. *Health Behavior and Health Education: Theory, Research, and Practice.* 2nd ed. San Francisco: Jossey-Bass Publishers; 1997:60–84.

22. Institute of Medicine. *The Second Fifty Years: Promoting Health and Preventing Disability.* Washington, DC: National Academy Press; 1992.

23. Woolf SH, Kamerow DB, Lawrence RS, Medalie JH, Estes EH. The periodic health examination of older adults: The recommendations of the US Preventive Services Task Force: Part I. Counseling, immunizations, and chemoprophylaxis. *J Am Geriatr Soc.* 1990; 38:817–823.

24. Woolf SH, Kamerow DB, Lawrence RS, Medalie JH, Estes EH. The periodic health examination of older adults: The recommendations of the US Preventive Services Task Force: Part II. Screening tests. *J Am Geriatr Soc.* 1990;38:933–942.

25. Klinkman MS, Zazove P, Mehr DR, Ruffin MT. A criterion-based review of preventive health care in the elderly: Part 1. Theoretical framework and development of criteria. *J Fam Pract.* 1992;34:205–224.

26. Patterson C, Chambers LW. Preventive health care. *Lancet.* 1995;345:1611–1615.

27. Canadian Task Force on Preventive Health Care. *The Canadian Guide to Clinical Preventive Health Care.* Ottawa, Canada: Canadian Government Publishing; 1994.

28. US Preventive Services Task Force. *Guide to Clinical Preventive Services: An Assessment of the Effectiveness of 169 Interventions.* 2nd ed. Baltimore: Williams & Wilkins; 1996.

29. US Preventive Services Task Force. *Guide to Clinical Preventive Services: An Assessment of the Effectiveness of 169 Interventions.* Baltimore: Williams & Wilkins; 1989.

30. Rochon PA, Dickinson E, Gordon M. The Cochrane Field in Health Care of Older People: Geriatric medicine's role in the collaboration. *J Am Geriatr Soc.* 1997;45:241–243.

31. Clark K, Bowers M, Wallace RB, et al. The accuracy of self-reported hearing loss in women aged 60–85 years. *Am J Epidemiol.* 1991;134:704–708.

32. Mandel JS. Colorectal cancer screening. *Cancer Metastasis Rev.* 1997;16:263–279.

33. Harris KM, Vogel VG. Breast cancer screening. *Cancer Metastasis Rev.* 1997;16: 231–262.

34. Mandelblatt J, Gopaul I, Wistreich M. Gynecological care of elderly women: Another look at Papanicolaou smear testing. *JAMA.* 1986;256:367–371.

35. Celentano DD, Shapiro S, Weisman CS. Cancer preventive screening behavior among elderly women. *Prev Med.* 1982;11:454–463.

36. Weintraub NT, Violi E, Freedman ML. Cervical cancer screening in women aged 65 and over. *J Am Geriatr Soc.* 1987;35:870–875.

37. Ruchlin HS. Prevalence and correlates of breast and cervical cancer screening among older women. *Obstet Gynecol.* 1997;90:16–21.

38. Costa PT, Williams TF, Somerfield M. *Early Identification of Alzheimer's Disease and Related Dementias.* Rockville, MD: US Dept of Health and Human Services, Public Health Service, Agency for Health Care Policy and Research; 1996. Clinical Practice Guideline, No. 19. AHCPR Publication Number 97–0703.

39. Cooper B, Bickel H. Population screening and the early detection of dementing disorders in old age: A review. *Psychol Med.* 1984;14:81–95.

40. Jones TV, Williams ME. Are mental status questionnaires of clinical value in everyday office practice? An opposing view. *J Fam Pract*. 1990;30:197–200.

41. Reding M, Haycox J, Blass J. Depression in patients referred to a dementia clinic: A three-year prospective study. *Arch Neurol*. 1985;42:894–896.

42. Rabins PV, Merchant A, Nestadt G. Criteria for diagnosing reversible dementia caused by depression: Validation by 2-year follow-up. *Br J Psychiatry*. 1984;144:488–492.

43. Emery VO, Oxman TE. Update on the dementia spectrum of depression. *Am J Psychiatry*. 1992;149:305–317.

44. Devanand DP, Sano M, Tang MX, et al. Depressed mood and the incidence of Alzheimer's disease in the elderly living in the community. *Arch Gen Psychiatry*. 1996;53: 175–182.

45. Rabins PV. Prevention of mental disorders in the elderly: Current perspectives and future prospects. *J Am Geriatr Soc*. 1992;40:727–733.

46. Warshaw G. Are mental status questionnaires of clinical value in everyday office practice? An affirmative view. *J Fam Pract*. 1990;30:194–197.

47. American Diabetes Association. Report of the Expert Committee on the Diagnosis and Classification of Diabetes Mellitus. *Diabetes Care*. 1998;21(Suppl 1):55–119.

48. Bemben DA, Hamm RM, Morgan L, Winn P, Davis A, Barton E. Thyroid disease in the elderly: Part 2. Predictability of subclinical hypothyroidism. *J Fam Pract*. 1994; 38:583–588.

49. Bemben DA, Winn P, Hamm RM, Morgan L, Davis A, Barton E. Thyroid disease in the elderly: Part 1. Prevalence of undiagnosed hypothyroidism. *J Fam Pract*. 1994; 38:577–582.

50. Livingston EH, Hershman JM, Sawin CT, et al. Prevalence of thyroid disease and abnormal thyroid tests in older hospitalized and ambulatory persons. *J Am Geriatr Soc*. 1987;35:109–114.

51. Cooper DS. Subclinical hypothyroidism. *JAMA*. 1987;258:246–247.

52. Helfand M, Crapo LM. Screening for thyroid disease. *Ann Intern Med*. 1990;112: 840–849.

53. Jajich CL, Ostfeld AM, Freeman DH. Smoking and coronary heart disease mortality in the elderly. *JAMA*. 1984;252:2831–2834.

54. Wallace P, Cutler S, Haines A. Randomized controlled trial of general practitioner intervention in patients with excessive alcohol consumption. *Br Med J*. 1988;297: 663–668.

55. Fleming MF, Barry KL, Manwell LB, Johnson K, London R. Brief physician advice for problem alcohol drinkers: A randomized controlled trial in community-based primary care practices. *JAMA*. 1997;277:1039–1045.

56. Goldberg HI, Mullen M, Ries RK, et al. Alcohol counseling in a general medicine clinic: A randomized controlled trial of strategies to improve referral and show rates. *Med Care*. 1991;29(7 Suppl):49–56.

57. Simonsick EM, Lafferty ME, Phillips CL, et al. Risk due to inactivity in physically capable older adults. *Am J Public Health*. 1993;83:1443–1450.

58. Morey MC, Cowper PA, Feussner JR, et al. Evaluation of a supervised exercise program in a geriatric population. *J Am Geriatr Soc*. 1989;37:348–354.

59. Stones MJ, Dawe D. Acute exercise facilitates semantically cued memory in nursing home residents. *J Am Geriatr Soc*. 1993;41:531–534.

60. Ford DE. Principles of screening applied to psychiatric disorders. *Gen Hosp Psychiatry.* 1988;10:177–188.

61. Broadhead WE, Blazer DG, George LK, Tse CK. Depression, disability days, and days lost from work in a prospective epidemiologic survey. *JAMA.* 1990;264:2524–2528.

62. Wells KB, Stewart A, Hays RD, et al. The functioning and well-being of depressed patients: Results from the Medical Outcomes Study. *JAMA.* 1989;262:914–919.

63. Johnson J, Weissman MM, Klerman GL. Service utilization and social morbidity associated with depressive symptoms in the community. *JAMA.* 1992;267:1478–1483.

64. Fava GA, Kellner R. Prodromal symptoms in affective disorders. *Am J Psychiatry.* 1991;148:823–830.

65. Horwath E, Johnson J, Klerman GL, Weissman MM. Depressive symptoms as relative and attributable risk factors for first-onset major depression. *Arch Gen Psychiatry.* 1992;49:817–823.

66. Gallo JJ, Rabins PV, Lyketsos CG, Tien AY, Anthony JC. Depression without sadness: Functional outcomes of nondysphoric depression in later life. *J Am Geriatr Soc.* 1997;45:570–578.

67. Rose G. Mental disorder and the strategies of prevention. *Psychol Med.* 1993;23:553–555.

68. Sartorius N, Henderson AS. The neglect of prevention in psychiatry. *Aust N Zealand J Psychiatry.* 1992;5:548–553.

69. Blumer D, Heilbronn M. Chronic pain as a variant of depressive disease: The pain-prone disorder. *J Nerv Ment Dis.* 1982;170:381–414.

70. Parmelee PA, Katz IR, Lawton MP. The relation of pain to depression among the elderly. *J Gerontol.* 1991;46:15–21.

71. Cadoret RJ, Widmer RB. The development of depressive symptoms in elderly following the onset of severe physical illness. *J Fam Pract.* 1988;27:71–76.

72. Morris PLP, Robinson RG, Raphael B. Prevalence and course of post-stroke depression in hospitalized patients. *Int J Psychiatry Med.* 1990;20:327–342.

73. Schubert DSP, Taylor C, Lee S, Mentari A, Tamaklo W. Physical consequences of depression in the stroke patient. *Gen Hosp Psychiatry.* 1992;14:69–76.

74. Stern RA, Bachman DL. Depressive symptoms following stroke. *Am J Psychiatry.* 1991;148:351–356.

75. Turner RJ, Beiser M. Major depression and depressive symptomatology among the physically disabled: Assessing the role of chronic stress. *J Nerv Ment Dis.* 1990;178:343–350.

76. Endicott J. Measurement of depression in patients with cancer. *Cancer.* 1984;53:2243–2249.

77. Ford DE, Kamerow DB. Epidemiologic study of sleep disturbances and psychiatric disorders: An opportunity for prevention? *JAMA.* 1989;262:1479–1484.

78. Harlow SD, Goldberg EL, Comstock GW. A longitudinal study of risk factors for depressive symptomatology in elderly widowed and married women. *Am J Epidemiol.* 1991;134:526–538.

79. Ames D. Depressive disorders among elderly people in long-term institutional care. *Aust N Zealand J Psychiatry.* 1993;27:379–391.

80. Rovner BW, German PS, Brant LJ, Clark R, Burton L, Folstein MF. Depression and mortality in nursing homes. *JAMA.* 1991;266:215–216.

81. Gallo JJ, Franch MS, Reichel W. Dementing illness: The patient, caregiver, and community. *Am Fam Physician.* 1991;43:1669–1675.

82. Gallo JJ. The effect of social support on depression in caregivers of the elderly. *J Fam Pract.* 1990;30:430–436.

83. Murrell SA, Himmelfarb S, Wright K. Prevalence of depression and its correlates in older adults. *Am J Epidemiol.* 1983;117:173–185.

84. Kaplan GA, Roberts RE, Camacho TC, Coyne JC. Psychosocial predictors of depression: Prospective evidence from the Human Population Laboratory Studies. *Am J Epidemiol.* 1987;125:206–220.

85. Gallo JJ, Royall DR, Anthony JC. Risk factors for the onset of major depression in middle age and late life. *Soc Psychiatry Psychiatr Epidemiol.* 1993;28:101–108.

86. Rutz W, Walinder J, von Knorring L, Rihmer Z, Pihlgren H. Prevention of depression and suicide by education and medication: Impact on male suicidality. An update from the Gotland Study. *Int J Psychiatry Clin Pract.* 1997;1:39–46.

87. Rutz W, Von Knorring L, Walinder J. Frequency of suicide on Gotland after systematic postgraduate education of general practitioners. *Acta Psychiatr Scand.* 1989;80: 151–154.

88. Tinetti ME, Baker DI, McAvay G, et al. A multifactorial intervention to reduce the risk of falling among elderly people living in the community. *N Engl J Med.* 1994;331: 821–827.

89. Wolf-Klein GP, Silverstone FA, Basavaraju N, et al. Prevention of falls in the elderly population. *Arch Phys Med Rehabil.* 1988;69:689–691.

90. Rubenstein L, Robbins A, Josephson R, et al. The value of assessing falls in an elderly population. *Ann Intern Med.* 1990;113:308–316.

91. American Medical Association Council on Scientific Affairs. Elder abuse and neglect. *JAMA.* 1987;257:966–971.

92. Bourland MD. Elder abuse: From definition to prevention. *Postgrad Med.* 1990;87: 139–144.

93. Pillemer K, Finkelhor D. The prevalence of elder abuse: A random sample survey. *Gerontologist.* 1988;8:51–57.

94. Andrew CC, Reichman WE, Berbig LJ. The relationship between dementia and elder abuse. *Am J Psychiatry.* 1993;150:643–646.

95. Kurrle SE, Sadler PM, Cameron ID. Patterns of elder abuse. *Med J Aust.* 1992;157:673–676.

96. Douglass RL. *Domestic Mistreatment of the Elderly—Towards Prevention.* Washington, DC: American Association of Retired Persons; 1992.

97. McDowell JD, Kasselbaum DK, Strombos SE. Recognizing and reporting victims of domestic violence. *J Am Dent Assoc.* 1992;123:44–50.

98. All AC. A literature review: Assessment and intervention in elder abuse. *J Gerontol Nurs.* 1994;20:25–32.

99. Ehrlich F. Patterns of elder abuse. *Med J Aust.* 1993;158:292–293.

100. Bendik MF. Reaching the breaking point: Dangers of mistreatment in elder caregiving situations. *J Elder Abuse Negl.* 1992;4:39–59.

101. Fisher B, Costantino JP, Wickerham DL, et al. Tamoxifen for Prevention of Breast Cancer: Report of the National Surgical Adjuvant Breast and Bowel Project P-1 Study. *J Natl Cancer Inst.* 1998;90:1371–1388.

102. Breitner JCS, Welsh KA, Helms MJ, et al. Delayed onset of Alzheimer's disease with nonsteroidal anti-inflammatory and histamine H2 blocking drugs. *Neurobiol Aging.* 1995;16:523–530.

103. Rozzini R, Ferrucci L, Losonczy K, Havlik RJ, Guralnik JM. Protective effect of chronic NSAID use on cognitive decline in older persons. *J Am Geriatr Soc.* 1996;44: 1025–1029.

104. Fried LP, Guralnik JM. Disability in older adults: Evidence regarding significance, etiology, and risk. *J Am Geriatr Soc.* 1997;45:92–100.

105. Hadley EC, Ory MG, Suzman R, Weindruch R, Fried L. Physical frailty: A treatable cause of dependence in old age. *J Gerontol.* 1993;48:1–88.

106. Fried LP, Herdman SJ, Kuhn KE, Rubin G, Turano K. Preclinical disability: Hypotheses about the bottom of the iceberg. *J Aging Health.* 1997;3:285–300.

107. Hebert R, Bravo G, Korner-Bitensky N, Voyer L. Predictive validity of a postal questionnaire for screening community-dwelling elderly individuals at risk of functional decline. *Age Ageing.* 1996;25:159–167.

108. Gottheil E, Druley KA, Skoloda TE. *The Combined Problems of Alcoholism, Drug Addiction, and Aging.* Springfield, IL: Charles C Thomas; 1985.

109. Campbell AJ, McCosh L, Reinken J. Drugs taken by a population based sample of subjects 65 years and over in New Zealand. *N Zealand Med J.* 1983;96:378–380.

110. Desai TH, Rajput AH, Desai HB. Use and misuse of drugs in the elderly. *Prog Neuropsychopharmacol Biol Psychiatry.* 1990;14:779–784.

111. Finch J. Prescription drug abuse. *Primary Care.* 1993;20:231–239.

112. Law R, Chalmers C. Medications and elderly people: A general practice survey. *Br Med J.* 1976;1:565–568.

113. Thompson TL, Moran MG, Nies AS. Psychotropic drug use in the elderly: Part I. *N Engl J Med.* 1983;308:134–138.

114. Thompson TL, Moran MG, Nies AS. Psychotropic drug use in the elderly: Part II. *N Engl J Med.* 1983;308:194–199.

115. Williams P. Factors influencing the duration of treatment with psychotropic drugs in general practice: A survival analysis approach. *Psychol Med.* 1983;13:623–633.

116. Rosholm JU, Hansen LJ, Hallas J, Gram LF. Neuroleptic drug utilization in out-patients—A prescription database study. *Br J Clin Pharmacol.* 1993;36:579–583.

117. Takala J, Ryynanen OP, Lehtovirta E, Turakka H. The relationship between mental health and drug use. *Acta Psychiatr Scand.* 1993;88:256–258.

118. Larson EB, Kukull WA, Buchner D, Reifler BV. Adverse drug reactions associated with global cognitive impairment in elderly persons. *Ann Intern Med.* 1987;107:169–173.

119. O'Connor RD. Benzodiazepine dependence—A treatment perspective and an advocacy for control. In: Cooper JR, Czechowicz DJ, Molinari SP, Petersen RC, eds. *Impact of Prescription Drug Diversion Control Systems on Medical Practice and Patient Care.* Rockville, MD: Department of Health and Human Services; 1993:266–269. NIDA Research Monograph 131. DHHS Publication No. 93–3507.

120. Graham K. Identifying and measuring alcohol abuse among the elderly: Serious problems with existing instrumentation. *J Stud Alcohol.* 1986;47:322–326.

121. Ray WA, Griffin MR, Schaffner W, Baugh DK, Melton LJ. Psychotropic drug use and the risk of hip fracture. *N Engl J Med.* 1987;316:363–369.

122. Montamat SC, Cusack B. Overcoming problems with polypharmacy and drug misuse in the elderly. *Clin Geriatr Med.* 1992;8:143–158.

123. Spears R, Drinka PJ, Voeks SK. Obtaining a durable power of attorney for health care from nursing home residents. *J Fam Pract.* 1993;36:409–413.

124. Rubin SM, Strull WM, Fialkow MF, Weiss SJ, Lo B. Increasing completion of the durable power of attorney for health care: A randomized, controlled trial. *JAMA.* 1994; 271:209–212.

125. American College of Physicians. American College of Physicians Ethics Manual. Part 2: The physician and society; research; life-sustaining treatment; other issues. *Ann Intern Med.* 1989;111:327–335.

126. Davidson KW, Hackler C, Caradine DR, et al. Physicians' attitudes on advance directives. *JAMA.* 1989;262:2415–2419.

127. Steinbrook A. Decision making for incompetent patients by designated proxy. *N Engl J Med.* 1984;310:1598–1601.

128. Schneiderman LJ, Arras JD. Counseling patients to counsel physicians on future care in the event of patient incompetence. *Ann Intern Med.* 1985;102:693–698.

129. Buchanan A, Brock DW. Deciding for others. *Milbank Q.* 1986;64(suppl 2):17–94.

130. Danis M, Garrett J, Harris R, Patrick DL. Stability of choices about life-sustaining treatments. *Ann Intern Med.* 1994;120:567–573.

131. Danis M, Southerland LI, Garrett JM, et al. A prospective study of advance directives for life-sustaining care. *N Engl J Med.* 1991;324:882–888.

132. The SUPPORT Principal Investigators. A controlled trial to improve care for seriously ill hospitalized patients: The Study to Understand Prognoses and Preferences for Outcomes and Risks of Treatments (SUPPORT). *JAMA.* 1995;274:1591–1598.

133. Teno J, Lynn J, Wenger N, et al. Advance directives for seriously ill hospitalized patients: Effectiveness with the Patient Self-Determination Act and the SUPPORT intervention. *J Am Geriatr Soc.* 1997;45:500–507.

134. Stone R, Cafferata GL, Sangl J. Caregivers of the frail elderly: A national profile. *Gerontologist.* 1987;27:616–626.

135. George LK, Gwyther LP. Caregiver well-being: A multidimensional examination of family caregivers of demented adults. *Gerontologist.* 1986;26:253–259.

136. Drinka TJK, Smith JC, Drinka PJ. Correlates of depression and burden for informal caregivers of patients in a geriatric referral clinic. *J Am Geriatr Soc.* 1987;35:522–525.

137. Mace NL, Rabins PV. *The 36-Hour Day.* 3rd ed. Baltimore: Johns Hopkins University Press; 1999.

138. Gallagher-Thompson D, DeVries HM. "Coping with frustration" classes: Development and preliminary outcomes with women who care for relatives with dementia. *Gerontologist.* 1994;34:548–552.

139. Brodaty H, Peters KE. Cost effectiveness of a training program for dementia carers. *Int Psychogeriatr.* 1991;3:11–22.

140. Council on Scientific Affairs of the American Medical Association. Physicians and family caregivers: A model for partnership. *JAMA.* 1993;269:1282–1284.

141. Perry JR, Szalai JP, Norris JW. Consensus against both endarterectomy and routine screening for asymptomatic carotid artery stenosis. *Arch Neurol.* 1997;54:25–28.

142. Sauve JS, Laupacis A, Ostbye T, Feagan B, Sackett DL. Does this patient have a clinically important carotid bruit? *JAMA.* 1993;270:2843–2845.

143. Katz S, Branch LG, Branson MH, et al. Active life expectancy. *N Engl J Med.* 1983;309:1218–1224.

11

Assessment in Special Settings: Nursing Home, Home Care, and Hospice

Bruce E. Robinson

This chapter discusses issues of assessments offered in three settings: the nursing home, home care, and hospice. As comprehensive geriatric assessment is required in all of these settings and is discussed thoroughly in other chapters, only aspects of assessment unique to each special environment are discussed here.

ASSESSMENT IN THE NURSING HOME

Assessment of an older person for appropriate placement within the variety of home and institutional options for long-term care is the ideal indication for comprehensive geriatric assessment, and is discussed elsewhere in this book. This section will discuss the special issues relevant to assessment within the nursing home setting.

After a Health Care Financing Administration–sponsored investigation of quality in long-term care, the Institute of Medicine noted, "Providing high quality care requires careful assessment of each resident's functional, medical, mental, and psychosocial status upon admission, and reassessment periodically thereafter . . . ."[1] This investigation set the stage for the incorporation within the Omnibus Budget Reconciliation Act, 1987 (OBRA87) of a provision mandating that all

303

residents of Medicare- or Medicaid-participating facilities undergo comprehensive, multidisciplinary assessments, including the items on a national tool entitled the Minimum Data Set (MDS). Information from quasi-experimental research suggests that since the national implementation of the MDS in 1991 improvements have occurred in care process indicators, functional status, and health conditions, while hospitalization rates have declined.[2] While the contribution of the MDS to the improvements observed is not entirely known, the MDS is likely here to stay both as a mandatory resident evaluation and as a future reimbursement tool for long-term care facilities. MDS version 2.0 is discussed in this chapter.[3]

The MDS consists of a core set of screening, clinical, and functional measures. It is combined with the Resident Assessment Protocols (RAPs) and Utilization Guidelines (the rules for the use of the MDS and RAPs) into the Resident Assessment Instrument (RAI). The RAPs (Exhibit 11–1) are problem-oriented frameworks for organizing MDS information. They aim to identify social, medical, and psychological problems from the many items of the MDS to form the basis for care planning in the nursing home.

In the conceptual model for the RAI, specific diseases or dysfunction identified by the MDS act as "triggers" for the associated RAPs. Exhibit 11–2 provides the assessment domains and the RAPs triggered within specific domains. The actual questions will not be listed or discussed, but represent expert opinion on the best brief measures for the concepts to be assessed. The triggered RAPs then further direct the collection of information useful to developing a care plan for the targeted item, using a RAP Guideline or Key. For illustration purposes, Exhibit 11–3 outlines the RAP Key for RAP 2: Cognitive Loss/Dementia. Any plan for assessment of a nursing home resident should include the use and refinement of the data collected in the MDS.

The MDS is not a substitute for intelligent clinical evaluation. Accuracy of most items was found on only 49% of residents surveyed.[4] Experienced clinicians reviewing the RAP guidelines should quickly recognize the difficulty that any predetermined, structured assessment will have in dealing with the extraordinary complexity and variability of older adults. The MDS can be viewed as a start in acquiring the broad base of clinical information necessary to organize good long-term care. As the data are gathered, the staff of a long-term care facility processes the MDS information, gathers additional data from clinical nursing and other professional assessments, and develops care plans. Completing the assessment process requires that the geriatric clinician help identify the priority targets for additional assessment,

Exhibit 11–1 Resident Assessment Protocols

RAP	Supplemental Assessment
1. Delirium	Medical assessment, attention measure, selected laboratory tests
2. Cognitive loss/ Dementia	Cognitive screen Mini-Mental State Examination, Occupational Therapist (OT), or speech and language pathology (SLP) evaluation, functional staging
3. Visual Function	Optometric or ophthalmologic evaluation
4. Communication	SLP evaluation, audiology referral
5. ADL Functional/ Rehabilitation Potential	Performance-based assessment, physical therapist (PT)/OT/SLP evaluation, physiatric consult
6. Urinary Incontinence/ Indwelling Catheter	Genitourinary physical assessment, incontinence record
7. Psychosocial Well-Being	Social services assessment
8. Mood State	Clinical interview, depression screen, psychiatric or psychological evaluation
9. Behavioral Symptoms	Behavior monitoring record, psychiatric evaluation
10. Activities	Social services assessment
11. Falls	Direct gait assessment, PT/OT evaluation
12. Nutritional Status	Medical assessment, weight chart, dietary consultation
13. Feeding Tubes	SLP, dietary evaluation
14. Dehydration/ Fluid Maintenance	Dietary evaluation, intake and output record, calorie count, laboratory tests
15. Oral/Dental Care	Oral assessment, dental consultation
16. Pressure Ulcers	Braden* scale, enterostomal therapist, OT (positioning)
17. Psychotropic Drug Use	Psychiatric evaluation, psychological assessment
18. Physical Restraints	Medical assessment, OT/PT

*See Exhibit 8–2.

and evaluate them clinically. This clinical evaluation supplements the RAI with additional structured assessments chosen by evidence, experience, and consultations from other disciplines when warranted (see Exhibit 11–1). Many of the special evaluations and therapies require physician's orders to implement.

The targets of the geriatric clinician's initial assessment include an accurate list of all active and relevant past medical problems. An initial functional profile should be obtained, and opportunities for remediation identified. The goals of the care provided, particularly toward survival, function, and discharge, should be determined after careful

Exhibit 11-2 Minimum Data Set (MDS) Data Categories

Data Description	*Triggers RAP No.*
• Identification and background information	
• Cognitive patterns	1, 2, 5, 17*
• Communication/hearing problems	2, 4, 17*
• Vision patterns	3
• Mood and behavior patterns	
1. depression indicators	8
2. behavioral symptoms	1, 9, 11, 17*
• Psychosocial Well-Being	7
• Physical functioning and structural problems	
1. ADLs	5, 16
2. balance	17
3. bedfast	16
• Continence	
1. bowel incontinence	16
2. constipation, impaction	17*
3. urinary, indwelling catheter, briefs	6
• Disease diagnoses	
1. hypotension	17*
2. peripheral vascular disease	16
3. depression	17*
4. cataracts	3
5. glaucoma	3
6. urinary tract infection	14
7. dehydration	14
• Health conditions	
1. weight gain, insufficient fluid, fever, bleeding	14
2. hallucinations, dizziness, syncope, unsteady gait, aspiration	17*
3. falls, hip fracture	11, 17*
• Oral nutritional status	
1. mouth pain	15
2. weight down or change	12
3. poor intake, no taste	12
4. IV therapy	12, 14
5. feeding tube	13, 14
6. altered diet	12
• Oral/dental status	15
• Skin condition	12, 16
• Activity pursuit	10
• Medications	
1. antipsychotic, antianxiety, antidepressant	11,17*
2. diuretic	14
• Special treatment and procedures	
1. trunk restraint	11, 16, 18
2. limb restraint or chair prevents rising	18
• Discharge potential	
• Assessment information	

To trigger 17, one drug and one other 17 item must be present.

Source: Data from J.N. Morris et al., *Long-Term Care Facility Resident Assessment Instrument (RAI) Users Manual*, Briggs Health Care Products, © 1995.

Exhibit 11–3 Outline of RAP Key for RAP 2: Cognitive Loss/Dementia

---

The following factors should be reviewed for relationship to cognitive loss:
• Neurological
  1. mental retardation/developmental disability
  2. delirium
  3. cognitive decline
  4. Alzheimer's disease or other dementia

The following are confounding problems that may suggest reversible causes:
• Mood/behavior
  1. depression or mood decline
  2. behavioral symptoms
  3. anxiety disorder
  4. other psychiatric disorder
• Concurrent medical problems
  1. constipation
  2. diarrhea
  3. fecal impaction
  4. diabetes
  5. hypothyroidism
  6. congestive heart failure
  7. emphysema
  8. urinary tract infection
  9. pain
• Failure to thrive
  1. terminal prognosis
  2. low weight or weight loss
• Functional limitations
  1. ADL impairment or ADL decline
  2. decline in continence
• Sensory impairment
  1. hearing problems
  2. speech unclear
  3. visual problems
• Medications
  1. antipsychotics
  2. anti-anxiety medications
  3. antidepressants
  4. diuretics
• Involvement factors
  1. withdrawal
  2. restraints

Source: Data from J.N. Morris et al., *Long-Term Care Facility Resident Assessment Instrument (RAI) Users Manual,* Briggs Health Care Products, © 1995.

---

assessment by the interdisciplinary team and discussions with the resident and family.

A brief discussion of special elements of the general evaluation of the long-term care resident is warranted. The data available from the MDS should be reviewed. These data serve as a base of information and can suggest directions for useful evaluation. A complete medication list for both over-the-counter and prescription drugs is required, and an output of the evaluation is reasonable justification for each medication to be continued. Evaluation of an older person should include an assessment of functional mobility. Direct evaluation of gait, balance, endurance, and musculoskeletal performance is accomplished in those who can walk by the clinician's asking them to accompany him or her down the hall. Standing blood pressure should be measured. Near visual acuity can be easily tested with a pocket card. Examination of the eyes for cataracts as well as abnormalities of the lids and conjunctivae is simply done. Hearing should be adequate for communication. If the resident has difficulty hearing the clinician during the assessment, the clinician should consider conducting a more detailed evaluation. Oral evaluation is critical since oral and dental problems abound in residents of long-term care and may have an impact on both quality of life and nutrition.

Cardiopulmonary assessment should include estimation of adequacy of air exchange and endurance, when possible. While performing the abdominal examination, the clinician should be alert for the multiple movable masses of fecal stasis, bladder distention, and signs of abdominal aneurysm. During pelvic examination, he or she should routinely check for vaginitis and uterine prolapse. Rectal examinations are important in the detection of constipation and fecal impaction.

Musculoskeletal examination should begin with a brief assessment of the function of the upper extremities by asking the resident to grasp the hands behind the head and lower extremities by examining the gait or by employing manual muscle testing. Range of motion, particularly of the knees and hips, should be routinely assessed in those unable to walk. Disability or deformity evident on screening should be investigated with a full clinical assessment of the involved joint, nerve, and muscle groups.

Neurologic examination includes expanded mental status testing. Residents with reasonable communication skills can be tested for cognitive decline by using traditional cognitive screens, such as the Folstein Mini-Mental State examination. A substantial portion of long-term care residents will "bottom out" on cognitive screens designed for dementia detection. These residents can continue to be followed with observational measures, such as the Functional Assessment Staging scale, that record changes in advanced dementia (see Chapter 4, Functional Assessment). A depression screen is critical. "Are you sad or blue?" or "How are your spirits?" may suffice to detect depression. Detection of depression when dementia is advanced is particularly difficult. A high index of suspicion, sensitivity to depressive implications of behavior changes, and frequent therapeutic trials of low toxicity antidepressants may be the simplest approach. Skilled geropsychiatrists offer added resources in these areas. See Chapter 3, Mental Status Assessment, for more information.

In addition to the usual medical assessment, nursing home residents need more timely and extensive efforts in determining their philosophies toward medical treatments since life-threatening events are inevitable. The prevalence of dementia and depression requires that families must often become involved in these discussions. The most basic question of resuscitation in sudden death is a good place to start. The issue of artificial feedings in the event of loss of ability to orally nourish is a second issue that should always be discussed. The clinician can help by anticipating changes in mental or physical health that are predicted by age and conditions, and by exploring the resident's and the family's wishes for medical intervention. Other more restrictive philosophies that would reject hospitalization and even antibiotics are common in advanced illness. The clinician's goal is to offer information on the natural history of disease and the effectiveness of treatment to families, and listen to their preferences for intervention in current and future states. Thus, the final decisions may reflect both a complete understanding of illness and treatment held by the clinician and the perceptions of value of life states and burdens of interventions held by the resident.

ASSESSMENT IN HOME CARE

More than 10 million Americans currently need some type of care so that they can remain in their own homes or other noninstitutional settings, compared to the roughly 2 million living in nursing homes and chronic care hospitals.[5] The provision of services to functionally impaired, disabled, or ill individuals in the home begins with a comprehensive assessment. The link between assessment and effective home care is so strong that it is difficult to discuss home care process and outcomes without discussing comprehensive assessment in the home. The effectiveness of one is dependent on the other. Individuals requiring home care will generally demonstrate the highest potential for benefit of careful assessment and management when compared to persons in other settings. The problems that limit movement and access to services within the community suggest a high level of need. Despite problems, that they are still successfully living in their homes suggests the potential to benefit from carefully targeted services.

Precise definition of the goals of home care assessment is difficult since home care can be used as a substitute for entry into or retention in long-term care, hospital care, outpatient evaluation, or rehabilitative services. Persons in need of home care demonstrate high prevalence of impairments in multiple domains, a characteristic that makes them good candidates for comprehensive geriatric assessment. The goals of assessment are those generally accepted for comprehensive geriatric assessment: to improve diagnostic accuracy, guide the selection of interventions to restore or preserve health, recommend an optimal environment, predict outcomes, and monitor clinical change.[6] An additional goal is added when Medicare home health services are at issue: to determine eligibility for home health services. Medicare's expenditures for home health care increased from $2.4 billion in 1989 to $17.7 billion in 1996,[7] leading to changes in reimbursement policy that are causing many home nursing providers to leave the field. Medicare funding of home services can be provided only when a physician attests, under the threat of "fine, imprisonment or civil penalty,"[8] such services are permissible under the rules listed in Exhibit 11–4.

Information on the cost-effectiveness of home care services suggests that careful targeting is necessary to achieve a balance between cost and benefit.[9] Unmet needs abound in home care; for every institutionalized older person, there are additional equally disabled individuals living at home, often with little formal medical support. Geriatric assessment of the home care client can do much to improve the targeting of clinical services in the home.

Home medical assessment is useful, with new information gained in areas of behavioral problems, caregiver issues, safety, and medical diagnoses.[10] The structure of one in-home assessment program[11] that demonstrated a 60% reduction in functional disability and institutionalization is shown in Table 11–1. This assessment produced an average of 5.9 self-care recommendations and 5.6 other recommendations per person assessed. At present, such in-home assessment programs are an exception rather than the rule since geriatric clinician home visits remain pitifully underused.[12]

Exhibit 11–4 Medicare Requirements for Provision of Home Health Services

- Home bound
- Intermittent need for one or more of:
  1. skilled nursing care
  2. physical therapy
  3. speech therapy
- Under the care of the certifying physician
- Physician periodic review of care plan

In general, the medical practitioner is able to take advantage of multiple providers who are well compensated in their performance of evaluation in the home. Nurses, social workers, psychologists, physical therapists, occupational therapists, speech therapists, and others are funded by Medicare to perform their specific evaluations. The clinician is required to authorize visits by each of these providers and should ensure that reasonable goals exist to justify the costs of the providers' participation in the care plan. Reasonable supervision of these outside assessments includes a rational examination of the plan developed in light of the patient and his or her problems. The clinician should coordinate the plan with rational clinical and therapeutic expectations. Doing so is made more difficult because these patients are homebound, and physician visits are infrequent.

The MDS for Home Care (MDS-HC) has been through several iterations and is being adopted as a required assessment tool by several states. The MDS-HC is a sophisticated multidimensional assessment, similar to the long-term care MDS, and provides an excellent base from which comprehensive assessments can be developed. It is combined with the Clinical Assessment Protocols (CAPs) to form the RAI Home Care. The CAPs provide general guidelines for further assessment and individualized care planning of triggered problems, just as is found in their long-term care counterparts.

Table 11–1 UCLA In-Home Assessment Program

Domain	Measure
Physical health	History and physical
	Urinalysis
	Fecal occult blood test
	Medication review
	Height/weight
Mental health	Cognitive screen
	Depression screen
Social sources	Social network
	Quality of social support
Environment	Home safety check
	Access to outside
Function	Gait and balance
	Vision and hearing

Source: Data from A. Stuck et al., A Trial of Annual In-Home Comprehensive Geriatric Assessments for Elderly People Living in the Community, *New England Journal of Medicine*, Vol. 333, pp. 1184–1189, © 1995.

The MDS-HC includes measures in the areas listed in Exhibit 11–5. Reliability of the measures is generally excellent (weighted Kappa 0.74).[13] The MDS-HC could do much to expand the database available to providers in home settings.

ASSESSMENT IN HOSPICE CARE

In the United States in 1998, an estimated 564,800 deaths occurred due to cancer.[14] An increase of nearly 20% in the last decade, this number will continue to increase with the aging of the population. Hospice is a palliative and supportive home care system for coordinating the care of these persons at the end of life. Hospice care, provided by a diverse team of professionals, is focused on broad elements of health (ie, physical, mental, social, and spiritual), and offers assistance over long periods of time, compared to other Medicare-funded interventions. The goal of care is to support the quality of life of patient and family, while eventually accepting a comfortable death at the place of residence, be it home or nursing home.

The initial question requiring assessment is that of appropriateness of hospice care, and eligibility for hospice Medicare benefits. Medicare hospice coverage provides supportive care and financial benefits not avail-

---

Exhibit 11–5 Areas Included in the Minimum Data Set for Home Care (MDS-HC)

- Cognitive pattern
- Communication/hearing
- Vision
- Mood/behavior
- Social function
- Informal support
- Physical functioning
- Continence
- Diagnoses
- Health conditions
- Preventive health measures
- Nutrition/hydration
- Dental status
- Skin condition
- Environmental assessment
- Service utilization
- Medications

Source: Data from J.N. Morris et al., Comprehensive Clinical Assessment in Community Setting: Applicability of the MDS-HC, *Journal of the American Geriatric Society*, Vol. 45, pp. 1017–1024, © 1997, Lippincott Williams & Wilkins.

able in other programs. Home care does not have to be "skilled" to allow a variety of supportive services to be funded. No copayments are required, and drugs related to the terminal illness are funded by Medicare. Many other payers offer hospice benefits similar to that of Medicare.

Under the Medicare hospice benefit, "end of life" is defined as a life expectancy of 6 months or less if the terminal disease takes its usual course. The majority of hospice patients have cancer diagnoses, with fairly linear trajectories. While the exact timing of death is difficult to predict, functional status and the symptom constellation of dry mouth, dyspnea, eating problems or anorexia, dysphagia, and weight loss have prognostic value for mortality, regardless of tumor type or metastatic pattern. Exhibit 11–6 gives general criteria for appropriate hospice care.

A number of noncancer diseases have points at which median survival is 6 months or less. These noncancer, chronic progressive diseases, such as cardiopulmonary disease, organ failure, and progressive neurological diseases, are characterized by exacerbations and remissions on a background of a slow downward trajectory. Survival is uncertain at a given point in time and variability is pronounced, compared to cancer survival. Even among the most seriously ill hospitalized patients, prognosis is difficult.

Clinicians often overestimate life expectancy in these diseases, thereby limiting access of needy persons and families to an enhanced program of home support. Terminal patients with far-advanced heart, kidney, liver, lung, and neurologic diseases are eligible for care and constitute an increasing proportion of hospice referrals. The great difficulty in determining prognosis for these diseases has resulted in the development of guidelines for hospice referral (Table 11–2),[15] which are an attempt to develop some consistency within the hospice industry in standards for hospice eligibility. They also seek to resolve tension between the hospice providers and federal regulators, who have re-

---

Exhibit 11–6 National Hospice Organization General Criteria for Hospice Care

- Life-limiting condition, known to client and family
- Selection of treatment goals directed toward relief of symptoms
- Either:
  1. Clinical progression of disease (disease specific, multiple hospitalizations, or functional decline (eg, Karnofsky, ≤50%, dependent in 3 out of 6 ADLs))
  2. Severe nutritional impairment related to the disease (eg, unintended weight loss of >10% over 6 months or albumin <2.5 mg/dl)

Source: Data from B. Stuart et al., *Medical Guidelines for Determining Prognosis in Selected Non-Cancer Disease*, 2nd ed., © 1996, National Hospice Organization.

Table 11–2 National Hospice Organization Guidelines for Prognosis in Chronic Diseases

Condition	Criteria
Heart disease	NYHA IV, EF <20%, refractory to optimal treatment, including vasodilators. Other factors suggesting poor prognosis: symptomatic arrhythmias resistant to antiarrhythmic therapy, history of cardiac arrest, unexplained syncope, cardiogenic brain embolism
Pulmonary disease	Disabling dyspnea, FEVI <30%, frequent emergencies, cor pulmonale, hypoxemia on O_2, hypercapnea, resting tachycardia, unintended weight loss
Dementia	Bed or chair bound, ADL dependent, incontinent, unable to communicate, severe medical comorbidity, nutritional compromise, tube feedings refused or impaired nutrition on tube feedings
Stroke	Acute phase, beyond 3 days: coma, abnormal brain stem response, absent verbal response, absent withdrawal to pain
	Dysphagia precluding nutrition when artificial feedings refused Post stroke dementia, Karnofsky <50%, nutritional compromise Recurrent aspiration pneumonia, urinary infection, sepsis, decubitus ulcers
Renal disease	Meet criteria for transplant or dialysis but refused, CCr <15cc/min, serum creatine >8 mg/dl (6mg/dl for diabetics)
Liver disease	Not considered for transplant, albumin <2.5, prothrombin time >5 sec over control, recurrent variceal bleeding, cachexia, alcohol use At least one of: refractory ascites, SBP, hepatorenal syndrome, hepatic encephalopathy, coma

Note: NYHA IV, New York Heart Association Stage IV; EF, ejection fraction; FEV1, forced expiratory volume in 1s; CCr, creatinine clearance.
Source: Data from B. Stuart et al., *Medical Guidelines for Determining Prognosis in Selected Non-Cancer Disease*, 2nd ed., © 1996, National Hospice Organization.

cently begun to challenge admissions and, in some cases, demand large repayments from hospice organizations for unauthorized care.

The development of a plan of care for a hospice patient requires a comprehensive geriatric assessment. The assessment is generally accomplished by multiple categories of providers: only 33% of hospice staff are skilled nursing personnel, and about 15% are counselors or social workers.[16] Assessment generally includes a spiritual assessment, in addition to the traditional physical, psychological, social, and functional elements. Structured assessments of pain and other symptoms targeted for palliation are recommended.

A cluster of signs and symptoms often precedes death, and indicates, in hospice language, that a person is "actively dying." These are listed in Exhibit 11–7.

Exhibit 11-7 Signs of Impending Death

* Cool, mottled extremities
* Somnolence
* Delirium
* Incontinence
* Decreased appetite and thirst
* Decreased urine output
* Congestion (death rattle)
* Restlessness
* Cheyne–Stokes respiration

CONCLUSION

This chapter has called attention to the special considerations for effective implementation of geriatric assessment in the nursing home, home care, and hospice. Geriatric assessment constitutes an essential component of care when nursing home placement is considered and after admission, to avoid unnecessary functional and cognitive limitations. In home care, geriatric assessment provides the information that can inform clinicians about how to support the older person at home. The domains of geriatric assessment pertain to developing a care plan in hospice care because persons with advanced illness may be at increased risk for uncontrolled pain and other unpleasant symptoms. Older adults in the settings of care discussed in this chapter are particularly vulnerable to functional impairment or other threats to quality of life that might be ameliorated if assessed and treated.

REFERENCES

1. Institute of Medicine. *Improving the Quality of Care in Nursing Homes.* Washington, DC; National Academy Press; 1986:74.

2. Ouslander JG. The Resident Assessment Instrument (RAI): Promise and pitfalls. *J Am Geriatr Soc.* 1997;45:975–976.

3. Morris JN, Murphy K, Nonemaker S. *Long-Term Care Facility Resident Assessment Instrument (RAI) Users Manual.* Des Moines, IO: Briggs Health Care Products; 1995.

4. Hawes C, Mor V, Phillips CD, et al. The OBRA-87 nursing home regulations and implementation of the Resident Assessment Instrument: Effects on process quality. *J Am Geriatr Soc.* 1997;45:975–985.

5. Feasley JC, ed. *Best at Home: Assuring Quality Long-Term Care in Home and Community-Based Settings.* Washington, DC: Institute of Medicine, National Academy Press; 1996.

6. Solomon D. National Institutes of Health Consensus Development Conference Statement: Geriatric assessment methods for clinical decision-making. *J Am Geriatr Soc.* 1988;36:342–347.

7. Scanlon WJ. *Home Health Cost Growth and Administration's Proposal for Prospective Payment.* Washington, DC: US General Accounting Office; 1997. GAO/T-HEHS-97–92.

8. Health Care Financing Administration (form 485). Washington, DC: Dept of Health and Human Services; February 1994: OMB No 0938–0357.

9. Kemper P. The evaluation of the National Long Term Care Demonstration: 10. Overview of the findings. *Health Serv Res.* 1988;23:161–174.

10. Ramsdell JW, Swart JA, Jackson JE, Renvall M. The yield of a home visit in the assessment of geriatric patients. *J Am Geriatr Soc.* 1989;37:17–24.

11. Stuck A, Aronow HU, Steiner A, et al. A trial of annual in-home comprehensive geriatric assessments for elderly people living in the community. *N Engl J Med.* 1995; 333:1184–1189.

12. American Medical Association Council on Scientific Affairs. Educating physicians in home health care. *JAMA.* 1991;265:769–771.

13. Morris JN, Fries BE, Steel K, et al. Comprehensive clinical assessment in community setting: Applicability of the MDS-HC. *J Am Geriatr Soc.* 1997;45:1017–1024.

14. Landis SH, Murray T, Bolden S, Wingo PA. Cancer Statistics. 1998; CA48(1):6–9.

15. Stuart B, Alexander C, Arenella C, et al. *Medical Guidelines for Determining Prognosis in Selected Non-Cancer Disease.* 2nd ed. Arlington, VA: National Hospice Organization; 1996.

16. *Hospice Facts and Statistics.* Washington, DC: Hospice Association of America; 1995.

Geriatric Assessment Program: The University Hospital Geriatric Evaluation Center, Cincinnati, Ohio

Irene Moore and Gregg Warshaw

Older persons and their families are often seriously affected when cognitive impairment, functional decline, financial difficulties, or medical conditions arise. Late life is frequently associated with multisystem medical and psychosocial problems, situations that may particularly benefit from comprehensive assessment.[1] This chapter will present geriatric assessment as a response to the natural threats in aging, both normal and pathological, and will describe The University Hospital Geriatric Evaluation Center (GEC) affiliated with the Health Alliance of Greater Cincinnati and the University of Cincinnati. Geriatric assessment may be implemented as a consultation or as a second opinion with the goal of increasing diagnostic accuracy, improving long-term placement options, consolidating medications, decreasing hospital or nursing home stays, contributing to family proactive planning, and promoting independence for older adults.

GERIATRIC EVALUATION CENTER STRUCTURE

The GEC is located on the campus of Maple Knoll Village (MKV), a nationally accredited, continuing-care retirement community in north Cincinnati. Every aspect of MKV is specifically designed and uniquely

317

suited to meet the needs of older adults. Since 1848, MKV has developed a leading geriatric care reputation. In 1987, The University Hospital, a tertiary care center in cooperation with the University of Cincinnati Department of Family Medicine, initiated the GEC. The GEC is organized as an outreach, ambulatory service of The University Hospital located on the MKV campus.

The success of the University of Cincinnati and MKV affiliation is attributable to a previous strong working relationship. First, the University of Cincinnati College of Nursing and Health and MKV collaborated in 1982, sharing a Robert Wood Johnson Teaching Nursing Home grant, based at the MKV nursing facility. MKV and the college received national recognition for this initiative. Secondly, the MKV medical director, a full-time University of Cincinnati faculty member, is also the GEC medical director. This established working partnership strengthened the MKV endorsement of the innovative approach to affiliate with The University Hospital and to house the GEC.

A formal affiliation agreement exists between The University Hospital and MKV. The agreement includes five key components:

1. There is an established mutual understanding of the GEC design and philosophy.
2. The University Hospital employs and designates staff; MKV maintains the right, however, to dismiss any university employee with sufficient cause.
3. Dedicated space of 800 ft^2 is adapted for the GEC suite.
4. Equipment, laundry, mailing, photocopying, and assistance for efficient center operation are included in a monthly rent.
5. GEC client billing is performed by The University Hospital for technical charges, and by the Department of Family Medicine for professional charges.

Medically, the GEC is largely self-sufficient. The geriatrician draws labs, which are taken by courier to the University laboratory. Physical exams are primarily accomplished by the medical team with minimal nursing assistance.

Promotional strategies, including publicity, advertisement, and a brochure, reinforce MKV and The University Hospital's combined mission of service to older adults. Ancillary services, such as physical therapy and occupational therapy, already established at MKV, are readily available to GEC clients. The GEC maintains responsibility to The University Hospital in preparing budgets. Although the GEC requests only a small budget each year, primarily for partial support of the staff and to cover office rental, the limited revenue generated from client care reimbursement means that the GEC has a difficult time defending its budget to the hospital. The GEC program has an educational and research mission and is a significant asset to the hospital for public relations. The labor intensive efforts combined with the specialized skills necessary to provide optimal assessment for at-risk older adults continue to be undervalued. Unfortunately, insurance payers have yet to appreciate the long-term advantages of multidisciplinary, comprehensive geriatric assessment.[2]

GERIATRIC EVALUATION CENTER PROFILE

The University Hospital and the GEC share three interrelated missions that emphasize clinical care of, education for, and research about older adults and their families.

Clinical Mission

GEC activity emphasizes four interrelated clinical strategies that allow for a unique assessment. These strategies include an interdisciplinary team, a multidimensional evaluation, a family approach, and adequate time and flexibility to discuss assessments and planned treatments with the client and the family.

Core Interdisciplinary Team

No single discipline can meet the multiple needs of geriatric clients and their family members. Every client seen in the GEC meets with a geriatrician and a nurse or a social worker, who serve as the core team members. This core geriatrics team is often supplemented by additional health care professionals in a wide variety of disciplines including psychiatry, pharmacy, physical therapy, and occupational therapy. Such consultations are available as required and specifically designated by the core geriatrics team.

Multidimensional Evaluation

All GEC assessments include a collection of data in the five dimensions of social, economic, psychological, medical, and functional status.

Family-Centered Approach

The GEC emphasizes the involvement of family and other caregivers in the assessment and treatment plans for older adults. The clinical encounter frequently involves independent and simultaneous interviews with family members during the assessment. A large number of cognitively impaired clients are seen at the GEC. Since cognitively impaired clients sometimes cannot provide accurate information, informant interviews are required. An important service of the GEC concerns the education of the client and family about clinical diagnosis and available services.

Adequate Time and Flexibility

To accomplish comprehensive outpatient assessment, 3-hour appointments are scheduled. This extended appointment allows for adequate clinical assessment and time to discuss in-depth assessments and identified problems with the client and the family.

Educational Mission

The GEC is a valuable interdisciplinary educational site. The Ohio Board of Regents mandates that each Ohio medical school provide geriatrics training for its medical students. The GEC serves as a primary teaching setting for third-year family practice clerkship students and fourth-year medical students who choose geriatric medicine as an elective. The University of Cincinnati Department of Family Medicine requires all second-year family practice residents to participate in a month-long geriatric medicine rotation that includes time at the GEC. Geriatric medicine fellows spend a year-long longitudinal care experience in the GEC as part of the requirement for geriatric medicine fellowship accreditation. In addition, graduate students from the University of Cincinnati College of Medicine and the College of Nursing and Health as well as learners from other disciplines and universities may request an elective rotation in the GEC. Several general educational strategies are utilized to ensure positive learning experiences.

Team Integration and Supervision

New learners are oriented to the procedures of the clinic and exposed to all the facets of team function. The trainees work with colleagues from their own disciplines as well as with faculty from other disciplines. When involved with client assessment, the learners are frequently given considerable responsibility for data collection and follow-up. Learners present cases at the team conferences.

Standard Database

Although the clinical approach of the GEC is client-oriented and flexible, with so many learners and part-time providers a standard database and assessment sequence are utilized. Using a standardized assessment protocol is essential for learners as a guide to the assessment process, and ensures that novice providers do not omit important components of the assessment.

Case/Intake Conference

The case/intake conference is a weekly review of the new cases seen at the GEC, and also provides an opportunity to review ongoing cases. For learners the conference is an occasion to ask questions of the multidisciplinary team and to learn about the many additional cases in which they do not directly participate. Complex cases are presented in depth to senior faculty, providing an opportunity for discussion and problem solving.

Research Mission

Part of the outcome of a GEC comprehensive assessment is the gathering of a rich database that contains information about multiple domains of the older person. The database provides an excellent opportunity for research protocols and chart-review analysis. While geriatric clinics are perceived as improving care by providing more specialized evaluation, these services need to be evaluated by criteria similar to those being developed for other types of medical services. Do all clients benefit equally, or do some (eg, those with multiple disabilities) have a greater possibility of an improved outcome? Does such an outpatient service recognize more diagnoses, decrease the number of unnecessary medications, improve the accuracy of diagnoses, or improve the delivery of health care services? Is client care improved by making more diagnoses or by managing existing diagnoses more effectively? How can team function be evaluated, and how should team composition be determined? What are the optimal assessment parameters and instruments to be employed? For example, is the best strategy to use comprehensive assessment instruments for all clients, or is it more productive to use narrow protocols for specific clinical problems such as dementia protocols or incontinence assessment instruments? The future development of specialized outpatient geriatric services will depend on the evaluation of questions such as these. The GEC is an ideal site for research in these areas.

GERIATRIC EVALUATION CENTER

Telephone Referrals

GEC patients are referred from a variety of sources. Generally, a family member contacts the GEC to arrange a diagnostic evaluation due to a medical change or home safety issues. Many calls result from media coverage enhancing public awareness of the GEC's consultation service. Increasingly, despite sensitive territorial issues, primary care providers are referring their patients for a second opinion or consultation. Health maintenance organization limitations create barriers for some older adults who are restricted to using specific hospitals.

The referral criteria for GEC clients are broadly defined. Referred persons are generally community-dwelling Medicare recipients aged 65 years and older. Exceptions occur for mentally retarded/developmentally disabled, middle-aged adults who display symptoms of early aging or Alzheimer's disease, or younger adults with an early diagnosis of Alzheimer's disease. Furthermore, homebound or physically ill older adults may request a GEC home visit or nursing facility consult.

The geriatric assessment begins with the first telephone call requesting an appointment. At that point, the interviewer elicits the main problem, the subjective perception of concerns regarding the older adult. The range of services is reviewed with the caller to be certain the GEC is the appropriate site to address his or her concerns (Exhibit 12–1). During the telephone intake, the interviewer clearly reviews the GEC process and what to expect. The concept of working with a medical and psychosocial team focusing on the whole person is a new and unfamiliar idea for many callers. The necessity of a reliable informant or an identifiable primary caregiver to attend the appointment is emphasized so that maximum benefit may be derived from the assessment.

Preparatory strategies are reviewed with the caller. The family is urged to compose a prioritized list of concerns to guide the appointment and to be sure that specific questions are answered. In particular, many family members express anxiety about disclosing the appointment to a demented or paranoid older adult. Family members are encouraged to maintain a matter of fact and calm manner when discussing the appointment, as any anxious emotion can needlessly agitate and alarm some people. Families are also encouraged to explain

Exhibit 12–1 What Geriatric Assessment Can Offer

- Comprehensive medical/social assessments and diagnostic evaluation
- Special guidance with problems of memory loss
- Assistance with proactive planning
- Assessment of complications caused by multiple medications
- Help with problems of falling
- Social work or nursing counseling
- Telephone information service to identify and locate community services and other resources useful to older adults and their families
- Guidance with long-term living arrangements or in-home or relocation alternatives

---

the appointment as an experience to relieve the family member's mind regarding the older adult's health, medications, and overall well-being, rather than emphasizing the deteriorating condition of the relative. In addition, the family member is encouraged to ask for the support from someone the older person respects, such as his or her primary care provider, priest, or a specific family member. Finally, it is suggested that the family utilize its vantage point of knowing the older adult and capitalizing on strategies to which the older adult may respond favorably, for example, by pointing out that the appointment will be completely covered by insurance.

The GEC interviewer reminds the caller during the telephone intake process that the GEC does not provide primary care. The older adult maintains his or her relationship with a primary care provider, who has the overall responsibility and treatment decision-making authority.

Intake Procedures

Upon confirming the appointment, a letter is sent to the responsible family member as a reminder to bring insurance information, medications, eyeglasses, hearing aids, and a snack. A release of medical information is included requesting that a copy of the client's records be sent to the GEC prior to the appointment. An insurance sheet is also included. The GEC brochure is sent to assist in building confidence in GEC expertise and to reiterate what to expect from the appointment. One week prior to the appointment, a telephone call is made to the family confirming the appointment and notifying the family of the receipt of medical records, or if further follow-up is needed, to obtain requested medical information.

Registration

Upon arrival at the GEC, releases for financial status and treatment are signed by the client or power of attorney to fulfill billing requirements. Family members are encouraged to request a copy of the GEC assessment for their own education and to use in further appointments with other health care providers. The interviewer verifies demographic information and photographs the older adult. The photograph is maintained in the client's chart for future identification. Also, clients are photographed upon follow-up visits looking for comparative changes in their appearance. Exhibit 12–2 provides an outline of an appointment schedule.

The Assessment

Core interdisciplinary team members meet simultaneously with the older adult and with family members. The medical team spends interpretive time correcting misconceptions regarding the etiology of geri-

---

Exhibit 12–2 Geriatric Evaluation Center Appointment Outline

1:30 PM–1:45 PM	• Client/family registers, insurance information is completed, demographics are verified.
	• Core team meets to review records, clarifies chief complaint, and orients and assigns learners to assessment process.
1:45 PM–1:50 PM	• Core team greets patient and family.
1:50 PM–2:50PM	• Medical team meets with family.
	• Psychosocial team meets with client.
2:50 PM–3:05 PM	• Client and family take a break.
	• Teams and learners consult.
3:05 PM–4:00 PM	• Medical team meets with client.
	• Psychosocial team meets with family.
4:00 PM–4:15 PM	• Client and family take a break.
	• Teams and learners consult.
4:15 PM–4:45 PM	• Core team confers with family to review findings and make recommendations.

Exhibit 12–3 Communication Checklist for Interviewing Older Adults

- Establish rapport—smile
- Manner—be calm
- Body position—face older adult
- Setting—use quiet, relaxing setting
- Lighting—avoid darkness and glare
- Hearing—use amplifier headphones if needed
- Voice—speak clearly and in a low tone
- Repetition—repeat the same phrase exactly
- Terms—don't use jargon, be culturally sensitive
- Language barrier—be observant for problems

atric illnesses with the family. A review of the chief complaint, past medical and surgical history, social history including level of education attainment, occupation, exposures to health hazards, family history, and durable power of attorney are reviewed with the family.

Concomitantly, the nurse or social worker meets with the older adult, keeping in mind strategies that facilitate communication with older adults (Exhibit 12–3). Beginning with the older adult's main concerns regarding his or her health and living situation, the interview leads into educational attainment, employment history, social resources, and the individual's plan of care in the event of disabling physical or mental illness. Cognitive and affective screening batteries are administered (Exhibit 12–4).[3–6] Also, the patient's perception of physical and instrumental activities of daily living (ADL) are reviewed. The family genogram and financial status information are begun.

Following the initial one-hour interview by the medical and psychosocial teams, the professionals meet privately to compare notes and review information collected to begin formulation of an initial diagnostic impression. The teams then transpose and the older adult

Exhibit 12–4 Components of the Geriatric Evaluation Center (GEC) Cognitive Testing

- Folstein Mini-Mental State exam[3]
- Word list generation (determines verbal fluency)[4]
- Clock drawing (evaluates constructional ability)[5]
- Paired associate learning[4(p82)]
- Verbal story for immediate recall[5]
- Higher cognitive functions, calculations[4(pp124,125)]
- Geriatric Depression Scale[6]

meets with the medical team for further history and a comprehensive, focused physical and neurologic examination. Simultaneously, the nurse or social worker meets with the family after receiving verbal permission from the identified client to share the interview information. A review of the cognitive screening results with the family members provides objective evidence regarding cognitive abilities. Background information and a brief problem-oriented review of antecedents leading up to the appointment are reviewed. A description of the older adult's premorbid personality is obtained as well as validation of information given by him or her, especially regarding ADL.

The discussion recommending that the family link to community services and resources may be sensitive. Most caregivers believe they will use services as soon as they feel they are needed.[7] Considerations related to legal, financial, and medical planning are essential, but the family members often need time to absorb the diagnosis and results of the evaluation before they can attempt to obtain community resources. Providing families with written take-home information may be one of the most important services practitioners offer.[8]

The construction of the client's genogram may reveal family strengths for additional care or bring to light unpleasant family memories of previous disease and sickness. Preparing a family genogram provides a review of the family system and may reveal potential additional support members. The genogram includes all family members, both living and deceased. In preparing the genogram in partnership with the family members, the health care provider may provide a comfortable forum to discuss difficult topics. A predictor of how the family will react emotionally to caregiving responsibilities is often apparent from its previous response to similar crisis situations. The family genogram, including the family members' geographic locations, may also elicit discussion of alternative ways (eg, financial) family members might contribute to the well-being of the frail relative. Asymmetric responsibilities are commonly encountered. Inequity in shared obligations for caregiving often results in conflict. For example, health care providers commonly hear something similar to, "My brother doesn't do anything for mom, yet he is still her favorite." Listing the alternative ways to be a caregiver and exploring previous family relationships may provide support and direction for the caregiver. An additional appointment specifically for a family conference may result in a better response to issues of longstanding family conflict and a more informed family with regard to coping with the needs of the older relative. Family members are encouraged to maintain a notebook of referral information and contacts. Assisting the family with organizing and interpreting referral information is one of the goals of geriatric assessment (Exhibit 12–5).

Upon completion of the medical examination with the older adult and the psychosocial interview with the family, the clinicians meet privately to develop individualized recommendations to assist with client care strategy planning and to determine what additional tests may be required.

Family Conference

Finally, a conference, attended by the interdisciplinary core team members, family members, and the older adult, is held to review the diagnostic impression and deliver written recommendations. Meeting with the family and client to discuss recommendations in the GEC may increase compliance with those recommendations. The team ensures sustained professional availability. A written preliminary report is given to the family and, with the client's permission, is forwarded to the primary care provider.

Exhibit 12–5 Resource and Referral Information for Older Adults and Family Members

Caregiver support services
Companionship and support services
Driving evaluation programs
Eldercare Locator National Services (anywhere in United States: 1-800-677-1116)
Family support services (counseling)
Financial
   Medicare (1-800-772-1213)
   Social Security benefits (1-800-772-1213)
Health-related agencies/services
   Alzheimer's Association (1-800-442-3322)
   Arthritis Foundation (1-800-283-7800)
   Parkinson's Foundation (1-800-457-6676)
   Foundation for Health in Aging (1-212-421-1513)
Home health care
Housing options
Legal assistance
Medical emergency response services
Primary information and referral agencies
Transportation

Case/Intake Conference

The case/intake conference is a review of the new clients seen over the previous week in the GEC. The case/intake conference also provides a chance to reexamine ongoing cases. At the conference, a decision can be made whether to refer or follow up with persons that have been assessed. Specific recommendations might include, for example, a referral to the Alzheimer's Association or to adult protective services. Some individuals will return for follow-up visits, while most will be contacted via telephone regarding implementation of plans with the family and the primary care provider.

CONCLUSION

The GEC illustrates an ambulatory outpatient service, utilizing an interdisciplinary team approach as a broad-based response to complex geriatric clinical challenges. Because of the location of the GEC on the campus of the MKV, rather than at the hospital, the GEC typifies a model for medical care that is provided as an outreach activity in a community setting.

REFERENCES

1. Rubenstein L. Clinical effectiveness of multidimensional geriatric assessment. *J Am Geriatr Soc.* 1983;31:758.

2. Greganti MA, Hanson LC. Comprehensive geriatric assessment: Where do we go from here? [editorial]. *Arch Intern Med.* 1996;156:16.

3. Folstein MF, Folstein S, McHugh PR. Mini-Mental state: A practical method for grading the cognitive state of patients for the clinician. *J Psychiatr Res.* 1975;12:189–198.

4. Strub RL, Black FW. *The Mental Status Exam in Neurology.* Philadelphia: FA Dan's Co; 1993:51–53.

5. Sutherland P, Hill JL, Mellow AM, et al. Clock drawing in Alzheimer's disease: A novel measure of dementia severity. *J Am Geriatr Soc.* 1989;37:725–729.

6. Yesavage JA, Brink TL, Rose TL, et al. Development and validation of a geriatric depression screening scale: A preliminary report. *J Psychiatr Res.* 1983;17:37–49.

7. Christenson D, Moore I. Intensive case management in Alzheimer's disease home care: An interim report on the Cincinnati (Ohio) Medicare Alzheimer's Project. *J Long-Term Home Health Care.* 1994;13:43–52.

8. Agency for Health Care Policy and Research. *Recognition and Initial Assessment of Alzheimer's Disease and Related Dementias: Clinical Practice Guidelines.* Rockville, MD: US Dept of Health and Human Services, November 1996. AHCPR publication 97–0702:72.

13

Putting Geriatric Assessment into Practice

In this final chapter, two perspectives on practicing multidimensional geriatric assessment will be highlighted: (1) integrating the assessment components into primary health care; and (2) establishing the geriatric assessment program. Before addressing these practical concerns, ethical issues in geriatric assessment will be discussed. Next, a review of the evidence will suggest which components of geriatric assessment programs improve geriatric care and outcomes. The goal is to tie together the various aspects of geriatric assessment in a way that will facilitate the use of geriatric assessment concepts in the clinical care of older adults by physicians, nurses, social workers, and other professionals.

Interdisciplinary geriatric assessment programs or teams are ideal if they are available. Although more of these units continue to be developed, it is not practical to expect that every older person requires a formal assessment by a team. But the usefulness of assessment instruments described in earlier chapters for the primary physician cannot be overemphasized. Indeed, the primary care physician is in the best position to be a case finder, coordinator, and manager for older persons. In the same way, the visiting nurse can use these tools in nursing assessment to help identify the older adult at risk of functional decline, hospitalization, or adverse effects from therapeutic intervention. Other health care professionals such as social workers will value brief mental status examinations and the systematic approach to eliciting values regarding treatment for assessing clients. Geriatric assessment teams may cover more ground than individual practitioners, but even the finest assessment must be linked to services and ongoing monitoring to be useful to the client and to the family. Delineating the appropriate boundaries between practices and teams needs to be worked out, particularly given the current emphasis on managed care.

The use of instruments and questionnaires for systematic clinical observation in medicine is not unprecedented. Assessment forms and instruments are widely used by clinicians who care for children. Examples of clinical instruments are the Apgar score to assess newborn health, the Dubowitz forms for estimation of gestational age, and the Denver Developmental Screening Examination for assessment of developmental milestones. The instruments for assessing multiple domains in the older adult, the "new technology of geriatrics,"[1] can be employed in the same way. The everyday use of computers to record responses from the patient and caregiver may someday facilitate the assessment and reevaluation process.

ETHICAL ISSUES IN GERIATRIC ASSESSMENT

Ethical dilemmas arise in seeking and performing a comprehensive geriatric assessment. Two important ethical principles that should guide clinicians are: (1) beneficence that asserts clinicians have a duty to help others (beneficence includes nonmaleficence, that one ought not inflict harm), and (2) respect for the autonomy of patients (or self-governance, being one's own person, without constraints imposed by another's actions or by psychological or physical limitations).

The General Practice contract in the United Kingdom mandates that the general practitioner offer a home visit (either by the physician or by a member of the primary health care team, such as a nurse clinician) to citizens aged 75 years and older for the purpose of assessing the patient's total health care needs.[2,3] The home visit is viewed as an ideal means to assess health including sensory functions, mobility, mental condition, physical condition including continence, social environment, and use of medicines. Under the contract, the general practitioner is required to discuss the conclusions and recommendations of the assessment, "unless to do so would, in the opinion of the doctor, be likely to cause serious harm to the physical or mental health of the patient."[2]

American clinicians and patients might take the point of view of the older person who may ask, "Who is coming into my home to examine me? Why must I be subjected to intrusion and loss of privacy? What right does this doctor or nurse have to come snooping in my home just because I have reached 75 years of age?" Yet the patient's autonomy is respected because, while the doctor is required to offer the home visit, the patient may decline the offer. British doctors say that beneficence is the overriding reason for this requirement, while autonomy is respected. The doctor shows beneficence and nonmaleficence in judging what knowledge would be likely to seriously harm the physical or mental health of the patient. Although there are ethical concerns, particularly in regard to respecting the British patient's autonomy, there is much that is attractive in guaranteeing that important dimensions are assessed in an older adult's home as part of good medical practice.

Even though what is described above sounds well thought out and even ideal, much thought must be given to the complex dilemmas that sometimes arise, requiring a great deal of wisdom in providing answers. For example, there might be a doctor or geriatrician and a caregiver who both know that a certain patient's problems are very complicated. Hence, the clinician turns to a geriatric assessment program for a more thorough multidimensional assessment. The assessment team concludes that the patient's state is precarious, and that unless certain recommendations are accepted, the team must report the case to governmental protective agencies. Perhaps the clinician has known the patient and the caregiver or family on an intimate basis for the past decade. The recommendations of the team who knows the patient less well may be an anathema to both the clinician and the family. Although the current situation may not be ideal because only the wife is available in case of problems during night hours, the family has managed, and there have thus far been no falls or adverse incidents other than loss of control of bladder in bed. The family is terrified by the recommendation that a nursing home is required, and the family cannot afford additional home health aides. Now the situation has suddenly become a legal one with hard feelings on all sides. Situations like this have occurred in comprehensive geriatric assessments, and the members of the assessment program feel certain of their beneficent actions, not aware of the ways in which their recommendations may cause harm in the long run. In pressing the issue, the team may not respect the patient's or family's autonomy. There are many situations in which there are no perfect solutions, but only compromises. The multidimensional assessment framework at least provides a reminder that recommendations directed at one problem may have adverse consequences on other areas. Additional ethical issues related to the search for unidentified conditions or risk factors were discussed in Chapter 10.

EVIDENCE OF THE EFFECTIVENESS OF GERIATRIC ASSESSMENT

The National Institutes of Health Consensus Statement on Geriatric Methods for Clinical Decision-Making set the stage for stating the goals of assessment.[4] Soon after, another Consensus Conference on Geriatric Assessment sponsored by the Department of Veterans Affairs, the National Institute on Aging, and the Robert Wood Johnson Foundation stressed the need for research on content and efficacy of geriatric evaluation and management interventions, measuring outcomes of care in geriatric evaluation and management units, and targeting criteria for geriatric evaluation and research.[5] In the years that followed, there have been conflicting results from different studies concerning the value of geriatric assessment, who should be involved, and how assessment results should be communicated to primary health care. Reuben and colleagues,[6] working in a managed care setting, found that comprehensive geriatric assessment by a consultative team did not improve the health or survival of hospitalized patients who were selected on the basis of 13 screening criteria. Rubenstein and coworkers[7] found significant reduction in mortality when inpatient consultation services and home assessment services were provided, but no significant effect on survival was found for outpatient geriatric assessment programs. Siu et al[8] did not find significant improvement in outcomes for comprehensive geriatric assessment for frail older patients that was carried out prior to hospital discharge and continued at home.

In contrast, Stuck and associates,[9] in a trial of annual in-home comprehensive geriatric assessments for older adults living in the community, found that such a program of in-home assessments could delay the development of disability and reduce the need for nursing home placements among older persons living at home. Alessi and coworkers[10] demonstrated a continued yield of discovered problems when comprehensive geriatric assessment was repeated on an annual basis for 3 years. Comprehensive geriatric assessment with home-based follow-through by advance practice nurses resulted in better outcomes and fewer recurrent hospitalizations among persons aged 65 years and older.[11]

A meta-analysis on 28 controlled trials demonstrated that geriatric assessment programs with control over medical recommendations and extended ambulatory follow-up were more likely to be effective than consultative programs that only provided feedback of recommendations to physicians.[12,13] In other words, the key elements of programs showing the benefit of comprehensive geriatric assessment were improved communication and the use of additional strategies designed to enhance physician implementation of recommendations and patient adherence.[8,14–22] Collaborative care models of primary health care for chronic medical conditions such as diabetes are an emerging paradigm with a number of features[23]:

1. mutual delineation of problems
2. goal setting and planning in which patients and providers work together on a specific problem and develop an action plan that is compatible with the patient's preferences and values
3. creation of a patient education program in which patients can be taught those skills necessary to take an active role in the treatment or action plan
4. active and ongoing follow-up, in which patients are monitored at specific intervals with regard to health status, possible adverse effects or complications, and as a means of checking on the patient's adherence to the treatment plan and the need for modification of the treatment plan

All of these collaborative efforts are possible. Although practitioners should develop a relationship with a special geriatric assessment program or unit, professionals working individually may arrive at the same recommendations as a multidisciplinary team.[24,25] Geriatric assessment imposes a methodological approach that can be learned and carried out by primary care physicians alone and assisted by trained health professionals such as nurses, nurse practitioners, social workers, and nutritionists. Changes in education at medical schools, residencies, continuing medical education programs, and educational programs for other health professionals will lay the foundation for geriatric assessment to be a standard for primary care physicians and other health professionals.

INTEGRATING GERIATRIC ASSESSMENT INTO PRIMARY CARE

This section concerns incorporating geriatric assessment into clinical practice from the perspective of individual practitioners. Later, the organization of the geriatric assessment team composed of several professionals working together will be discussed. As an adjunct to the clinical examination, use of geriatric assessment tools has the potential to improve the quality of the evaluation of the older person. In a classic early study of the unmet needs of older persons, Williamson and colleagues[26] found many important but unrecognized impairments. Barber and Wallis[27] employed multidimensional assessment forms to enable general practitioners to screen elderly patients for social, functional, and economic difficulties, finding many previously unknown conditions. Pinholt and colleagues[28] showed how using instruments such as the ones discussed in this book improved the evaluation process for older patients. In that study, 79 older persons were assessed with simple measures of cognitive functioning (Cognitive Capacity Screening Examination), nutritional state (history, physical examination, and serum albumin), visual acuity (reading the newspaper), gait (observation), and evaluation of function in activities of daily living (ADL). The assessment was compared with unassisted evaluation. Assuming the assessment instruments are correct, the study's physicians and nurses detected impairment at a low rate: mental impairment, 32%; vision impairment, 33%; nutritional deficiency, 58%; and incontinence, 65%. Miller and coworkers[29] examined 183 medical outpatients aged 70 years and older. While over half of the patients had at least one meaningful impairment in cognitive function (Mini-Mental State Examination), affect (Geriatric Depression Scale), gait (Tinetti test of gait and balance), or nutritional status (serum albumin), few abnormalities had been recognized and addressed by the medical care team.[29] In the United Kingdom, mandated health checks for persons aged 75 years and older, often carried out by the practice nurses, resulted in high rates of previously unrecorded problems.[30] The multidomain framework with standardized evaluation provides useful clinical information that otherwise gets lost in the focus on a particular presenting problem.

Standard use of such instruments would facilitate the development of a common language of assessment, thereby leading to improved communication among professionals caring for older persons. Description of a client by functional ability complements the medical problem list. When a client is reported to have a certain score on a mental status examination, everyone would understand its interpretation. Questions prompting consultation might be more clearly defined, thereby facilitating communication of generalists with specialists. Making observations with standard instruments could lead to a better understanding of the relationships among the mental, affective, functional, social, economic, and physical spheres. Multidimensional assessment can be a tool to appreciate a holistic view that is often espoused, but frequently ignored in actual practice.

Developing the Geriatric Assessment Interview

Several considerations guide the selection of the content, sequence, and format of geriatric assessment in primary care. The domains of multidimensional geriatric assessment wax and wane in importance, depending on the specific situations the older patient and family are grappling with at the time. A major issue in designing the primary care assessment relates to the time that assessments take to perform. No firm estimates for the time to carry out a complete assessment can be given, but the more impaired the older adult, the more time the assessment will take. In ambulatory primary care practice, functional status, mental status, depression, and the use of alcohol and medicines are highly salient to care, and assessment would be facilitated if the needed forms were easily available when the care is provided in the office or other settings. Computers may facilitate information management. When appropriate, assessment can be extended to include more detailed evaluation that might involve referral to a geriatric assessment team. In the case of most of the instruments discussed in this book, minimal clinical training is probably sufficient. In the review of the domains that follow, areas to consider in developing a customized assessment repertoire for primary care practice are highlighted.

The Domains of Geriatric Assessment

When older persons are evaluated and treated, the consequences of each medical problem on each domain of multidimensional assessment should be considered.[31] How will the treatment of a medical condition such as hypertension affect cognitive or functional status? At the same time, what are the implications of the patient's cognitive, functional, or economic status for treatment of medical conditions?

Mental Status

All health care professionals who deal with older adults should make themselves familiar with one short mental status examination. With an attitude that evaluation of cognitive function is a matter of course, the mental status examination will not be offensive to the patient or embarrassing for the examiner. At hospital admission, nursing home admission, within the first few visits of a new patient to the practice, or any time that cognitive status is an issue because of behavior or memory complaints, a clinician should assess mental status. A periodic evaluation among the oldest of patients may be warranted in order to detect early signals of medication side effects or medical problems. Clinicians should remember that patients with a diagnosis of Alzheimer's disease or other dementia may improve if a coexisting depression or delirium is treated.

Older persons have significant developmental work to do, especially in dealing with loss. Although health care professionals are unable to solve all the problems of older persons, good listening skills can be used to advantage in helping older persons come to terms with feelings like helplessness. Depression is often a treatable cause of disability. Because of physiologic changes with age, older persons may be particularly vulnerable to the adverse effects of excessive use of alcohol or other substances, including medications.

Functional Assessment

Functional assessment helps set priorities around which the medical, social, and economic resources available for problem solving can be rallied. Functional assessment also helps maintain a perspective not considered in a traditional diagnosis-centered approach. Functional assessment is central to understanding how the older person may remain independent. Changes in function signal a problem whose source should be addressed and whose solution may be found not in a medically remedial condition but rather with a realignment of the social situation. It may be most useful to ask ambulatory older patients about their driving habits and instrumental ADL, while for patients in assisted living facilities or in nursing homes, the focus should be on the more basic ADL.

Social Assessment

Is the older person engaged in any social activity, whether with family, friends, faith community, or senior citizen organizations? Does the older adult leave home to enjoy coffee with a friend, attend a church service, or participate in a senior citizen center? Who visits the patient—family members, meals-on-wheels, neighbors, or visiting home nurses? For those with disability, most long-term care is provided by the family. Regardless of the mental, functional, and physical status of the patient, the need for nursing home placement may hinge on the availability of willing and capable caregivers. Access to health care for the older person may depend on transportation provided by a caregiver. The caregiver should be involved when recommendations are developed for the older client. Dementia may be associated with behavioral or psychiatric symptoms that are difficult to deal with and will require the emotional and instrumental support of the caregiver.

The domains of geriatric assessment may usefully be applied to evaluating the ability of the caregiver to provide support.

Values Assessment

The treatment plan must consider the goals of autonomy, informed consent, and quality of life. Clinicians are in a position to help the client and family clarify the ethical dilemmas that face them in health care decision making. The Values History can assist the practitioner in this process. If the older adult is impaired in decision-making capacity, it is best to discuss treatment issues with the family in advance of a crisis.

Physical Assessment

Older persons take longer to examine than younger patients. The increased amount of time in disrobing and getting dressed, problems of hearing impairment and unstable gait, and the propensity of some older persons to be garrulous and not focused in conversation may lead to shortcuts in physical examination. Effective geriatric care requires that the physician expend more effort than with most adult patients. The presenting symptom may involve the most poorly compensated organ system, so that pneumonia or congestive heart failure presents as delirium. Issues like sexual functioning, urinary incontinence, and nutritional problems may not be brought directly to the physician's attention, further confusing the diagnostic picture.

Health Promotion and Disease Prevention

Preventive strategies may be divided into standard disease prevention and geriatric-oriented prevention; both should be considered in formulating a plan for prevention. Preventive medicine strategies have to be tailored to the individual older adult, taking into account the local conditions of practice as well as the functional and cognitive status of the patient. Practice should also be informed by the evidence-based guidelines and recommendations that are available. Physicians must decide which protocols are most salient for the older persons in their practice since general recommendations may not account for local circumstances.

Computers in Geriatric Assessment

Computer technology promises the possibility of an effective, efficient, and standardized means of assessing an older patient's status on a visit-by-visit basis as well as detecting changes. The practical limitations of information handling without using computers makes noncomputer approaches unwieldy and slow, as well as limits the quality of the information. Computers can provide standardized presentation, rapid processing of responses, maximum test reliability, and minimum data errors.[32] Longitudinal assessments are of great value in monitoring various populations for health problems—for instance, those due to dementia, depression, chronic illness, or negative drug interactions. For such a system to be used in a significant portion of general medical settings, it must be relatively inexpensive, easily implemented, user friendly, reliable, and deemed as providing valid information by clinicians.

Computer-based assessment has been employed in clinical settings[33-45] and appears to be acceptable to patients.[46-48] Individuals over the age of 65 years appear to be receptive to the use of computer technology.[49,50] Older adults with previous experience with computers have more favorable attitudes toward computers,[51] and prior experience should be considered in evaluating response to the use of computer technology by older adults. Although older adults with sensory or motor impairments may find computers more difficult to use, software and hardware can be adapted to facilitate the interaction with the computer, compensating, for example, for hearing loss or impaired vision with louder or larger stimuli. Anticipating the needs of older adults can be expected to increase willingness to use computers.[52,53] In any case, future cohorts of older adults will have had more exposure to computers than have prior generations and should be comfortable with them.

The computer assists the practitioner not only by reminding him or her and the patient of the need for a screening mammogram or an influenza vaccine, but also by helping the practitioner perform the comprehensive geriatric assessment across all the relevant domains. Perhaps in the 21st century, the patient will interact visually or vocally with a computer in English, Spanish, Vietnamese, or German at different levels of literacy. The end result may be a more efficient, effective, and useful geriatric assessment.

Reimbursement

In this section, some issues related to reimbursement for geriatric assessment activities that apply to individual practitioners and teams will be discussed. Some institutions bill separately for components of the geriatric assessment (eg, the comprehensive history and physical examination, the nursing examination, the physical therapy assessment, and the nutritional assessment). Physicians and institutions will have to carefully follow the results of billing for prolonged evaluation and management services. There are now codes for prolonged services (99354–99357). These services involve direct (face-to-face) physician/patient contact that is beyond the usual in either the inpatient or outpatient setting, which may be appropriate for many aspects of geriatric assessment. Codes 99358 and 99359 are for prolonged physician service without direct (face-to-face) patient contact. In Current Procedural Terminology (CPT™), Modifier 21 can be applied to indicate the highest level in a given category of service, when the criteria for prolonged service is not met. In the changing health system, the professional will have to follow what reimbursements are made for the prolonged and comprehensive efforts of complicated geriatric assessment. On a positive note, codes for prolonged services did not exist at the time of previous editions of this book.

Reimbursement for geriatric assessment in primary care practice will change with new fee codes that will be granted for clinical effort that exceeds what has been traditional office or clinic care. The assessment is already mandated in the long-term care setting.[54] In the meantime, components of the assessment can be carried out over a period of outpatient visits scheduled one or two weeks apart. Using the assessment instruments described in this book may ensure completeness. When a problem is detected by thorough assessment, it can then be explored in greater detail. Nurses and other staff can capably complete parts of the evaluation.[31]

ORGANIZATION OF GERIATRIC ASSESSMENT PROGRAMS

The purpose of this section is to discuss organizing geriatric assessment teams, using selection criteria to identify older adults who may benefit most from geriatric assessment, establishing the geriatric assessment program, reporting results of assessment, and expanding services around a geriatric assessment program. A model geriatric assessment program, the Geriatric Assessment Program of the University Hospital Geriatric Evaluation Center of the University of Cincinnati Medical Center in Cincinnati, Ohio, was described in Chapter 12. The five essential components of a model program are:

1. the targeting of high-risk patients for geriatric assessment
2. a collaborative and interdisciplinary process
3. a patient-centered focus of evaluation and care
4. implementation of diagnostic and care plans through empowerment of primary care providers

5. active participation in the management and coordination of treatment and services along a continuum of care over time and place

Geriatric assessment programs have been described with different purposes, criteria for admission, referral patterns, organization of team members, and location. Goals of assessment may include, for example, comprehensive evaluation, appropriate placement, rehabilitation, education, or research. Sometimes evaluation in a geriatric assessment unit is required prior to nursing home placement to determine whether some less intensive care would be more appropriate. Evaluations often are performed on an elective basis to link patients to the proper community resources.

Geriatric assessment programs vary in organization and staff, partly reflecting the purposes and goals of the program. For example, a team organized for the evaluation of dementia might be primarily oriented to neurology or psychiatry. Most assessment teams have a core team of a physician, nurse, and social worker, especially when outpatient-based. Specialists may participate in the assessment process routinely or may be used on a consultative basis. Professional support such as occupational therapy, physical therapy, or audiology may also be routine for all patients or may be consulted as deemed appropriate by the core evaluation team. The use of specialists routinely for all patients can be expensive and inefficient, and a smaller team can probably evaluate most problems adequately.[55-57]

The roles of team members in the multidisciplinary approach to geriatric assessment vary, but typically, the physician performs a history and physical examination, evaluates mental status and mood, orders the appropriate tests, and communicates with other health care professionals. Within the multidisciplinary team format, the nurse evaluates functional ability, nutrition, and use of free time and usually is the professional who performs the home visit when this is part of the assessment. Social workers explore family dynamics, examine financial and living arrangements, may be the professionals who make the home visit, and act as liaison for the team between the client and various support agencies. Other professionals (eg, dietitians, occupational therapists, physical therapists, dentists, and medical and surgical subspecialists) may be part of the core team or may be used in a consultative capacity.

Inpatient units follow a similar arrangement except that often rehabilitation is stressed rather than overall evaluation or assessment for placement. Gerontologic nurse specialists (ie, gerontologic clinical nurse specialists and gerontologic nurse practitioners) are trained to perform a complete health assessment, including the assessment of functional status. Nurse specialists may perform broadly defined tasks, which cross interdisciplinary boundaries when other professionals are unavailable. For example, a nurse specialist may be called on to determine the need and eligibility for support services and benefits. Nutrition assessment and counseling may be performed by a gerontologic nurse or nutritionist specialist. In some practice settings, the nurse may need to make decisions about medical diagnosis and treatment. Indeed, nurses often assume the role of case manager, by performing the assessment, establishing a working nursing diagnosis, providing appropriate nursing care, and seeing to the patient's medical and social needs. A survey of geriatric assessment teams showed that 75% followed a standard protocol and 65% employed printed forms; 75% of the outpatient teams surveyed used published instruments such as the ones found in this book.[1]

Selection Criteria

Selection criteria for acceptance into a geriatric assessment program vary, and over the past decade, there has been much research effort to define such criteria.[58] If certain patients are excluded because there is no predicted benefit from comprehensive assessment, might health care professionals be denying help to some patients and encouraging a self-fulfilling prophecy? Criteria for exclusion from comprehensive geriatric assessment have included documented disorders indicating imminent death (eg, malignancy or end-stage congestive heart failure), long-standing psychotic disorders, well-evaluated irreversible dementia progressed to a degree that the patient can perform no more than three ADL, and long-term nursing home patients.[59,60] Criteria of inclusion have involved requirements that at least one family member or surrogate be willing to participate with the patient in the program, that nursing home placement is contemplated, functional impairment is present, the patient is clinically stable, and a personal physician is available.[61] Screening questionnaires for stratification of older persons according to risk of hospitalization have been designed and tested in managed care populations in order to direct more intensive efforts at assessment and treatment.[62,63]

Establishing the Geriatric Assessment Program

One of the first questions to be answered in establishing a geriatric assessment team is the composition of the core team. In part, this depends on the primary function of the team. If the objective is rehabilitation, for example, occupational therapists and physical therapists may form a regular part of the team. If diagnosis is the major goal, the team may be set up differently. Each institution must decide what resources are available and what it can offer. A geriatric assessment program might ideally use a team of physician, nurse, and social worker and may include a home visit, but the standard protocol may have to be modified in some circumstances. Sometimes the assessment will be carried out by the physician as well as a nurse or social worker and only one of the professional staff will perform the home visit, or, in certain instances, the home visit will be skipped. An institution may vary its protocol within certain standards, based on the resources that are generally available as well as taking into account day-to-day variations in staffing.

Referral to geriatric assessment programs may originate from families who are concerned about their older family members, seeking advice on such issues as alternatives to institutional care, decisions about placement in a nursing home, or polypharmacy. In many cases, families are seeking a second opinion. The staff person receiving the first phone contact will discover that not every family is seeking a geriatric assessment but may be searching for a primary care physician to take charge of an older family member's care. The geriatric assessment program should work hand in hand with some other type of primary care resource. A geriatric assessment program might work with a family health center, outpatient medical clinic, a geriatric clinic, or selected family physicians or internists.

The examining physician must spend ample time with the patient, listening and observing and providing warmth, sensitivity, and concern. It is helpful to give the family ample time alone with the physician or nurse or social worker, or some combination, to discuss the family's concerns in the absence of the client. The practitioner must be aware of the conflict that sometimes develops between the patient's autonomy and the beneficence of the family. Discussions with family members or caregivers must not be allowed to interfere with the autonomy of the competent older adult.

A home visit can be invaluable. The home visit yields important insights into the patient's situation and interaction with family members. The team can get quite a different impression of the situation and of the therapeutic possibilities when a demented patient is seen in his or her own home, surrounded by concerned family members, telling of children whose pictures are over the mantel, compared with the demented elderly person living in an apartment alone. How well the patient manages with ADL, that is, functional status, may be directly evaluated. Home visits are rewarding because rapport is established with both patient and family members when the team meets them in a familiar environment. The team who has evaluated the patient at home is also better informed when prescribing home health services and when dealing with service agencies. Visiting older persons in their homes is a superb learning experience for trainees as well.

Not every geriatric assessment program may be able to provide home visits. Although the home visit enhances and facilitates the process of geriatric assessment, it may not always be practical or feasible. A program that does not routinely provide home visits might carry out a home visit as the only means of answering specific questions that are raised in the office evaluation. The principal concern may be related to architecture or safety. For example, in the case of an older woman with osteoarthritis, the chief issue may be giving up her home because of the lack of a bathroom on the downstairs level. A home visit may provide the solution of building a bathroom on that level.

In a typical outpatient evaluation, any consultations required are arranged, radiographic tests ordered, and laboratory investigations obtained at the initial meeting. Following the evaluation, the team members meet to discuss the information gathered. Once all these results are compiled, recommendations are made to the patient and family at a summary meeting. A letter summarizing findings is sent to the patient's primary care physician if one has been identified by the patient or caregiver.

Formal consultative agreements with a neurologist, psychiatrist, urologist, physical medicine and rehabilitation specialist, cardiologist, and other specialists will assist in obtaining consultations rapidly. Other professionals also have key roles, such as nutritionists, either as part of the core team or as readily available consultants. Occasionally, the team may have to wait three to four weeks for a consultation. Frequently, however, families or, indeed, the patient's circumstances demand a rapid disposition or decision, so having to wait is an undesirable situation.

It is imperative that the geriatric assessment team maintain good ties with community physicians by sending the patient back to the referring physician. Some patients do not have a physician, and many are able to be followed in a collaborative fashion with the primary care physician. Since many patients are referred for evaluation by social agencies, early contact and familiarization with the professionals and services available in the community are important for smooth interactions across disciplines.

Reporting the Results and Recommendations of Geriatric Assessment

To increase effectiveness, the results of assessment need to be tied to services. Clear reporting of assessment findings should facilitate communication with primary care physicians, and an outline is provided in Exhibit 13–1. In addition to the topic areas of the report keyed to the domains of multidimensional geriatric assessment, the report

Exhibit 13–1 Report Outline for Geriatric Assessment

- Reason for current evaluation
  - who made the contact
  - stated reason for contact
  - where the patient has been seen previously
- Medical history
  - current symptom presentation
  - when symptoms were first noted
  - pace of progression and change of symptoms
  - resolved and ongoing medical conditions and treatments
  - health promotion and disease prevention activities (eg, Pap smear)
- Functional status
  - activities of daily living
  - instrumental activities of daily living
  - driving status, including adaptations to driving
  - summary of functional status and unmet need for care
- Social assessment
  - caregiver description
  - list of the major caregivers
  - expressed caregiver burden
  - social support available to caregivers
  - family income and its perceived adequacy
  - living environment and arrangements
- Current health status
  - nutritional risk
  - health behaviors
  - tobacco use
  - alcohol consumption
  - exercise
- Current psychiatric status
  - depression
  - cognitive impairment
- Preferences for care in the event of serious illness
- Summary statement
- Care plan

should conclude with a summary statement and a care plan. The summary statement should highlight the most pressing issues. To increase effectiveness, the summary statement should have a format of a single paragraph with a set of bullets that allows the reader to grasp the critical clinical issues of the care plan. The care plan should parallel the summary statement, with suggestions for dealing with each bulleted point. The care plan should be specific about who will provide a recommended service (eg, an agency or family members), how often it will be provided, how long it will be provided, and what financing arrangements will pay for it.

Expanding Services around Geriatric Assessment

A geriatric assessment program can be the focal point for an entire range of services devoted to geriatrics and long-term care as components of a hospital or health care system. The geriatric assessment team can serve as a starting point for developing an umbrella for many programs on aging, such as a center or an interdisciplinary program. An institution might develop many services around the centerpiece of a geriatric assessment program (Exhibit 13–2). The geriatric assessment program can be an initial demonstration of institutional commitment. Then, the institution would create services that the patients need, while working closely with the agencies or persons already providing services in the community. As managed care organizations, hospitals, and other health care groups coalesce through corporate merger or reorganization, professional teams that perform comprehensive geriatric assessment will serve not just a few clinical practices or hospitals, but larger integrated systems. For example, if five hospitals are part of a health system, one assessment team might be available to serve three to five of the participating hospitals.

CONCLUSION

Since the first edition of this book was published in 1988, there has been significant progress and growing interest in the technology of geriatric assessment. It is hoped that geriatric assessment will become not only a specialized area of knowledge and skill, but an area of competency that will be the professional and community standard for all primary care physicians and other health care professionals who care for older persons.

Exhibit 13–2 Services for Which the Geriatric Assessment Program May Be a Centerpiece

 1. Respite care
 2. Homemaker services
 3. Caretakers' support group
 4. Caretakers' educational program
 5. Information and referral hot line
 6. Transportation services
 7. Geriatric day care
 8. Widows' or widowers' support group
 9. Inpatient geriatric assessment team
10. Geriatric assessment inpatient unit
11. Osteoporosis clinic
12. Retirement and insurance counseling
13. Legal and financial services for older persons
14. Educational programs and lectures for older persons
15. Alzheimer's disease assessment and treatment program
16. Intermediate care facilities
17. Skilled nursing facilities
18. Alzheimer's disease day care
19. Case management program
20. Upgraded rehabilitation including inpatient services
21. Newsletter for older persons
22. Hospice
23. Retirement center and life care facilities
24. Satellite geriatric primary care clinics
25. Geriatric psychiatric unit
26. Travel services for older persons
27. Seniors' membership plan

Multidimensional assessment of the older person is a challenging clinical task. Geriatric medicine melds the art and science of medicine because ethical and judgment issues frequently accompany treatment issues. There may be a time when benign neglect is appropriate (the principle of minimal interference[64]). In other situations, the clinician should go all out regardless of age. Considerable wisdom and clinical experience are needed to weigh the multidimensional factors that go into such decisions. Practitioners who can assess the physical, mental, social, economic, and ethical issues affecting the well-being of the older person can be more effective, more realistic, and, it is hoped, wiser, in evaluating and managing care of older adults.

REFERENCES

1. Epstein AM, Hall JA, Besdine R, et al. The emergence of geriatric assessment units: The "new technology of geriatrics." *Ann Intern Med.* 1987;106:299–303.

2. Fowler G, Gray M, Anderson P. *Prevention in General Practice.* Oxford, England: Oxford University Press; 1993.

3. Iliffe S, Patterson L, Gould MM. *Health Care for Older People.* London, England: BMJ Books; 1998.

4. National Institutes of Health Consensus Development Conference. National Institutes of Health Consensus Development Conference Statement: Geriatric assessment methods for clinical decision-making. *J Am Geriatr Soc.* 1988;36:342–347.

5. Dego R, Applegate WB, Kramer A, Meehan S. Report of a consensus conference on geriatric assessment. *J Am Geriatr Soc.* 1991;39:1S-59S.

6. Reuben DB, Borok GM, Wolde-Tsadik G. A randomized clinical trial of comprehensive geriatric assessment in the care of hospitalized patients. *N Engl J Med.* 1995; 332:1345–1350.

7. Rubenstein LZ, Stuck AE, Siu AL, Wieland D. Impacts of geriatric evaluation and management programs on defined outcomes: Overview of the evidence. *J Am Geriatr Soc.* 1991;39:8–16.

8. Siu AL, Kravitz RL, Keeler E, et al. Postdischarge geriatric assessment of hospitalized frail elderly patients. *Arch Intern Med.* 1996;156:76–81.

9. Stuck AE, Aronow HU, Steiner A, et al. A trial of annual in-home comprehensive geriatric assessments for elderly people living in the community. *N Engl J Med.* 1995; 333:1184–1189.

10. Alessi CA, Stuck AE, Aronow HU, et al. The process of care in preventive in-home comprehensive geriatric assessment. *J Am Geriatr Soc.* 1997;45:1044–1050.

11. Naylor MD, Brooten D, Campbell R, et al. Comprehensive discharge planning and home follow-up of hospitalized elders: A randomized clinical trial. *JAMA.* 1999;281: 613–620.

12. Stuck AE, Siu AL, Wieland GD, Adams J, Rubenstein LZ. Comprehensive geriatric assessment: A meta-analysis of controlled trials. *Lancet.* 1993;342:1032–1036.

13. Stuck AE, Wieland D, Rubenstein LZ, Siu AL, Adams J. Comprehensive geriatric assessment: Meta-analysis of main effects and elements enhancing effectiveness. In: Rubenstein LZ, Wieland D, Bernabei R, eds. *Geriatric Assessment Technology: The State of the Art.* Milan, Italy: Editrice Kurtis; 1995:11–26.

14. Shah PN, Maly RC, Frank JC, Hirsch SH, Reuben DB. Managing geriatric syndromes: What geriatric assessment teams recommend, what primary care physicians implement, what patients adhere to. *J Am Geriatr Soc.* 1997;45:413–419.

15. Maly RC, Abrahamse AF, Hirsch SH, Frank JC, Reuben DB. What influences physician practice behavior? An interview study of physicians who received consultative geriatric assessment recommendations. *Arch Fam Med.* 1996;5:448–454.

16. Reuben DB, Frank JC, Hirsch SH, McGuigan KA, Maly RC. A randomized clinical trial of outpatient comprehensive geriatric assessment coupled with an intervention to increase adherence to recommendations. *J Am Geriatr Soc.* 1999;47:269–276.

17. Bula CJ, Alessi CA, Aronow HU, et al. Community physicians' cooperation with a program of in-home comprehensive geriatric assessment. *J Am Geriatr Soc.* 1995;43: 1016–1020.

18. Boult C, Boult L, Murphy C, Ebbitt B, Luptak M, Kane RL. A controlled trial of out-patient geriatric evaluation and management. *J Am Geriatr Soc.* 1994;42:465–470.

19. Boult C, Boult L, Morishita L, Smith SL, Kane RL. Outpatient geriatric evaluation and management. *J Am Geriatr Soc.* 1998;46:296–302.

20. Silverman M, Musa D, Martin DC, Lave JR, Adams J, Ricci EM. Evaluation of out-patient geriatric assessment: A randomized multi-site trial. *J Am Geriatr Soc.* 1995;43:733–740.

21. Valenstein M, Kales H, Mellow A, et al. Psychiatric diagnosis and intervention in older and younger patients in a primary care clinic: Effect of a screening and diagnostic instrument. *J Am Geriatr Soc.* 1998;46:1499–1505.

22. Maly RC, Hirsch SH, Reuben DB. The performance of simple instruments in de-tecting geriatric conditions and selecting community-dwelling older people for geriatric assessment. *Age Ageing.* 1997;26:223–231.

23. Von Korff M, Gruman J, Schaefer J, Curry SJ, Wagner EH. Collaborative manage-ment of chronic illness. *Ann Intern Med.* 1997;127:1097–1102.

24. Lachs MS, Feinstein AR, Cooney LM, et al. A simple procedure for general screen-ing for functional disability in elderly persons. *Ann Intern Med.* 1990;112:699–706.

25. Applegate WB. Use of assessment instruments in clinical settings. *J Am Geriatr Soc.* 1987;35:45–50.

26. Williamson J, Stokoe IH, Gray S, et al. Old people at home: Their unreported needs. *Lancet.* 1964;1:1117–1120.

27. Barber JH, Wallis JB. Assessment of the elderly in general practice. *J Royal College Gen Pract.* 1976;26:106–114.

28. Pinholt EM, Kroenke K, Hanley JF, et al. Functional assessment of the elderly: A comparison of standard instruments with clinical judgement. *Arch Intern Med.* 1987;147:484–488.

29. Miller DK, Morley JE, Rubenstein LZ, Pietruszka FM, Strome LS. Formal geriatric as-sessment instruments and the care of older general medical outpatients. *J Am Geriatr Soc.* 1990;38:645–651.

30. Brown K, Williams EI, Groom L. Health checks on patients aged 75 years and over in Nottinghamshire after the new GP contract. *Br Med J.* 1992;305:19–21.

31. Levy SM. Multidimensional assessment of the older patient. In: Gallo JJ, Busby-Whitehead J, Rabins PV, Silliman R, Murphy J, eds. *Reichel's Care of the Elderly: Clinical Aspects of Aging.* 5th ed. Baltimore: Lippincott Williams & Wilkins; 1999:20–38.

32. Kennedy RS, Baltzley DR, Wilkes RL, Kuntz LA. Psychology of computer use: IX. A menu of self-administered microcomputer-based neurotoxicology tests. *Percept Motor Skills.* 1989;68:1255–1272.

33. Steer RA, Rissmiller DJ, Ranieri WF, Beck AT. Dimensions of suicidal ideation in psychiatric inpatients. *Behav Res Ther.* 1993;31:229–236.

34. Mathisen KS, Evans FJ, Meyers K. Evaluation of a computerized version of the Diagnostic Interview Schedule. *Hosp Community Psychiatry.* 1987;38:1311–1315.

35. Greist JH, Klein MH, Erdman HP, et al. Comparison of computer- and interviewer-administered versions of the Diagnostic Interview Schedule. *Hosp Community Psychiatry.* 1987;38:1304–1311.

36. Adang RP, Vismans FJ, Ambergen AW, Talmon JL, Hasman A, Flendrig JA. Evalua-tion of computerised questionnaires designed for patients referred for gastrointestinal endoscopy. *Int J Biomed Comput.* 1991;29:31–44.

37. Erdman HP, Greist JH, Gustafson DH, Taves JE, Klein MH. Suicide risk prediction by computer interview: a prospective study. *J Clin Psychiatry.* 1987;48:464–467.

38. Allen CC, Ellinwood E Jr., Logue PE. Construct validity of a new computer-assisted cognitive neuromotor assessment battery in normal and inpatient psychiatric samples. *J Clin Psychol.* 1993;49:874–882.

39. Spinhoven P, Labbe MR, Rombouts R. Feasibility of computerized psychological testing with psychiatric outpatients. *J Clin Psychol.* 1993;49:440–447.

40. Farrell AD, Camplair PS, McCullough L. Identification of target complaints by computer interview: Evaluation of the computerized assessment system for psychotherapy evaluation and research. *J Consult Clin Psychol.* 1987;55:691–700.

41. Steer RA, Rissmiller DJ, Ranieri WF, Beck AT. Structure of the computer-assisted Beck Anxiety Inventory with psychiatric inpatients. *J Pers Assess.* 1993;60:532–542.

42. Erdman HP, Klein MH, Greist JH, et al. A comparison of two computer-administered versions of the NIMH Diagnostic Interview Schedule. *J Psychiatr Res.* 1992;26: 85–95.

43. Bucholz KK, Robins LN, Shayka JJ, et al. Performance of two forms of a computer psychiatric screening interview: Version I of the DISSI. *J Psychiatr Res.* 1991;25:117–129.

44. Roizen MF, Coalson D, Hayward RS, et al. Can patients use an automated questionnaire to define their current health status? *Med Care.* 1992;30:MS74–MS84.

45. Blouin AG, Perez EL, Blouin JH. Computerized administration of the Diagnostic Interview Schedule. *Psychiatry Res.* 1988;23:335–344.

46. French CC, Beaumont JG. The reaction of psychiatric patients to computerized assessment. *Br J Clin Psychol.* 1987;26:267–278.

47. Clayer JR, McFarlane AC, Wright G. Epidemiology by computer. *Soc Psychiatry Psychiatr Epidemiol.* 1992;27:258–262.

48. Anonymous. Blood donors more likely to reveal HIV risks to computer. *Del Med J.* 1992;64:649.

49. Ansley J, Erber JT. Computer interaction: Effect on attitudes and performance in older adults. *Educ Gerontol.* 1988;14:107–119.

50. Ryan EB, Szechtman B, Bodkin J. Attitudes toward younger and older adults learning to use computers. *J Gerontol.* 1992;47:P96–101.

51. Kerschner PA, Hart KC. The aged user and technology. In: Dunkle RE, Haug MR, Rosenberg M, eds. *Communication Technology and the Elderly.* New York: Springer Publishing Co; 1984:135–144.

52. Hoot JL, Hayslip B. Microcomputers and the elderly: New directions for self-sufficiency and life-long learning. *Educ Gerontol.* 1983;9:493–499.

53. Hartley AA, Hartley JT, Johnson SA. The older adult as a computer user. In: Robinson PK, Livingston J, Birren JE, eds. *Aging and Technology Advances.* New York: Plenum Press; 1984:347–348.

54. Levenson SA. *Medical Direction in Long-Term Care.* 2nd ed. Durham, NC: Carolina Academic Press; 1993.

55. Lefton E, Bonstelle S, Frengley D. Success with an inpatient geriatric unit: A controlled study of outcome and follow-up. *J Am Geriatr Soc.* 1983;31:149–155.

56. Moore JT, Warshaw GA, Walden LD, et al. Evolution of a geriatric evaluation clinic. *J Am Geriatr Soc.* 1984;32:900–905.

57. Rubenstein LZ, Rhee L, Kane RL. The role of geriatric assessment units in caring for the elderly: An analytic review. *J Gerontol.* 1982;37:513–521.

58. Reuben DB. Defining and refining targeting criteria. In: Rubenstein LZ, Wieland D, Bernabei R, eds. *Geriatric Assessment Technology: The State of the Art.* Milan, Italy: Editrice Kurtis; 1995:265–269.

59. Rubenstein LZ, Abrass JB, Kane RL. Improved care for patients on a new geriatric evaluation unit. *J Am Geriatr Soc.* 1981;29:531–536.

60. Liem PH, Chernoff R, Carter WJ. Geriatric rehabilitation unit: A 3-year outcome evaluation. *J Gerontol.* 1986;41:44–50.

61. Applegate WB, Akins D, Zwaag RV, et al. A geriatric rehabilitation and assessment unit in a community hospital. *J Am Geriatr Soc.* 1983;31:206–210.

62. Boult C, Dowd B, McCaffrey D, Boult L, Hernandez R, Krulewitch H. Screening elders at risk of hospital admission. *J Am Geriatr Soc.* 1993;41:811–817.

63. Pacala JT, Boult C, Boult LB. Predictive validity of a questionnaire that identifies elders at risk for hospital admission. *J Am Geriatr Soc.* 1995;43:374–377.

64. Seegal D. The principle of minimal interference in the management of the elderly patient. *J Chronic Dis.* 1964;17:299–300.

Index

A

Abdomen
  pain assessment, 256–257
  physical examination, 240–241
Abdominal aortic aneurysm,
  293–294
Actinic keratosis, 225
Activities of daily living
  Barthel Index, 107–109
  ceiling or threshold effects, 106
  determination of need assess-
    ment, 112–113, 114–115
  instrumental activities of daily
    living
  combined assessments,
    112–116
  components, 105
  Katz Index of Activities of Daily
    Living, 107, 108
  measures, 106
  Medical Outcomes Study Short
    Form 36, 113–116, 117–120
Acute pain, 251
Advance care planning, 22
Advance directives, 7, 292
  communication, 195–204
  conditions for applicability,
    197–198
Age-associated memory impairment, 36
Alcohol abuse, 81, 282
  measures, 81–82, 83–84
Alcohol Use Disorder Identification
  Test, 81–82, 83–84

Alzheimer's disease
  diagnostic criteria, 45, 46
  differential diagnostic considera-
    tions, 133–134
  Functional Assessment Staging of
    Alzheimer's Disease, 131–134
  symptomatology, 133–134
Anxiety disorder, 82
Aphasia, 38–39
Arcus senilis, 230
Arrhythmia, 238
Aspirin, 288
Attention, mental status examina-
  tion, 37
Attitudes, ethnicity, 18
Auscultation, 237

B

Balance, physical examination,
  244, 245–247
Barthel Index, activities of daily liv-
  ing, 107–109
Basal cell carcinoma, 225
Beck Depression Inventory, 77–79
Beliefs, ethnicity, 18
Benign senescent forgetfulness, 36
Bike helmet, 283
Binswanger dementia, 47–48
Blessed Dementia Score, dementia,
  123, 124
Blood pressure
  disease prevention, 275
  health promotion, 275
  hypertension, 221

Blood pressure—(*continued*)
  low, 221–222
  physical examination, 220–222
Body mass index, 223
Breast
  disease prevention, 278
  health promotion, 278
  physical examination, 241
Broca's aphasia, 40

C

Calcium, 287
Carbon monoxide detector, 286
Care setting, 8
Caregiver
  caregiver burden, 167–169
  depression, 168
  knowledge, 293
  stress, 293
Category fluency test, 62–63
Center for Epidemiologic Studies
  Depression Scale, 79–81
Chemoprophylaxis
  disease prevention, 287–288
  health promotion, 287–288
Chest, pain assessment, 256–257
Chronic pain, 251
  barriers to management, 251–252
  defined, 251
Clinical breast examination
  disease prevention, 278
  health promotion, 278
Clinical Dementia Rating Scale,
  dementia, 134–135, 136–137, 138
Clock-drawing task, 64–65, 66
Cognitive assessment, ethnicity,
  19–20
Cognitive Capacity Screen, 59–60, 61
Cognitive impairment
  disease prevention, 279–280
  etiology, 30–31
  health promotion, 279–280
  pain assessment, 258–259
Communication
  advance directives, 195–204

ethnicity, 17
physical assessment, 214–216
Comprehension, 38, 39
Computer, geriatric assessment,
  337–338
Conduction aphasia, 40
Conductive hearing loss, 232
Consciousness level, mental status
  examination, 37
Cortical dementia, 42–47

D

Decubitus ulcer, physical examination, 226, 227–228
Delirium, defined, 42
Dementia
  affective component, 49
  Blessed Dementia Score, 123, 124
  characterized, 42
  Clinical Dementia Rating Scale,
    134–135, 136–137, 138
  components, 42
  defined, 42
  differential diagnosis, 42–50
  disease prevention, 279–280
  driving, 150–151
  endocrine abnormality, 49–50
  etiology, 42–50
    classification, 42–43
  Functional Assessment Staging of
    Alzheimer's Disease, 131–134
    differential diagnostic consid-
      erations, 133–134
    symptomatology, 133–134
  Functional Dementia Scale,
    124–125
  Functional Rating Scale for the
    Symptoms of Dementia,
    128–130
  Global Deterioration Scale for
    Primary Degenerative
    Dementia, 131
  health promotion, 279–280
  infection, 50
  metabolic abnormality, 49

O

Older Americans Resources and Services (OARS) Multidimensional Functional Assessment Questionnaire, economic assessment, 178, 179–180
Orientation-Memory-Concentration Test, 62, 64
Osteoarthritis, 239

P

Pain assessment, 8, 251–259
abdomen, 256–257
chest, 256–257
cognitive impairment, 258–259
ears, 256
extremities, 256–257
eyes, 256
genitalia, 256–257
head, 256
historical assessment, 252–255
multidimensional pain scales, 253
musculoskeletal system, 257–258
neck, 256
neurological system, 258
nose, 256
pelvis, 256–257
physical assessment, 255–258
skin, 256
throat, 256
unidimensional pain scales, 252–253
Pain diary, 254–255
Pap smear
disease prevention, 278–279
health promotion, 278–279
Parkinson's disease, dementia, 48–49
Patient Self-Determination Act, 195–196
Pelvis, pain assessment, 256–257
Physical activity, 283
Physical assessment, 213–247

communication, 214–216
dementia, 216
geriatric review of systems, 218
history taking, 216–219
primary care, 337
rapport, 214–216
Physical examination, 7, 219–247
abdomen, 240–241
balance, 244, 245–247
blood pressure, 220–222
breast, 241
components, 219–247
decubitus ulcer, 226, 227–228
ears, 231–233
eyes, 229–231
gait, 244, 245–247
genitourinary system, 242–243
hair, 226–229
head, 229
heart, 236–239
height, 222–224
lungs, 236–239
mouth, 234
musculoskeletal system, 239–240
nails, 226–229
neck, 235–236
nervous system, 243–244
nose, 233–234
nutrition, 222–224
pulse, 219
respiration, 222
skin, 224–226
teeth, 235
temperature, 222
weight, 222–224
Physical Performance Test, functional assessment, 120
Pick's disease, 45
Pneumococcal vaccine, 289
Polypharmacy, 291
Predictive value
Mini-Mental State Examination, 54–55
Short Portable Mental Status Questionnaire, 56–57, 58
Primary care